# Pediatric Endocrinology: Part II

*Guest Editor*

ROBERT RAPAPORT, MD

ENDOCRINOLOGY AND METABOLISM CLINICS OF NORTH AMERICA

www.endo.theclinics.com

*Consulting Editor*
DEREK LEROITH, MD, PhD

December 2009 • Volume 38 • Number 4

SAUNDERS an imprint of ELSEVIER, Inc.

**W.B. SAUNDERS COMPANY**
*A Division of Elsevier Inc.*

1600 John F. Kennedy Boulevard • Suite 1800 • Philadelphia, Pennsylvania 19103-2899

http://www.theclinics.com

**ENDOCRINOLOGY AND METABOLISM CLINICS OF NORTH AMERICA Volume 38, Number 4 December 2009 ISSN 0889-8529, ISBN-13: 978-1-4377-1214-8, ISBN-10: 1-4377-1214-2**

Editor: Rachel Glover
Developmental Editor: Theresa Collier



*Endocrinology and Metabolism Clinics of North America* (ISSN 0889-8529) is published quarterly by Elsevier Inc., 360 Park Avenue South, New York, NY 10010-1710. Months of issue are March, June, September, and December. Periodicals postage paid at New York, NY and additional mailing offices. Subscription prices are USD 271.00 per year for US individuals, USD 457.00 per year for US institutions, USD 139.00 per year for US students and residents, USD 340.00 per year for Canadian individuals, USD 560.00 per year for Canadian institutions, USD 394.00 per year for international individuals, USD 560.00 per year for international institutions, and USD 206.00 per year for international and Canadian and foreign students/residents. To receive student/resident rate, orders must be accompanied by name of affiliated institution, date of term, and the signature of program/residency coordinator on institution letterhead. Orders will be billed at individual rate until proof of status is received. Foreign air speed delivery is included in all *Clinics* subscription prices. All prices are subject to change without notice. **POSTMASTER:** Send address changes to *Endocrinology and Metabolism Clinics of North America*, Elsevier Health Sciences Division, Subscription Customer Service, 3251 Riverport Lane, Maryland Heights, MO 63043. **Customer Service: Telephone: 1-800-654-2452** (U.S. and Canada); **1-314-447-8871** (outside U.S. and Canada). **Fax: 1-314-447-8029. E-mail: journalscustomerservice-usa@elsevier.com** (for print support); **journalsonlinesupport-usa@elsevier.com** (for online support).

*Reprints.* For copies of 100 or more, of articles in this publication, please contact the Commercial Rights Department, Elsevier Inc., 360 Park Avenue South, New York, NY 10010-1710; phone: (+1) 212-633-3813; fax: (+1) 212-462-1935; e-mail: reprints@elsevier.com.

*Endocrinology and Metabolism Clinics of North America* is covered in *MEDLINE/PubMed (Index Medicus), EMBASE/Excerpta Medica, Current Contents/Clinical Medicine, Current Contents/Life Sciences, Science Citation Index, ISI/BIOMED, BIOSIS,* and *Chemical Abstracts*.

Printed in the United States of America.

# Contributors

## CONSULTING EDITOR

**DEREK LeROITH, MD, PhD**
Chief, Division of Endocrinology, Metabolism, and Bone Diseases, Mount Sinai School of Medicine, New York, New York

## GUEST EDITOR

**ROBERT RAPAPORT, MD**
Professor of Pediatrics, Emma Elizabeth Sullivan Professor of Pediatric Endocrinology and Diabetes; Director, Division of Pediatric Endocrinology and Diabetes, Mount Sinai School of Medicine, New York, New York

## AUTHORS

**DENIS DANEMAN, MBBCH, FRCPC**
Division of Endocrinology, Department of Pediatrics, The Hospital for Sick Children and University of Toronto, Toronto, Ontario, Canada

**BRADLEY N. DELMAN, MD**
Associate Professor of Radiology, Department of Radiology, Mount Sinai School of Medicine, New York, New York

**ERICA A. EUGSTER, MD**
Professor of Pediatrics and Director of Pediatric Endocrinology, Department of Pediatrics, Riley Hospital for Children, Indiana University School of Medicine, Indianapolis, Indiana

**CHRISTOPHER P. HOUK, MD**
Associate Professor of Pediatrics, Department of Pediatrics, Medical College of Georgia, Augusta, Georgia

**MICHELLE KLEIN, MD**
Fellow, Division of Pediatric Endocrinology and Diabetes, Mount Sinai Hospital, New York, New York

**PETER A. LEE, MD, PhD**
Professor of Pediatrics, Department of Pediatrics, Penn State College of Medicine, Milton S. Hershey Medical Center, University Drive, Hershey, Pennsylvania; Department of Pediatrics, Indiana University School of Medicine, Riley Hospital for Children, Indianapolis, Indiana

**KAREN LIN-SU, MD**
Adrenal Steroid Disorders Program, Division of Pediatric Endocrinology, Mount Sinai School of Medicine, New York, New York

**MARIA I. NEW, MD**
Professor of Pediatrics, Professor of Genetics and Genomic Sciences and the Director of Adrenal Steroid Disorders Program, Division of Pediatric Endocrinology, Mount Sinai School of Medicine, New York, New York

**EURICO CARMAGO NETO, PhD**
Laboratorio Nobel and Centro de Triagem Neonatal, Porto Alegre, RS, Brazil

**SAROJ NIMKARN, MD**
Adrenal Steroid Disorders Program, Division of Pediatric Endocrinology, Mount Sinai School of Medicine, New York, New York

**YERAY NOVOA, MD**
Division of Pediatric Endocrinology and Diabetes, Mount Sinai Hospital, New York, New York

**KENNETH A. PASS, PhD**
Senior Research Scientist, Biggs Laboratory, Wadsworth Center, NYS Department of Health, Albany, New York

**SAYALI A. RANADIVE, MD**
Department of Endocrinology, Children's Hospital and Research Center Oakland, Oakland, California

**ROBERT RAPAPORT, MD**
Professor of Pediatrics, Emma Elizabeth Sullivan Professor of Pediatric Endocrinology and Diabetes; Director, Division of Pediatric Endocrinology and Diabetes, Mount Sinai School of Medicine, New York, New York

**ALAN ROGOL, MD**
Professor of Pediatrics, Department of Pediatrics, Indiana University School of Medicine, Riley Hospital for Children, Indianapolis, Indiana; Department of Pediatrics, University of Virginia, Charlottesville, Virginia

**HENRIETTA KOTLUS ROSENBERG, MD, FACR, FAAP**
Director of Pediatric Radiology, Department of Radiology, Mount Sinai Medical Center, Professor of Radiology and Pediatrics, The Mount Sinai School of Medicine, New York, New York

**STEPHEN M. ROSENTHAL, MD**
Professor of Pediatrics, Department of Pediatrics, Division of Endocrinology, University of California San Francisco, San Francisco, California

**ANPALAKAN SATHASIVAM, MD**
Fellow, Division of Pediatric Endocrinology and Diabetes, Mount Sinai Hospital, New York, New York

**SOFIA SHAPIRO, MD**
Fellow, Division of Pediatric Endocrinology and Diabetes, Mount Sinai School of Medicine, New York, New York

**VIDHYA VISWANATHAN, MD**
Fellow in Pediatric Endocrinology, Section of Pediatric Endocrinology, Department of Pediatrics, Riley Hospital for Children, Indiana University School of Medicine, Indianapolis, Indiana

**DIANE K. WHERRETT, MD, FRCPC**
Division of Endocrinology, Department of Pediatrics, The Hospital for Sick Children and University of Toronto, Toronto, Ontario, Canada

# Contents

**Foreword** xi

Derek LeRoith

**Preface** xv

Robert Rapaport

**Pediatric Disorders of Water Balance** 663

Sayali A. Ranadive and Stephen M. Rosenthal

Fluid homeostasis requires adequate water intake, regulated by an intact thirst mechanism and appropriate free water excretion by the kidneys, mediated by appropriate secretion of arginine vasopressin (AVP, also known as antidiuretic hormone). AVP exerts its antidiuretic action by binding to the X chromosome-encoded V2 vasopressin receptor (V2R), a G protein-coupled receptor on the basolateral membrane of renal collecting duct epithelial cells. After V2R activation, increased intracellular cyclic adenosine monophosphate mediates shuttling of the water channel aquaporin 2 to the apical membrane of collecting duct cells, resulting in increased water permeability and antidiuresis. Clinical disorders of water balance are common, and abnormalities in many steps involving AVP secretion and responsiveness have been described. This article focuses on the principal disorders of water balance, diabetes insipidus, and the syndrome of inappropriate antidiuretic hormone secretion.

**Imaging of Pediatric Pituitary Abnormalities** 673

Bradley N. Delman

Evaluation of the sella and surrounding structures in pediatric endocrinopathies is best performed with high-resolution magnetic resonance imaging. Adequate assessment relies not only on determining the size and shape of the gland but also on confirming normal signal characteristics and homogeneous parenchymal enhancement. Surrounding structures, including the hypothalamus-infundibulum-stalk and the skull base and midline structures about the cerebral hemispheres, warrant careful attention to identify any associated abnormalities. Tumors, whether they arise in the gland or affect gland function through mass effect, are usually well resolved on today's scanners and imaging provides accurate characterization of these lesions.

**Steroid 21 Hydroxylase Deficiency Congenital Adrenal Hyperplasia** 699

Saroj Nimkarn, Karen Lin-Su, and Maria I. New

Steroid 21 hydroxylase deficiency is the most common form of congenital adrenal hyperplasia (CAH). The severity of this disorder depends on the extent of impaired enzymatic activity, which is caused by various mutations of the 21 hydroxylase gene. This article reviews adrenal steroidogenesis and the pathophysiology of 21 hydroxylase deficiency. The three forms of CAH are then discussed in terms of clinical presentation, diagnosis and treatment, and genetic basis. Prenatal diagnosis and treatment are also reviewed. The goal of therapy is to correct the deficiency in cortisol secretion and suppress androgen overproduction. Glucocorticoid replacement has been the mainstay of treatment for CAH, but new treatment strategies continue to be developed and studied.

**Etiology and Treatment of Hypogonadism in Adolescents** **719**

Vidhya Viswanathan and Erica A. Eugster

Adequate functioning at all levels of the hypothalamic-pituitary-gonadal axis is necessary for normal gonadal development and subsequent sex steroid production. Deficiencies at any level of the axis can lead to a hypogonadal state. The causes of hypogonadism are heterogeneous and may involve any level of the reproductive system. This review discusses various causes of hypogonadism, describes the evaluation of hypogonadal states, and outlines treatment options for the induction of puberty in affected adolescents. Whereas some conditions are clearly delineated, the exact etiology and underlying pathogenesis of many disorders is unknown.

**Sonography of the Pelvis in Patients with Primary Amenorrhea** **739**

Henrietta Kotlus Rosenberg

Duplex/color Doppler sonography (US) is the imaging modality of choice for the evaluation of patients with primary amenorrhea. Careful correlation with clinical history, physical examination and laboratory findings significantly narrows the diagnostic possibilities thus allowing for a more precise diagnosis. This article discusses the wide gamut of etiologies of primary amenorrhea, the US appearance of pathologic processes that result in primary amenorrhea, and helps the reader understand when additional higher tech imaging is indicated.

**Optimizing Potential for Fertility: Fertility Preservation Considerations for the Pediatric Endocrinologist** **761**

Peter A. Lee, Alan Rogol, and Christopher P. Houk

Whether for the prepubertal or pubertal child, the goal of fertility preservation is to obtain cells or tissues to be used to produce future children. For the prepubertal child, preservation efforts involve germ cells, earlier forms of sperm, and immature follicles, rather than mature spermatozoa or follicles. Options for prepubertal children include for boys freezing testicular tissue and extracting testicular sperm or for girls obtaining ovarian cortical or follicular tissue for storage. These procedures involve extraction and storage of immature gametes for subsequent in vitro maturation, although attempts for sperm currently involve only animal studies. For adolescent subjects who have sufficient gonadal development and reserve, sperm, oocytes, and ovarian cortex can be retrieved as among adults.

**Prevention of Type 1 Diabetes** 777

Diane K. Wherrett and Denis Daneman

Prevention of loss of β cells in type 1 diabetes is a major goal of current research. Knowledge of the genetic susceptibility, increasing ability to predict who may be at risk, recognition of the potential clinical impact of residual insulin secretion after diagnosis, and development of new immunomodulatory agents have supported an increasing number of clinical trials to prevent β-cell loss. Interventions can be targeted at 3 stages: before the development of autoimmunity (primary prevention), after autoimmunity is recognized (secondary prevention), or after diagnosis when significant numbers of β cells remain (tertiary prevention). Thus far, several agents show promise when given shortly after diagnosis, but no interventions before diagnosis have shown benefit. Knowledge in this area has grown quickly in recent years and will continue to grow rapidly with several international collaborative efforts underway.

**The Role of Complementary and Alternative Therapies in Pediatric Diabetes** 791

Sofia Shapiro and Robert Rapaport

Complementary and alternative medicine (CAM), also referred to as holistic, or integrative, medicine, are terms that describe a heterogeneous collection of nontraditional therapies, from chemical substances, to biofeedback, to prayer. This review focuses on CAM in pediatric patients with type 1 and type 2 diabetes. CAM prevalence in this population and the specific modalities that have been studied in children are described. Randomized, placebo-controlled, prospective studies in young adults are evaluated for their applicability to pediatric patients. CAM's "complementary" role is emphasized, as there is evidence of significant morbidity when CAM replaces standard-of-care therapy.

**Recent Consensus Statements in Pediatric Endocrinology: A Selective Review** 811

Michelle Klein, Anpalakan Sathasivam, Yeray Novoa, and Robert Rapaport

Clinical guidelines and consensus statements serve to summarize and organize current knowledge on diverse subjects, and provide practical guidelines for proper clinical management. Recommendations should be based on research and evidence derived from appropriate sources. In 2008, more than 20 consensus statements were published in the pediatric literature alone. This article summarizes the salient points of the latest consensus statements jointly developed by multiple endocrine societies including the Lawson Wilkins Society for Pediatric Endocrinology and the European Society for Pediatric Endocrinology. As much as possible, the original intent and language of the statements was respected and paraphrased.

**Update: Newborn Screening for Endocrinopathies** 827

Kenneth A. Pass and Eurico Carmago Neto

Congenital hypothyroidism and congenital adrenal hyperplasia are included in many newborn screening (NBS) panels worldwide and in all state-sponsored programs in the United States. Both conditions meet the fundamental prerequisites for NBS: high incidence in the population; biomarkers in the dried blood specimen that are easily detected; and, effective therapies to lessen, if not prevent, the sequelae of late or no treatment. In this review, the history of NBS is discussed for these 2 conditions. The technologies and protocols used in their detection, and related subjects such as genetics, and treatment and outcomes, are also discussed.

**Index** **839**

## FORTHCOMING ISSUES

***March 2010***

**Hormones and the Science of Athletic Performance**

Primus-E. Mullis, MD, *Guest Editor*

***June 2010***

**Vitamin D**

Sol Epstein, MD, *Guest Editor*

***September 2010***

**Type 1 Diabetes**

Desmond Schatz, Mark Atkinson, and Michael Haller, *Guest Editors*

## RECENT ISSUES

***September 2009***

**Pediatric Endocrinology: Part I**

Robert Rapaport, MD, *Guest Editor*

***June 2009***

**Autoimmune Endocrine Disorders**

Simon H.S. Pearce, MD, *Guest Editor*

***March 2009***

**Lipids**

Donald A. Smith, MD, MPH, *Guest Editor*

**RELATED INTEREST**

***Pediatric Clinics of North America***
Volume 56, Issue 4 (August 2009)
**Pediatric Quality**
Leonard G. Feld, MD, PhD, MMM, FAAP and Shabnam Jain, MD, FAAP, *Guest Editors*

# Foreword

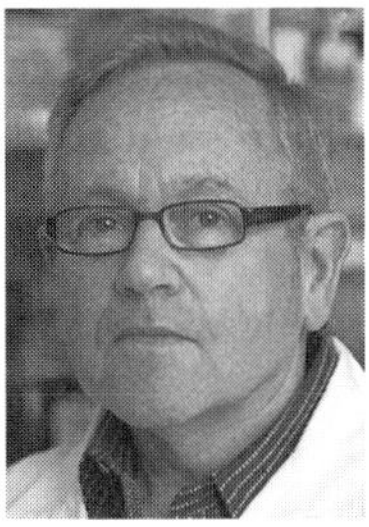

Derek LeRoith, MD, PhD
*Consulting Editor*

The problems of water and electrolyte imbalance are well described in the article by Drs. Ranadive and Rosenthal. First, they describe the normal physiology of water and electrolyte homeostasis. They follow with a discussion of the two common abnormalities, hyponatremia and hypernatremia, and the mechanisms causing these disorders. The authors describe the syndrome of inappropriate secretion of antidiuretic hormone and diabetes insipidus, central and nephrogenic. Diagnostic dilemmas and the established and newer therapies are also discussed in detail.

Dr. Delman, in his article, describes the embryology and anatomy of the hypothalamic-pituitary axis. He then discusses the imaging of this region, beginning with the normal appearance of structures, such as the sella, including changes to expect in the developmental period. This is followed by the appearance of various pathologic states. Pituitary adenomas, cystic lesions, and suprasellar lesions are some of the common lesions that are imaged using high-resolution MRI technology.

21-Hydroxylase deficiency is the most common genetic disorder causing and congenital adrenal hyperplasia (CAH). As described by Dr. New, the world's expert on this topic, there are three forms: salt-wasting, simple virilizing, and nonclassical. The clinical manifestations depend on lack of cortisol and mineralocorticoid and on androgen excess. Clinical diagnosis and laboratory testing help in diagnosis, and the mainstay of therapy is the replacement of corticosteroids and the reduction in adrenal androgen excess. The earlier the diagnosis is made, the better the outcome. The article includes an introduction to steroid synthesis and metabolism, an essential component required for the understanding how the enzyme defects lead to cortisol deficiency, corticotropin excess, and androgen excess in some cases of CAH.

Hypogonadism in adolescents is a devastating situation, regarding making the correct diagnosis, instituting appropriate and successful therapy, and the psychologic aspects that health care professionals need to be aware of. Viswanathan and Eugster discuss this condition of hypogonasim and how in boys, it manifests as a complete lack of secondary sexual development or failure of normal pubertal progression, whereas in girls, it presents as failure of pubertal initiation, pubertal progression, or menstrual irregularities. The hypogonadism may be hypergonadotropic or

Endocrinol Metab Clin N Am 38 (2009) xi–xiii
doi:10.1016/j.ecl.2009.09.006 endo.theclinics.com

hypogonadotropic in origin, and the diagnosis relies on measurements of circulating gonadotrophins and other specific manifestations of each specific syndrome, such as anosmia in Kallmann syndrome. In both cases, there are genetic and acquired syndromes. Sex steroid replacement therapy is the mainstay of treatment.

Dr. Rosenberg discusses the use of duplex/color Doppler sonography of the pelvis as an important diagnostic tool for evaluating primary amenorrhea. It avoids invasive technologies and can be used specifically to study the ovaries and uterus. Investigation starts with history and physical examination and includes hormonal measurements, chromosomal evaluation. Sonography is an important adjunct to these criteria and can be used in correlation with the other modalities.

A provocative and thought-provoking article on preservation of fertility by Dr. Lee and colleagues is included. Preserving tissue for later attempts at fertilization can occur from early developmental stages and from prepubertal ages. This can be considered in patients with gonadal failure or polycystic ovarian syndrome and, in particular, children undergoing treatment for cancer who will become infertile. Gonadal tissue, sperm, and oocyte samples can be obtained and stored appropriately. With these modern techniques perfected, pediatricians need to become comfortable enough to advise patients who may consider the necessary steps involved.

Type 1 diabetes mellitus is a classic autoimmune disorder with destruction of the beta cells of the pancreatic islets attacked by T cells and then by autoantibodies from B cells. Drs. Wherrett and Daneman discuss the various national and international trials that have been and are currently being carried out in an attempt to prevent the autoimmune destruction of the beta cells before the disease begins or soon after the diagnosis. Primary prevention trials are for those stages long before the disease is diagnosed clinically and are for predisposed individuals. Secondary prevention is intended to delay the progression of the destruction before total loss of beta cell function, and tertiary prevention is for those type 1 diabetics who, despite months of having the disease, still have some beta cell function and possibly some regenerative ability.

In a scholarly article on the use of complementary and alternative medicine use in type 1 diabetes mellitus, Drs. Shapiro and Rapaport discuss many of the popular compounds. These range from vitamin D or nicotinamide for prevention of the disease to vitamin E, cinnamon, vitamin B, zinc, chromium, α-lipoic acid, and omega-3 for improving diabetes control. After many trials, there is no convincing evidence that any of the agents tested has significant effects, although, on the positive side, if used in reasonable doses, they have proved safe.

The article by Drs. Klein and colleagues discusses consensus statements for various pediatric endocrinopathies by the major internationally recognized pediatric endocrine societies. Etiology, pathophysiology, and clinical manifestations of diabetic ketoacidosis are covered, followed by management. Management of idiopathic short stature, an important issue for practicing pediatric endocrinologists, is presented with the accepted definition, clinical assessment, and a discussion focusing on growth hormone therapy and the occasional use of recombinant human insulin-like growth factor 1. Children born small for gestational age are similarly discussed because consensus statements by the major pediatric societies have issued their reports. Finally, the problem of intersex disorders is discussed in-depth, covering definition, diagnosis, and management.

The focus of the article by Drs. Pass and Neto is on screening for two important, common, and treatable conditions: congenital hypothyroidism and CAH. With congenital hypothyroidism, some advocate using thyrotopin for screening, although it may miss cases of central hypothyroidism; others use a thyroxine/thyrotopin combination or one followed by the other; apparently, neither program is superior, although the thyroxine/thyrotopin combination, albeit expensive, is probably preferable. CAH is due to genetic mutations in hydroxylase enzymes and is generally screened for using the measurement of 17-hydroxyprogesterone, common to all downstream steroids that may be affected by the various hydroxylase deficiencies. As discussed, screening is essential, to allow for early intervention and prevention of the devastating complications associated with these serious conditions.

These two parts of "Pediatric Endocrinology" cover many topics, but each one gives readers adequate coverage of the subject matter, and the issue editor, Dr. Rapaport, is to be credited for the choice of topics and the experts who contributed.

Derek LeRoith, MD, PhD
Division of Endocrinology, Metabolism, and Bone Diseases
Mount Sinai School of Medicine
One Gustave L. Levy Place
Box 1055, Altran 4-36
New York, NY 10029, USA

E-mail address:
derek.leroith@mssm.edu

# Preface

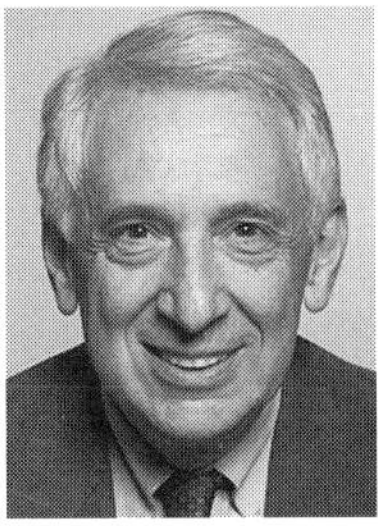

Robert Rapaport, MD
*Guest Editor*

Part II of the issue of *Endocrinology and Metabolism Clinics of North America* focusing on Pediatric Endocrinology contains contributions that reflect some of the more recent advances in the field. New thoughts on diabetes insipidus and its diagnosis are coupled with newer insights on imaging of the brain with MRI. Updates on congenital adrenal hyperplasia and gonandal disorders are coupled with findings on ultrasonographic visualization of the gonands along with current and future prospects for fertility preservation.

In as much as type 1 diabetes mellitus is still the most common form of diabetes seen in pediatrics, attempts at preventing it are under way. Many initiatives worthy of consideration are reviewed. At the same time, I want to acknowledge a trend that has become more prevalent in medicine today in the United States and worldwide, namely, the use of complimentary and alternative medicine. Therefore, a section critically reviewing evidence-based facts relevant to type 1 diabetes mellitus in childhood is included. A summary of recent consensus conference statements pertinent to pediatric endocrinology concludes the volume.

I hope readers gain an informative glimpse into selected aspects of the continually evolving field of pediatric endocrinology.

Thank you.

Robert Rapaport, MD
Division of Pediatric Endocrinology and Diabetes
Mount Sinai School of Medicine
One Gustave L. Levy Place, Box 1616
New York, NY 10029, USA

E-mail address:
robert.rapaport@mountsinai.org

Endocrinol Metab Clin N Am 38 (2009) xv
doi:10.1016/j.ecl.2009.09.005
endo.theclinics.com

# Pediatric Disorders of Water Balance

Sayali A. Ranadive, MD[a], Stephen M. Rosenthal, MD[b,*]

KEYWORDS

• Hyponatremia • Hypernatremia • Diabetes insipidus • SIADH

## PEDIATRIC DISORDERS OF WATER BALANCE

Under normal circumstances, plasma osmolality is maintained within a relatively narrow range (280–295 mOsm/kg). This homeostasis requires adequate water intake, regulated by an intact thirst mechanism and appropriate free water excretion by the kidneys, mediated by appropriate secretion of arginine vasopressin (AVP, also known as antidiuretic hormone). AVP is produced by a subset of magnocellular neurons in the paraventricular nuclei (PVN) and supraoptic nuclei (SON) of the hypothalamus. Axons from these neurons project via the pituitary stalk to the posterior pituitary gland.[1] The terminals of these axons contain neurosecretory granules that store AVP for release.[2] A gene on chromosome 20p13 encodes AVP and its carrier protein, neurophysin II (NPII). AVP and NPII are synthesized as a single polypeptide, cleaved within the neurosecretory granules and then reassembled into AVP-NPII complexes before secretion.[3] Stores of preformed AVP in the posterior pituitary can last for 30 to 50 days under basal circumstances or for 5 to 10 days during maximal stimulation.[4] This significant storage capacity explains why a defect in AVP synthesis may not become clinically apparent until weeks after a causal insult, and a partial defect may only be revealed after prolonged water deprivation.

AVP synthesis, transport, and secretion are regulated primarily by changes in plasma osmolality and, to a lesser degree, by changes in circulating volume.[1,5] Osmoreceptors in the hypothalamus (organum vasculosum of the lamina terminalis and anterior hypothalamus) stimulate secretion of AVP when plasma osmolality increases by as little as 1% in healthy individuals. Basal AVP levels are normally low, 0.5 to 2 pg/mL, and do not increase until plasma osmolality exceeds 280 mOsm/kg.[2] Maximum urine concentration (urine osmolality 900–1200 mOsm/kg) is attained at plasma AVP levels of 5 to 6 pg/mL. Although plasma AVP can continue to rise above 6 pg/mL with ongoing plasma hyperosmolality, further increases in urine

[a] Department of Endocrinology, Children's Hospital and Research Center Oakland, 747 52nd Street, Oakland, CA 94609, USA

[b] Department of Pediatrics, Division of Endocrinology, University of California San Francisco, 513 Parnassus Avenue, Room S672, San Francisco, CA 94143, USA

* Corresponding author.

*E-mail address:* rosenthals@peds.ucsf.edu (S.M. Rosenthal).

Endocrinol Metab Clin N Am 38 (2009) 663–672

doi:10.1016/j.ecl.2009.08.002

endo.theclinics.com

0889-8529/09/$ – see front matter 

osmolality cannot be achieved because of limits of the renal medullary gradient.[2] Changes in blood volume inversely affect AVP secretion such that 8% to 10% of decrease in circulating blood volume stimulates AVP secretion and increases in intravascular volume inhibit AVP release.[6] Baroreceptors in the carotid sinus and aortic arch (high-pressure baroreceptors) and in the atria and pulmonary venous circulation (low-pressure baroreceptors) relay pressure and volume information via the glossopharyngeal and vagus nerves, respectively, to the brain stem. These baroreceptors become activated when stretched by increases in intravascular volume, leading to inhibition of AVP secretion through fibers projecting from the brain stem to the PVN and SON of the hypothalamus.[6] In addition, many other factors affect AVP secretion; it is stimulated by pain, nausea, stress, and various drugs and is inhibited by multiple factors.[2,6]

Adequate water intake, governed by an intact thirst mechanism, is also regulated predominantly by changes in plasma osmolality, intravascular volume, and blood pressure. Thirst is consistently stimulated when plasma osmolality increases by 2% to 3% or when circulating blood volume decreases by 4% to 10%.[2,7] Because the thresholds that trigger thirst are higher than those that trigger AVP secretion, adequate thirst becomes essential during pathologic states of AVP deficiency or insensitivity.[2] Challenges in the management of adipsic diabetes insipidus, resulting from damage to thirst centers and to AVP-secreting neurons, highlight the critical role of thirst in the maintenance of plasma osmolality when AVP secretion or responsiveness is inadequate.

AVP exerts its antidiuretic action by binding to the X chromosome-encoded V2 vasopressin receptor (V2R), a G protein-coupled receptor on the basolateral membrane of renal collecting duct epithelial cells. After V2R activation, increased intracellular cyclic adenosine monophosphate (cAMP) mediates shuttling of the water channel aquaporin 2 (AQP-2) to the apical membrane of collecting duct epithelial cells, resulting in increased water permeability and antidiuresis (**Fig. 1**).[8]

Clinical disorders of water balance are common, and abnormalities in many steps involving AVP secretion and responsiveness have been described. This article focuses on the principal disorders of water balance, diabetes insipidus (DI), and the syndrome of inappropriate antidiuretic hormone secretion (SIADH).

## DIABETES INSIPIDUS

DI results from the inability to reabsorb free water. Polyuria, polydipsia, and hypo-osmolar urine are the hallmarks of this disorder, although hypernatremia may be present, particularly in infants, at the time of diagnosis. DI can be central, due to deficiency of AVP, or nephrogenic, due to a defect in AVP action in the kidneys (**Box 1**).[9,10]

Nephrogenic DI (NDI) may be genetic or acquired. The genetic causes are inactivating mutations of the *AVPR2* gene, located on the X chromosome (Xq28), or autosomal recessive or dominant mutations in the *AQP-2* gene, located on chromosome 12 (12q13). Acquired NDI can be caused by various conditions, including some forms of primary renal disease, obstructive uropathy, hypokalemia, hypercalcemia, sickle cell disease, and drugs such as lithium and demeclocycline.[2,9–11] Prolonged polyuria of any cause can also lead to some degree of NDI because of a reduction of tonicity in the renal medullary interstitium and a subsequent decrease in the gradient necessary to concentrate urine.

X-linked NDI (XNDI) is rare, affecting approximately 4 in 1,000,000 males worldwide, and it accounts for about 90% of the genetic causes of NDI. Of the 211 reported *AVPR2* mutations causing XNDI, approximately half are missense, and 31 of these

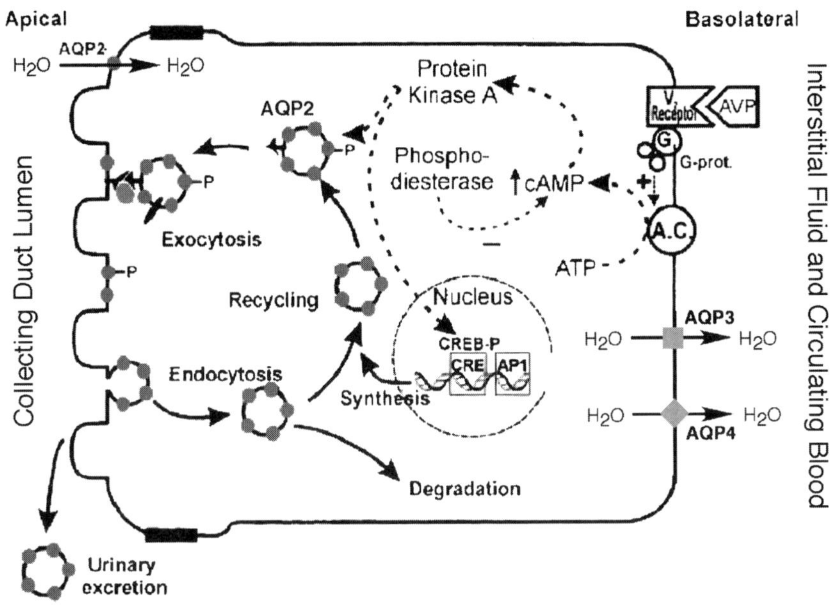


**Fig. 1.** Antidiurectic action of AVP on the renal collecting duct epithelial cell. AVP binding to the V2R, located on the basolateral membrane, results in an increase in cAMP and activation of protein kinase A (PKA). Ser256 on the C terminal of AQP-2 is phosphorylated by PKA, resulting in the shuttling of AQP-2 to the apical membrane, allowing the normally impermeable apical membrane to become permeable to water. In addition, acting through a cAMP-response element in the AQP-2 promoter, chronic exposure of these cells to AVP results in increased synthesis of AQP-2. AQP-3 and AQP-4, constitutively located on the basolateral border of the collecting duct membrane, provide channels for the transport of water out of the collecting duct cells and into the interstitium and circulation. ATP, adenosine triphosphate; CRE, cAMP response element; CREB, cAMP response element binding protein. *From* Nielsen S, Kwon TH, Christensen B, et al. Physiology and pathophysiology of renal aquaporins. J Am Soc Nephrol 1990;10:647–63; with permission.

have been characterized functionally.[12] Most *AVPR2* missense mutations result in a translated but misfolded V2R protein that remains trapped in the endoplasmic reticulum.[13–15] Pharmacologic chaperones can partially rescue the cell-surface expression and functional activity of misfolded mutant V2Rs that would otherwise be targeted for degradation.[16–18]

Infants with congenital (X-linked or autosomal) NDI typically present within the first several weeks of life with nonspecific symptoms, such as fever, vomiting, dehydration, and growth failure, associated with polyuria and hypo-osmolar urine (50–100 mOsm/kg). Mental retardation of variable severity and intracerebral calcifications of the frontal lobes and basal ganglia can result from repeated episodes of dehydration if the condition remains untreated.[19] Longstanding polyuria and polydipsia can lead to nonobstructive hydronephrosis, hydroureter, and megabladder.[20,21] Thiazide diuretics, along with low sodium intake, were historically used to treat NDI,[22] as this combination decreases glomerular filtration rate and results in decreased urine output. During the last 20 years, thiazide diuretics in combination with either amiloride or indomethacin have become the mainstay of congenital NDI treatment.[19,23,24] In vitro studies have demonstrated that pharmacologic chaperones, which are cell permeable, nonpeptide small molecules, can restore the cell-surface expression and function of misfolded

**Box 1**
**Causes of DI**

- Central DI
  - Congenital
    - Structural malformations affecting the hypothalamus or pituitary
    - Autosomal dominant (or rarely recessive) mutations in the gene encoding AVP-NPII
  - Acquired
    - Primary tumors or metastases
    - Infection (eg, meningitis, encephalitis)
    - Histiocytosis
    - Granulomatous diseases
    - Autoimmune disorders (lymphocytic infundibuloneurohypophysitis)
    - Trauma
    - Surgery
    - Idiopathic
- Nephrogenic DI
  - Congenital
    - X-linked: inactivating mutations in *AVPR2*
    - Autosomal: recessive or dominant mutations in *AQP-2*
  - Acquired
    - Primary renal disease
    - Obstructive uropathy
    - Metabolic causes (eg, hypokalemia, hypercalcemia)
    - Sickle cell disease
    - Drugs (eg, lithium, demeclocycline)
    - Prolonged polyuria of any cause

mutant V2Rs.[16–18,25] One such compound is orally active, well tolerated, and effective in decreasing urine volume in adults with severe XNDI.[18,26] Thus, pharmacologic chaperones represent a new, safe, and targeted therapy for XNDI caused by protein misfolding due to missense mutations of *AVPR2*.

Central DI is rarely congenital and more frequently, acquired. Congenital central DI may be caused by structural malformations affecting the hypothalamus or by autosomal dominant or recessive mutations in the gene encoding AVP-NPII. The autosomal dominant causes are more common and result from heterozygous *AVP-NPII* gene mutations.[3] The proposed mechanism for the dominant negative effect is that the heterozygous mutation disrupts the processing of the mutant precursor.[27,28] The accumulation of this misfolded protein in the vasopressinergic neurons causes a gradual destruction of these neurons.[3,27] In such patients, clinical DI usually develops several months to years after birth. A rare autosomal recessive form of central DI has been reported in association with a mutation in the *AVP-NPII* gene, resulting in a biologically inactive AVP.[29]

Acquired forms of central DI occur in association with a variety of disorders in which there is destruction or degeneration of vasopressinergic neurons. Causes include primary tumors (eg, craniopharyngioma, germinoma) or metastases, infection (meningitis, encephalitis), histiocytosis, granuloma, vascular disorders, autoimmune disorders (lymphocytic infundibuloneurohypophysitis), and trauma or surgery.[9,10,30] Idiopathic DI is a diagnosis of exclusion, and one that is made with decreasing frequency as a result of improved sensitivity of magnetic resonance imaging (MRI) of the brain and of tests for cerebral spinal fluid (CSF) and serum tumor markers.[30,31]

The principal presenting sign of DI is polyuria, which, in addition to deficiency or impaired responsiveness to AVP, may result from an osmotic agent (eg, hyperglycemia in diabetes mellitus) or from excessive water intake (primary polydipsia). Hypernatremia usually does not occur if patients have an intact thirst mechanism, adequate access to fluids, and no additional ongoing fluid loss (eg, diarrhea). Infants with DI, in addition to polyuria and polydipsia, may be irritable and may have fever of unknown origin, growth failure secondary to inadequate caloric intake, and hydronephrosis. Older children may also have nocturia and enuresis. DI may not be apparent in patients with coexisting untreated anterior pituitary-mediated adrenal glucocorticoid insufficiency, as cortisol is required to generate normal free water excretion.[2]

A diagnosis of DI can be made if simultaneous screening laboratory studies reveal hyperosmolality concurrent with urine that is inappropriately dilute. If DI is present, it is more likely to be uncovered by these screening tests if they are obtained as soon as possible after awakening and before any fluid intake (assuming that the patient has not consumed fluids overnight). However, because most patients with DI have intact thirst and can drink to prevent hyperosmolality and hypernatremia, a standardized water deprivation test is often necessary to make the diagnosis. The patient is monitored with serial measurements of weight, serum sodium level, serum osmolality, urine volume, and urine osmolality while being fasted and deprived of water for 8 to 10 hours. If urine osmolality greater than 750 mOsm/kg is achieved with any degree of water deprivation, DI can be excluded.[6,9] The diagnosis of DI is established if serum osmolality rises above 300 mOsm/kg and urine osmolality remains below 300 mOsm/kg. Urine osmolality in the 300 to 750 mOsm/kg range during water deprivation may indicate partial DI.[9] If DI is suspected, a plasma sample should be obtained for AVP radioimmunoassay. AVP or a synthetic analog (desmopressin) should then be administered to distinguish AVP deficiency from AVP unresponsiveness.

MRI of the brain, with particular attention to the hypothalamic-pituitary region, is indicated in patients with central DI. The posterior pituitary hyperintensity ("bright spot") on T1-weighted magnetic resonance images is often absent in central DI.[30,32–35] However, the bright spot can be absent in normal individuals,[36] and conversely, children with central DI can have a normal bright spot at the time of diagnosis.[37–39] Therefore, the presence of the bright spot does not establish neurohypophyseal integrity, and its absence does not always indicate central nervous system (CNS) pathology. In central DI patients with or without the posterior pituitary bright spot, an otherwise normal MRI warrants close follow-up with CSF tumor markers and cytology, serum tumor markers, and serial contrast-enhanced brain MRIs for early detection of an evolving occult hypothalamic-stalk lesion.[31]

The management of central DI includes treating the primary disease, correction of a fluid deficit, if present, and normalization of urine output with desmopressin. This AVP analog has markedly reduced pressor activity in comparison with native AVP, has a prolonged half-life, and can be administered orally, intranasally, or by subcutaneous injection. In infancy, if polyuria is not excessive, DI may be best managed with

**Box 2**
**Causes of SIADH**

1. Neurologic and psychiatric disorders
   a. Infections: meningitis, encephalitis, brain abscess
   b. Vascular: thrombosis, subarachnoid or subdural hemorrhage, temporal arteritis, cavernous sinus thrombosis, stroke
   c. Neoplasm: primary or metastatic
   d. Skull fracture, traumatic brain injury
   e. Psychosis, delirium tremens
   f. Other: Guillain-Barré syndrome, acute intermittent porphyria, autonomic neuropathy, postpituitary surgery, multiple sclerosis, epilepsy, hydrocephalus, lupus erythematosus.
2. Drugs
   a. Intravenous cyclophosphamide
   b. Carbamazepine
   c. Vincristine or vinblastine
   d. Thiothixene
   e. Thioridazine, other phenothiazines
   f. Haloperidol
   g. Amitriptyline, other tricyclic antidepressants or serotonin-reuptake inhibitors
   h. Monoamine oxidase inhibitors
   i. Bromocriptine
   j. Lorcainide
   k. Clofibrate
   l. General anesthesia
   m. Narcotics, opiate derivatives
   n. Nicotine
   o. Desmopressin overtreatment of DI or eneuresis
3. Lung diseases and interventions
   a. Pneumonia
   b. Tuberculosis
   c. Lung abscess, empyema
   d. Acute respiratory failure
   e. Positive pressure ventilation
4. Non-CNS tumors with ectopic production of AVP
   a. Carcinoma of lung (small cell, bronchogenic), duodenum, pancreas, thymus, olfactory neuroblastoma, bladder, prostate, uterus
   b. Lymphoma
   c. Sarcoma
   d. Leukemia

5. Miscellaneous
   a. AIDS
   b. Postoperative state
   c. Glucocorticoid deficiency
   d. Hypothyroidism
   e. Idiopathic

fluid intake alone to avoid a potential risk of hyponatremia with desmopressin treatment.

## SYNDROME OF INAPPROPRIATE ANTIDIURETIC HORMONE SECRETION

SIADH, caused by the inability to excrete free water, is characterized by hyponatremia and hypo-osmolality with inappropriately concentrated urine and natriuresis.[40–42] Following the original criteria established by Bartter and Schwartz,[40] a diagnosis of SIADH is made when the following occur: (1) plasma hypo-osmolality (<275 mOsm/kg), (2) less than maximally dilute urine (urine osmolality>100 mOsm/kg), (3) euvolemia (secondary to regulatory adaptations), (4) natriuresis, (5) normal renal function, and (6) no evidence of thyroxine or cortisol deficiency. Although most patients with SIADH have inappropriately measurable or elevated levels of plasma AVP relative to plasma osmolality, 10% to 20% of patients with SIADH do not have measurable AVP levels. This may reflect issues of assay sensitivity or may indicate a syndrome resembling SIADH, such as the recently described nephrogenic syndrome of inappropriate antidiuresis (NSIAD) associated with an activating mutation in the X-linked G protein-coupled V2R and unmeasurable circulating levels of AVP.[43]

Euvolemia in chronic SIADH is an important distinguishing factor in the evaluation of a patient with serum hypo-osmolality and has a bearing on treatment issues, as discussed subsequently. Euvolemia in chronic SIADH is thought to represent an adaptation to water overload. This adaptation is mediated, in part, at the cellular level through depletion of intracellular electrolytes (potassium) and organic osmolytes.[41] The loss of brain solutes is thought to allow effective regulation of brain volume during chronic hyponatremia and SIADH. Natriuresis, thought to be mediated in part through secretion of atrial natriuretic peptide, also contributes to volume regulation in chronic SIADH.[44] Cerebral salt wasting (CSW), associated with some intracranial diseases (eg, subarachnoid hemorrhage), is often considered in the differential diagnosis of SIADH. However, the hypo-osmolality, hyponatremia, and natriuresis in CSW are associated with volume contraction, which distinguishes this disorder from the euvolemic condition of SIADH.[41]

Several disorders and conditions are associated with SIADH and can be grouped into 5 categories (**Box 2**): (1) neurologic and psychiatric disorders, (2) a large variety of drugs (eg, phenothaiozines, tricyclic antidepressants), (3) various pulmonary disorders and interventions (eg, pneumonia, asthma, positive pressure ventilation), (4) non-CNS tumors with ectopic production of AVP, and (5) miscellaneous causes (eg, AIDS, postoperative state, glucocorticoid deficiency, severe hypothyroidism).[41,42]

Therapy for SIADH includes treatment of the underlying disorder (or discontinuation of an offending drug) and fluid restriction. Replacement of sodium loss may also be necessary, but it can usually be achieved through normal dietary salt intake. Severe hyponatremia (serum sodium<120 mEq/L) may be associated with CNS abnormalities, including seizures, and may require treatment with hypertonic (3%) intravenous sodium chloride solution. Concurrent use of a diuretic, such as furosemide, may be indicated when volume expansion is severe. Other therapeutic approaches include the use of agents that induce NDI, such as demeclocycline and lithium, although both are contraindicated particularly in younger pediatric patients because of untoward side effects. Urea has been used as an osmotic diuretic in pediatric SIADH and NSIAD.[45] A variety of nonpeptide V2R antagonists are in various stages of clinical trials or have been approved by the Food and Drug Administration for use in adults.[41]

If SIADH and hyponatremia are acute (<48 hours), it is thought that hyponatremia can be corrected quickly. However, if SIADH and hyponatremia are chronic (>48 hours), overzealous treatment can result in CNS damage, including central pontine myelinolysis (CPM).[41] Brain solute loss, although an important regulatory mechanism in chronic SIADH, may predispose to the development of CPM with rapid correction of serum osmolality. It is generally recommended that plasma sodium be corrected to a safe level of approximately 120 to 125 mEq/L at a rate of no greater than 0.5 mEq/L/h, with an overall correction that does not exceed 12 mEq/L in the initial 24 hours and 18 mEq/L in the initial 48 hours of treatment.[41]

## REFERENCES


1. Robertson GL. Antidiuretic hormone. Normal and disordered function. Endocrinol Metab Clin North Am 2001;30(3):671–94, vii.
2. Robinson AG, Verbalis JG. Posterior pituitary gland. In: Larsen PR, Kronenberg HM, Melmed S, et al, editors. Williams textbook of endocrinology. 10th edition. Philadelphia: Saunders; 2003. p. 281–329.
3. Rutishauser J, Kopp P, Gaskill MB, et al. Clinical and molecular analysis of three families with autosomal dominant neurohypophyseal diabetes insipidus associated with a novel and recurrent mutations in the vasopressin-neurophysin II gene. Eur J Endocrinol 2002;146(5):649–56.
4. Lederis K, Jayasena K. Storage of neurohypophysial hormones and the mechanism for their release. In: Heller H, Pickering BT, editors. Pharmacology of the endocrine system and related drugs. London: Pergamon; 1970. p. 111–54.
5. Roberts MM, Robinson AG, Hoffman GE, et al. Vasopressin transport regulation is coupled to the synthesis rate. Neuroendocrinology 1991;53(4):416–22.
6. Muglia LJ, Majzoub JA. Disorders of the posterior pituitary. In: Sperling MA, editor. Pediatric endocrinology. Philadelphia: Saunders; 2002. p. 289–322.
7. Baylis PH, Thompson CJ. Osmoregulation of vasopressin secretion and thirst in health and disease. Clin Endocrinol (Oxf) 1988;29(5):549–76.
8. Schrier RW, Cadnapaphornchai MA. Renal aquaporin water channels: from molecules to human disease. Prog Biophys Mol Biol 2003;81(2):117–31.
9. Baylis PH, Cheetham T. Diabetes insipidus. Arch Dis Child 1998;79(1):84–9.
10. Verbalis JG. Diabetes insipidus. Rev Endocr Metab Disord 2003;4(2):177–85.
11. Morello JP, Bichet DG. Nephrogenic diabetes insipidus. Annu Rev Physiol 2001; 63:607–30.
12. Spanakis E, Milord E, Gragnoli C. AVPR2 variants and mutations in nephrogenic diabetes insipidus: review and missense mutation significance. J Cell Physiol 2008;217(3):605–17.
13. Bichet DG, Birnbaumer M, Lonergan M, et al. Nature and recurrence of AVPR2 mutations in X-linked nephrogenic diabetes insipidus. Am J Hum Genet 1994; 55(2):278–86.

14. Wenkert D, Schoneberg T, Merendino JJ Jr, et al. Functional characterization of five V2 vasopressin receptor gene mutations. Mol Cell Endocrinol 1996; 124(1-2):43–50.
15. Pasel K, Schulz A, Timmermann K, et al. Functional characterization of the molecular defects causing nephrogenic diabetes insipidus in eight families. J Clin Endocrinol Metab 2000;85(4):1703–10.
16. Bernier V, Bichet DG, Bouvier M. Pharmacological chaperone action on G-protein-coupled receptors. Curr Opin Pharmacol 2004;4(5):528–33.
17. Morello JP, Salahpour A, Laperriere A, et al. Pharmacological chaperones rescue cell-surface expression and function of misfolded V2 vasopressin receptor mutants. J Clin Invest 2000;105(7):887–95.
18. Bernier V, Morello JP, Zarruk A, et al. Pharmacologic chaperones as a potential treatment for X-linked nephrogenic diabetes insipidus. J Am Soc Nephrol 2006; 17(1):232–43.
19. Kirchlechner V, Koller DY, Seidl R, et al. Treatment of nephrogenic diabetes insipidus with hydrochlorothiazide and amiloride. Arch Dis Child 1999;80(6): 548–52.
20. van Lieburg AF, Knoers NV, Monnens LA. Clinical presentation and follow-up of 30 patients with congenital nephrogenic diabetes insipidus. J Am Soc Nephrol 1999;10(9):1958–64.
21. Knoers NV, Deen PM. Molecular and cellular defects in nephrogenic diabetes insipidus. Pediatr Nephrol 2001;16(12):1146–52.
22. Kennedy GC, Crawford JD. Treatment of diabetes insipidus with hydrochlorothiazide. Lancet 1959;1(7078):866–7.
23. Alon U, Chan JC. Hydrochlorothiazide-amiloride in the treatment of congenital nephrogenic diabetes insipidus. Am J Nephrol 1985;5(1):9–13.
24. Knoers N, Monnens LA. Amiloride-hydrochlorothiazide versus indomethacin-hydrochlorothiazide in the treatment of nephrogenic diabetes insipidus. J Pediatr 1990;117(3):499–502.
25. Ranadive SA, Ersoy B, Favre H, et al. Identification, characterization and rescue of a novel vasopressin-2 receptor mutation causing nephrogenic diabetes insipidus. Clin Endocrinol (Oxf) 2009;71:388–93.
26. Serradeil-Le Gal C, Wagnon J, Valette G, et al. Nonpeptide vasopressin receptor antagonists: development of selective and orally active V1a, V2 and V1b receptor ligands. Prog Brain Res 2002;139:197–210.
27. Miller WI . Molecular genetics of familial central diabetes insipidus. J Clin Endocrinol Metab 1993;77(3):592–5.
28. Gagliardi PC, Bernasconi S, Repaske DR. Autosomal dominant neurohypophyseal diabetes insipidus associated with a missense mutation encoding Gly23→Val in neurophysin II. J Clin Endocrinol Metab 1997;82(11):3643–6.
29. Willcutts MD, Felner E, White PC. Autosomal recessive familial neurohypophyseal diabetes insipidus with continued secretion of mutant weakly active vasopressin. Hum Mol Genet 1999;8(7):1303–7.
30. Maghnie M, Cosi G, Genovese E, et al. Central diabetes insipidus in children and young adults. N Engl J Med 2000;343(14):998–1007.
31. Mootha SL, Barkovich AJ, Grumbach MM, et al. Idiopathic hypothalamic diabetes insipidus, pituitary stalk thickening, and the occult intracranial germinoma in children and adolescents. J Clin Endocrinol Metab 1997;82(5):1362–7.
32. Alter CA, Bilaniuk LT. Utility of magnetic resonance imaging in the evaluation of the child with central diabetes insipidus. J Pediatr Endocrinol Metab 2002; 15(Suppl 2):681–7.

33. Ghirardello S, Garre ML, Rossi A, et al. The diagnosis of children with central diabetes insipidus. J Pediatr Endocrinol Metab 2007;20(3):359–75.
34. Fujisawa I, Nishimura K, Asato R, et al. Posterior lobe of the pituitary in diabetes insipidus: MR findings. J Comput Assist Tomogr 1987;11(2):221–5.
35. Gudinchet F, Brunelle F, Barth MO, et al. MR imaging of the posterior hypophysis in children. AJR Am J Roentgenol 1989;153(2):351–4.
36. Brooks BS, el Gammal T, Allison JD, et al. Frequency and variation of the posterior pituitary bright signal on MR images. AJNR Am J Neuroradiol 1989;10(5):943–8.
37. Alonso G, Bergada I, Heinrich JJ. Magnetic resonance imaging in central diabetes insipidus in children and adolescents. findings at diagnosis and during follow-up. An Esp Pediatr 2000;53(2):100–5 [in Spanish].
38. Kubota T, Yamamoto T, Ozono K, et al. Hyperintensity of posterior pituitary on MR T1WI in a boy with central diabetes insipidus caused by missense mutation of neurophysin II gene. Endocr J 2001;48(4):459–63.
39. Maghnie M, Genovese E, Bernasconi S, et al. Persistent high MR signal of the posterior pituitary gland in central diabetes insipidus. AJNR Am J Neuroradiol 1997;18(9):1749–52.
40. Bartter FC, Schwartz WB. The syndrome of inappropriate secretion of antidiuretic hormone. Am J Med 1967;42(5):790–806.
41. Verbalis JG, Goldsmith SR, Greenberg A, et al. Hyponatremia treatment guidelines 2007: expert panel recommendations. Am J Med 2007;120(11 Suppl 1):S1–S21.
42. Baylis PH. The syndrome of inappropriate antidiuretic hormone secretion. Int J Biochem Cell Biol 2003;35(11):1495–9.
43. Feldman BJ, Rosenthal SM, Vargas GA, et al. Nephrogenic syndrome of inappropriate antidiuresis. N Engl J Med 2005;352(18):1884–90.
44. Cogan E, Debieve MF, Pepersack T, et al. Natriuresis and atrial natriuretic factor secretion during inappropriate antidiuresis. Am J Med 1988;84(3 Pt 1):409–18.
45. Huang EA, Feldman BJ, Schwartz ID, et al. Oral urea for the treatment of chronic syndrome of inappropriate antidiuresis in children. J Pediatr 2006;148(1):128–31.

# Imaging of Pediatric Pituitary Abnormalities

Bradley N. Delman, MD

**KEYWORDS**

- Pituitary imaging • Pituitary malformations
- Midline anomalies • Imaging of endocrinopathy

The normal pituitary is a bean-shaped gland that resides in the sella turcica, a fossa in the superior sphenoid bone within the central skull base. In humans, the gland has two dominant lobes, the posterior lobe (neurohypophysis, neural lobe) and the anterior lobe (adenohypophysis). The adenohypophysis is further comprised of: the pars distalis, which forms the most the anterior lobe; the pars tuberalis, which partially envelops the inferior stalk; and the pars intermedia, which correlates with the intermediate lobe in lower animals and which may secrete pro-opiomelanocortin (POMC) in the younger population, but is felt to involute by adulthood.[1] Anterior and posterior lobes are distinct embryologically and functionally. The hypothalamus, which is situated directly above, along the inferolateral aspect of the third ventricle, directs activity to each lobe by a different mechanism.

*Magnocellular pathway.* Hormonal supply to the posterior pituitary (neurohypophysis) is mediated through the magnocellular neurosecretory pathway. Because the posterior gland develops in contiguity with the hypothalamus, axons run continuously from the hypothalamic supraoptic and paraventricular nuclei into the neurohypophysis. The secretory mechanism relies on preserved axonal structure to transport oxytocin and vasopressin-containing vesicles from the cell bodies into the neurohypophysis.

*Parvocellular pathway.* The anterior pituitary (adenohypophysis) develops from an embryologic anlage that is distinct from the hypothalamus. As a result, no axonal contiguity exists between the hypothalamus and the anterior gland. This mechanism of hypothalamic-pituitary communication relies instead on the hypothalamic-hypophyseal portal system. The portal system transmits parvocellular messengers from the hypothalamic median eminence into the capillary bed of the anterior gland, where the messenger hormones can effect their influence to regulate adenohypophyseal secretion. Hormones secreted from the anterior gland include those that are derived from the basophilic population (follicle-stimulating

Department of Radiology, The Mount Sinai School of Medicine, One Gustave L. Levy Place, Box 1234, New York, NY 10029-6574, USA
*E-mail address:* bradley.delman@mountsinai.org

Endocrinol Metab Clin N Am 38 (2009) 673–698
doi:10.1016/j.ecl.2009.09.001
endo.theclinics.com

hormone, luteinizing hormone, corticotropin [ACTH], and thyroid-stimulating hormone) and those that are derived from the eosinophilic population (prolactin and growth hormone). In addition to these classic hormones, it is clear that the adenohypophysis also secretes many additional growth factors, cytokines, neurotransmitters, and other peptides.[2]

Both the hypothalamic axons and the hypophyseal portal system course through the hypothalamic infundibulum into the pituitary stalk. The stalk then inserts on the gland at or near its midline, at approximately the junction of the mid and posterior thirds. This position correlates roughly with the midpoint of the junction of the larger anterior and smaller posterior lobes. In practice, there can be significant variability even within the normal population in the overall size of the gland, the relative proportions of anterior and posterior lobes, the laterality of stalk insertion, and the overall bilateral symmetry of the gland.

Because of their differing embryologic origins, the anterior and posterior lobes have distinct arterial supplies.[3,4]

*Posterior pituitary supply.* The posterior pituitary derives its supply primarily from the inferior hypophyseal arteries, which arise bilaterally from the meningohypophyseal trunks. These meningohypophyseal trunks, which branch from the dorsal precavernous internal arteries, also give rise to local tentorial and meningeal branches. The inferior hypophyseal arteries may also supply portions of the superficial (peripheral) anterior pituitary lobe.

*Anterior pituitary supply.* Supply to the anterior gland is predominantly through the hypophyseal portal system on the surface of the pituitary stalk, which drains from the median eminence. Arterial supply to the median eminence itself is derived from the superior hypophyseal arteries, which may arise from either the posterior communicating arteries or from the supraclinoid internal carotid arteries directly. The superior hypophyseal arteries also supply portions of the superior stalk and optic chiasm.[5] The anterior lobe also receives venous blood from short portal vessels draining from the posterior lobe, accounting for up to one-third of the anterior pituitary supply.

*Venous drainage.* Venous blood drains from the anterior and posterior lobes into the cavernous sinuses. Blood draining from these sinuses may be sampled via simultaneous bilateral inferior petrosal sinus catheters to suggest laterality of secretory tumors when imaging is unable to resolve tumor location.

Although the sella itself is formed as a fossa within the central sphenoid bone, sellar margins are largely comprised of dura. Thus, the superior margin of the sella is defined by a dural plane, the diaphragma sella, with the infundibulum penetrating through the diaphragmatic hiatus to meet the gland below. The osseous anterior sellar wall, sellar floor, and posterior sellar wall are also lined by dura, which may consist of a thin sheet of fairly uniform thickness or it may be somewhat thicker, particularly around the anterosuperior and posterosuperior portions of the gland. Venous intercavernous sinuses may run within a thickened dural margin to communicate with one or both cavernous sinuses.[5] A dural plane also separates the sella from the cavernous sinuses laterally. Sinusoids within the cavernous sinuses contain venous drainage from not only the pituitary but also inflow from the ophthalmic veins, middle cerebral veins, and sphenoparietal sinuses. The sinuses further drain into the superior and inferior petrosal sinuses, pterygoid plexuses, and ophthalmic and angular veins of the face. It is the drainage into the inferior petrosal sinus that enables venous sampling via jugular catheters to determine the side of a hormone-secreting lesion.

Knowledge of surrounding structures is crucial for the surgical transsphenoidal endoscopic approach that has become widely used for exploration to the gland. Thus the floor and anterior wall of the sella may both abut the sphenoid sinus, offering a potential surgical window for resection of intrasellar pituitary tumors. Patients in whom tumors extend significantly into the suprasellar compartment may, in addition, require a subfrontal craniotomy for more complete tumor resection.

## EMBRYOLOGY

The pituitary gland, and indeed the entire hypothalamic-infundibular-pituitary axis, develop through a complex interplay between the developing diencephalon and the primitive oral stomodeum.[1,5–8] The process has been studied extensively in lower animals, and is believed to parallel the development in humans albeit at a different rate. Development and tropism proceed through opposing gradients of growth factors, transcription factors, and signaling proteins to encourage or discourage differentiation of specific cell types along what will become the infundibulum, stalk, and pituitary gland.

Development of the hypothalamic-pituitary axis is felt to proceed through 4 stages[1]

1. *Pituitary placode.* At approximately the fifth week of gestation, the anterior ridge of the neural plate displaces ventrally to form the roof of the developing oral cavity. The roof of the oral cavity thickens to compose the pituitary placode, which marks the onset of pituitary organogenesis.
2. *Rudimentary Rathke pouch.* As the oral cavity roof invaginates, it forms the rudimentary Rathke pouch. Because of a lack of overlying mesenchyme, when the roof invaginates it soon comes into contact with the evaginated diencephalon that will ultimately develop into the posterior pituitary. The contacting portion of the pouch develops into the pars intermedia.
3. *Definitive Rathke pouch.* Rathke pouch further deepens and folds on itself until it closes and the communication of the Rathke pouch cavity with the primitive oral cavity is lost. During this phase, the continued evagination of diencephalon results in development of the infundibulum.
4. *Adult Gland.* There is no further communication of the pouch with the oral cavity, and the specific cell types have developed in a specific spatial and temporal sequence.

Inherent in the development of the pituitary and associated structures is a well-orchestrated signaling system that allows cell differentiation and migration in specific orders. Thus, early in development the ventral diencephalon secretes several factors, including bone morphogenetic proteins (BMPs), Wnt5a, and fibroblastic growth factor (FGF) 10. Likewise, the oral ectoderm expresses Sonic Hedgehog (Shh) and Lhx3, ultimately thickening to form the pituitary placode. Gradations in signaling hormones such as BMP2 and FGFs provide for differentiation of specific pituitary cell types in their characteristic spatial and temporal arrangement. For example, there is a greater tendency for gonadotropes, thyrotropes, lactotropes, and somatotropes to develop ventrally (in this order, with gonadotropes most ventral), and melanotropes and corticotropes to develop dorsally.[9] Several factors are necessary to develop the posterior lobe, including Pit-1, Oct-1 and Oct-2, and Pit-Oct-Unc domain factors of the Brn family. Defects in specific genes may cause precise malformations. For example, a mutated or absent Brn-2 does not affect initial hypothalamic development, but it is associated with failed differentiation of the hypothalamic supraoptic and paraventricular nuclei; without these nuclei, the axons normally leading from them do not form and therefore the posterior gland will not form normally either. The reader is referred to several excellent reviews of the genetics of pituitary development and genetic basis of anomalies.[1,6,10–12]

## IMAGING TECHNIQUE

Preliminary evaluation of the sella is almost always performed using magnetic resonance imaging (MRI). Although an MRI examination takes considerably longer than computed tomography (CT) (at least 20 minutes for MRI and perhaps up to 35–40 minutes depending on the sequences obtained, compared with 5 minutes for CT), MRI offers markedly better parenchymal definition than CT, uses no ionizing radiation, and may be acquired in any orthogonal or oblique plane. MRI is not prone to the beam-hardening artifact from the surrounding sphenoid bone that is present on CT, but other artifacts can influence image quality, particularly metallic artifacts in dental braces or prostheses.

Sequences obtained for MRI vary significantly by institution, and choice of sequences depend on the specific scanner hardware available, field strength, and radiologist preference. In general, scans are obtained to survey the gland and surrounding tissue adequately, with coverage in at least 2 planes. Thus examinations might include sagittal and coronal T1-weighted and T2-weighted sequences, and gadolinium-enhanced sagittal and coronal T1-weighted sequences. Because sellar structures are so fine it is imperative to obtain thin-section images to limit the effects of partial volume averaging, a condition in which 2 adjacent structures cannot be clearly resolved because they lie within the same slice. Traditional imaging at 1.5 T employed 2 or 3 mm scan thickness with little or no gap (10% or less) between sections. With advances in scanner technology, and with the growing popularity and prevalence of 3 T scanners, many centers now obtain 1- or 1.5-mm sections or even volumetric scans to assess the sella. However, because increasing magnetic fields are associated with greater susceptibility artifacts, further advances in field strength may not offer similar gains in imaging resolution. Artifacts are of particular concern when scanning the sella, particularly in the peripubertal population in whom dental braces are common; technologists may be able to modify scanning parameters to minimize the effect of such metallic artifacts.

In addition to high-resolution sellar imaging, many institutions also obtain one or more survey sequences of the entire brain. As certain pituitary abnormalities can be associated with other midline defects, these larger field images should be scrutinized for congenital or developmental anomalies.

Some pituitary abnormalities, most notably microadenomas, are best or most reliably seen using T1-weighted sequences obtained with gadolinium chelate administration. Gadolinium is a lanthanide element that has 7 unpaired electrons, giving it paramagnetic properties.[13] This atom shortens the so-called T1 and T2 relaxation times of water. As a result, gadolinium that either remains in the blood pool or extravasates from the blood pool through a damaged blood-brain barrier causes the containing structure to appear bright, or hyperintense. This property distinguishes enhancing tissues from nonenhancing tissues.

It has long been known that free gadolinium is highly toxic to humans. However, when gadolinium is chelated to specific ligands it has a favorable safety profile. Ligands in clinical use include agents such as diethylene triamine pentaacetic acid (DTPA), which bind strongly to the gadolinium ion thereby minimizing release of free gadolinium into serum. Until about 2006, the approved gadolinium chelates were believed to have minimal potential side effects apart from the occasional allergic reaction. However, it has become clear that patients in dialysis-dependent kidney failure are at significant risk for a recently described and remarkably debilitating scleroderma-like disorder known as nephrogenic systemic fibrosis (NSF, formerly known as nephrogenic fibrosing dermopathy).[14] Although there is evidence that patients with a glomerular filtration rate <30 mL/min/1.73 $m^2$ are at greatest risk for NSF, particularly patients dependent on dialysis, many centers exercise caution in patients with even moderate renal failure (GFR = 30–59 mL/min/1.73 $m^2$). Depending on the degree of renal function remaining, these patients may be offered a half-dose preparation of a newer cyclic agent with greater T1-relaxivity, conferring improved contrast enhancement even at a lower dose. Alternatively, the contrast may be withheld entirely with recognition of the limitation on the diagnostic yield of the study.

## APPEARANCE OF THE NORMAL SELLA

The pituitary stalk extends inferiorly as a direct continuation of the hypothalamic infundibulum, projecting into the gland through a hiatus in the diaphragma sella. The stalk is broadest superiorly and tapers inferiorly to its insertion in the gland (**Figs. 1** and **2**). Although the upper limits of each segment of stalk have been defined in adults (3.5 mm at the median eminence, 2.9 mm at the midpoint and 1.9 mm at its insertion[15]) corresponding standards are scarce in children and assessment of pediatric stalk size tends to be based on experience rather than reference to age-appropriate measurement ranges. In children, as in adults, the stalk should taper from infundibulum to insertion on the gland, and caliber significantly less than 1 mm at any point should be regarded with suspicion.

In general the stalk is best seen on postgadolinium T1-weighted imaging because of the strong enhancement of the stalk. The stalk is moderately well seen on T2-weighted imaging because cerebrospinal fluid (CSF) acts as a natural source of contrast against the lower signal stalk. It is seen poorest on T1-weighted imaging because CSF and stalk are relatively close in inherent signal.

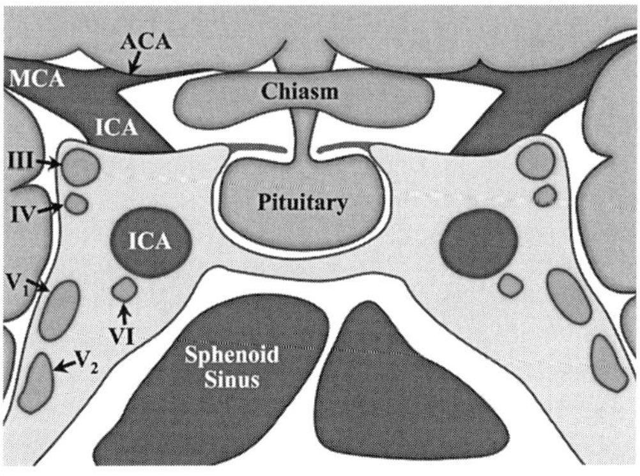


**Fig. 1.** A coronal section through the mid-sella. Note the tapering stalk that penetrates through the hiatus of diaphragma sella (not labeled) to insert on the central pituitary gland. The third (III), fourth (IV), ophthalmic trigeminal ($V_1$) and maxillary trigeminal ($V_2$) nerves sit in the lateral dural wall of the cavernous sinus; the sixth cranial nerve (VI) is the only nerve actually within the sinus, usually near the inferolateral margin of the internal carotid artery (ICA). The ICA continues anterior to the depicted plane before projecting intracranially, superiorly, and posteriorly back into plane, where it bifurcates into the middle cerebral artery (MCA) and anterior cerebral artery (ACA).

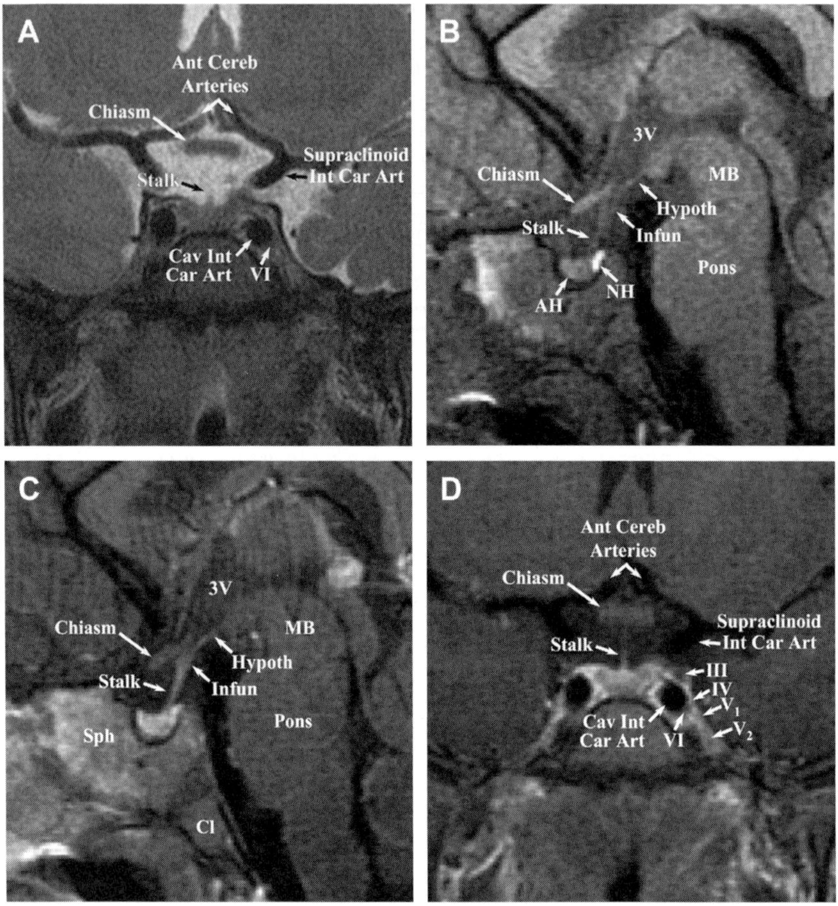


**Fig. 2.** Normal MR imaging through the sella. (*A*) Coronal T2-weighted image showing the stalk inserting on the central gland. Portions of the cavernous internal carotid artery (Cav Int Car Art) are shown, with the abducens nerve (VI) near the inferolateral vessel margin. The optic chiasm, supraclinoid internal carotid artery, and anterior cerebral arteries are also labeled. (*B*) Sagittal noncontrast T1-weighted midline image through the sella. The hypothalamus (Hypoth) and infundibulum (Infun) continue into the stalk, which inserts just anterior to the junction of the "bright spot" laden neurohypophysis (NH) and adenohypophysis (AH). The chiasm sits directly superior to the pituitary. The CSF-filled third ventricle (3V) is seen as a low signal fluid-filled structure. Portions of the brain stem including midbrain (MB) and pons are also labeled. (*C*) Sagittal postcontrast T1-weighted image. Distinction between AH and NH is lost, because the anterior gland is now enhanced. The infundibulum and stalk also enhance well. Portions of the sphenoid bone (Sph) and clivus (Cl) are also labeled. (*D*) Coronal postcontrast T1-weighted image shows many of the structures in (*A*). Note how well and homogeneously the gland enhances. In addition, with the benefit of contrast cranial nerves can be seen as nonenhancing foci in the lateral cavernous sinus wall: third (III), fourth (IV), ophthalmic trigeminal ($V_1$), and maxillary trigeminal ($V_2$).

CSF surrounding the stalk follows the properties of simple fluid, specifically low signal on T1-weighted imaging and high signal on T2-weighted imaging. Sometimes CSF pulsation artifacts reduce T2 signal in areas of greatest fluid motion, that is, displaced from other turbulence-causing structures such as the stalk and supraclinoid internal carotid arteries. Ordinarily the diaphragma sella is not well seen on routine sequences, however heavily T2-weighted sequences obtained at higher resolution (such as fast imaging employing steady-state acquisition [FIESTA] or constructive interference in steady state [CISS] imaging) may clarify the diaphragma in some patients by intensifying signal in the adjacent CSF.

Although the stalk must communicate with both the posterior and anterior lobes of the pituitary, it is frequently seen entering the gland near the midline above the posterior aspect of the anterior lobe, rather than at the junction of the anterior and posterior lobes. This apparently discordant configuration is likely related to the frequent anterior protrusion of the posterior lobe tissue in the midline that meets the stalk at its insertion. This lobule of posterior lobe, which is almost too thin to resolve by MRI but is clearly seen on gross specimens, is partially surrounded by the pars tuberalis of the anterior lobe.[5]

The gland is traditionally felt to be bilaterally symmetric, but within the normal population there exists considerable asymmetry even within normally functioning glands. Thus the pituitary stalk may normally insert slightly off midline, the configuration of the posterior pituitary bright spot may lie off-center, and even the gross contour of the gland may vary from side to side. In addition, the sella turcica itself may not be symmetric, either on a developmental basis or related to acquired factors such as tortuosity of the cavernous internal carotid artery.

Almost directly superior to the stalk's insertion on the gland sits the optic chiasm. On coronal images this may appear ovoid or slightly indented, such as the cross section of an erythrocyte. Signal tends to be isointense to white matter on T1-weighted imaging and T2-weighted imaging. It is ordinarily symmetric, and does not exhibit significant enhancement following gadolinium administration.

Lateral to the sella are the cavernous sinuses. Although they collect blood from discrete veins, instead of hollow central cavities the cavernous sinuses contain countless sinusoids, which together return venous blood to the petrosal sinuses. The sinusoids are isointense on T1-weighted imaging, slightly hyperintense on T2-weighted imaging, and enhance significantly with gadolinium because of the relatively large concentration of blood that fills them. The most conspicuous structure within each cavernous sinus is the cavernous segment of the internal carotid artery. The rapid flow of blood in these arteries leaves little magnetic signal, and thus normally flowing arterial blood appears dark. The cavernous carotid arteries loop anteriorly before continuing intracranially, ultimately bifurcating into the middle and anterior cerebral arteries.

Poorly seen about the sinuses, but of great clinical and surgical importance, are the third to sixth cranial nerves. Of these, only the abducens nerve (CN VI) actually sits within the sinusoids, usually near the inferolateral margin of the cavernous internal carotid artery. The remaining cranial nerves in this region, the oculomotor nerve (CN III), trochlear nerve (CN IV), ophthalmic trigeminal nerve (CN $V_1$), and maxillary trigeminal nerve (CN $V_2$), actually reside in the lateral cavernous sinus wall. Although the entire trigeminal nerve complex leaves the pons and enters Meckel cave together, the fibers of the mandibular portion (CN $V_3$) are the most inferiorly placed among all the trigeminal fibers, and are best seen on sella scans as they exit the foramen ovale.

## GLAND SIZE AND SIGNAL

Several large series of pediatric subjects have showed considerable variability in the size, shape, and signal of normal pediatric pituitary glands. Even among endocrinologically normal subjects of identical age and gender, gland measurements may vary significantly. Therefore the size of the gland must be considered within the clinical scenario, and assessment of gland function may be normal across a wide range of pituitary sizes and shapes.

The normal gland is hyperintense on T1-weighted imaging at birth, so that the anterior and posterior lobes are almost indistinguishable. The gland is also physiologically enlarged, with a corresponding concave superior margin. The high gland signal and prominent size are usually attributed to the lingering effects of maternal hormones. In the next 8 to 10 weeks the gland assumes the infant configuration: (1) the volume declines to a normal infant size; and (2) T1 signal in the anterior lobe drops to near isointensity with the posterior pons, the structure that is ordinarily used as an internal reference on pituitary studies (**Fig. 3**).

Signal in the posterior gland remains high on T1-weighted imaging in most patients. The source of this neurohypophyseal bright spot has been the subject of spirited debate. It is well known that fatty substances appear bright on T1-weighted imaging, so the lipid-rich secretory vesicle bilayer wall had historically been believed to account for the high T1 signal. However, it is also well known that concentrated protein solutions may also give a high T1 signal, and many investigators now believe that the neurophysin-vasopressin complex itself accounts for much of the high signal in the

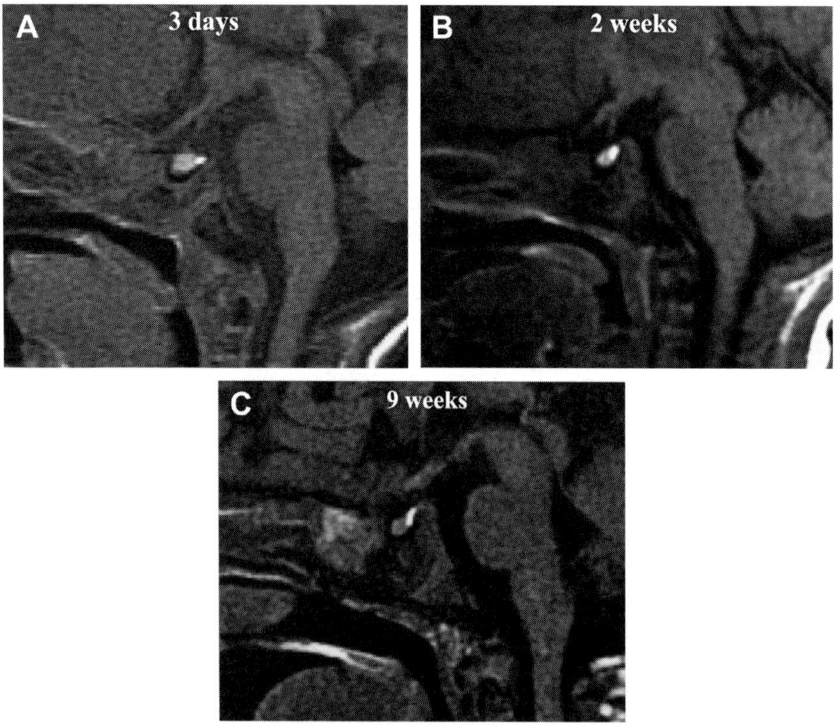


**Fig. 3.** Normal postnatal progression of the pituitary gland. All sagittal T1 noncontrast midline images. (*A*) At birth and through the early days of life the anterior lobe is hyperintense, and the gland is prominent with a convex superior margin. (*B*) After approximately 2 weeks the gland has begun to shrink and the anterior lobe is not quite as bright. (*C*) By approximately 2 months the gland assumes its normal infant state, with lower signal in the anterior gland and slight concavity of the superior gland margin.

posterior gland.[16] The relevance lies not in the source of the signal but its very presence. High signal in the posterior gland suggests a functioning hypothalamic-infundibular-pituitary axis, whereas the ectopic location of this signal (ie, hypothalamus, infundibulum, or stalk) suggests disruption of the normal axonal pathway leading into the posterior gland. This signal is characteristically absent in patients with central diabetes insipidus.[16]

The normal pituitary gland enhances symmetrically following administration of intravenous gadolinium. Intravenous gadolinium is used to characterize blood flow and tissue types within the sella. Dynamic contrast-enhanced sella scans, which require special preparation and are thus not included in the routine scanning protocol of most centers, have revealed the timing and pattern with which the hypothalamic-pituitary axis enhances. In general, the gland enhancement may take well over a minute, and with modern scanners many sets of images may be obtained in that time to chronicle temporal progression. The normal hypothalamus does not enhance well but the infundibulum does, reflecting the concentration of gadolinium in the blood filling the portal plexus that supplies the anterior gland. Enhancement then spreads down the pituitary stalk, with contrast especially intense at the diamond-shaped pituitary tuft at the stalk insertion. From the tuft, the contrast spreads centrifugally, first filling the central adenohypophysis and then incrementally enhancing to the outer margin. Anterior gland enhancement is considerably more robust than posterior gland enhancement, but because the posterior gland is intense even at baseline it also appears bright after contrast. Indeed, reference to unenhanced T1-weighted images is necessary for interpretation of postcontrast scans, because one must be sure that high signal on those scans actually reflects enhancement and not baseline signal. Many gland lesions enhance less than the anterior gland, but some sellar lesions (such as a diaphragma sella meningioma) may enhance quite prominently.

The simplest and earliest method used for measuring gland size was measurement of the maximum height in the midline. Gland height may indeed be the single most useful measurement in gland size determination, and it is still used for quick approximation of gland size. However, there is significant variability in the shapes of normal glands, and a gland that appears shallow may have a large width (transverse measurement) and/or depth (anterior-posterior measurement) resulting in normal volume overall. A more advanced technique uses the product of the maximal 3 orthogonal dimensions and a correction factor (0.524, or $\pi/6$), which is derived from the formula for the volume of a sphere ($4\pi r^3/3$); because glands are usually aspherical this formula is inaccurate in most situations. The most accurate formula based on current imaging technology adds the volume of the gland on each slice, either from a single plane (usually sagittal) or by averaging results from 2 or 3 planes. Indeed, investigators have found high correlation between measurements obtained in different planes, confirming the accuracy of both measurements.[17] From these studies, representative normal pituitary growth curves can be generated (**Fig. 4**). However, ranges of normal do vary among investigators, emphasizing the difficulty of relying on so-called normal ranges obtained using differing scanning techniques.

Glands of preterm infants are taller than those of normal term infants, even when correcting for gestational age. Preterm glands are so tall that preterm infants with a corrected postnatal age of up to 6 months have larger glands than even 2-year-old normal term children. The large gland size may relate to reduced insulin-like growth factor 1 and increased growth hormone in premature infants.[18]

In normal term children the pituitary height is fairly stable for the first 2 years of life, with some investigators measuring a modest decline in this period and others showing modest growth.[19,20] Much of the gland growth in the first 2 years is derived from

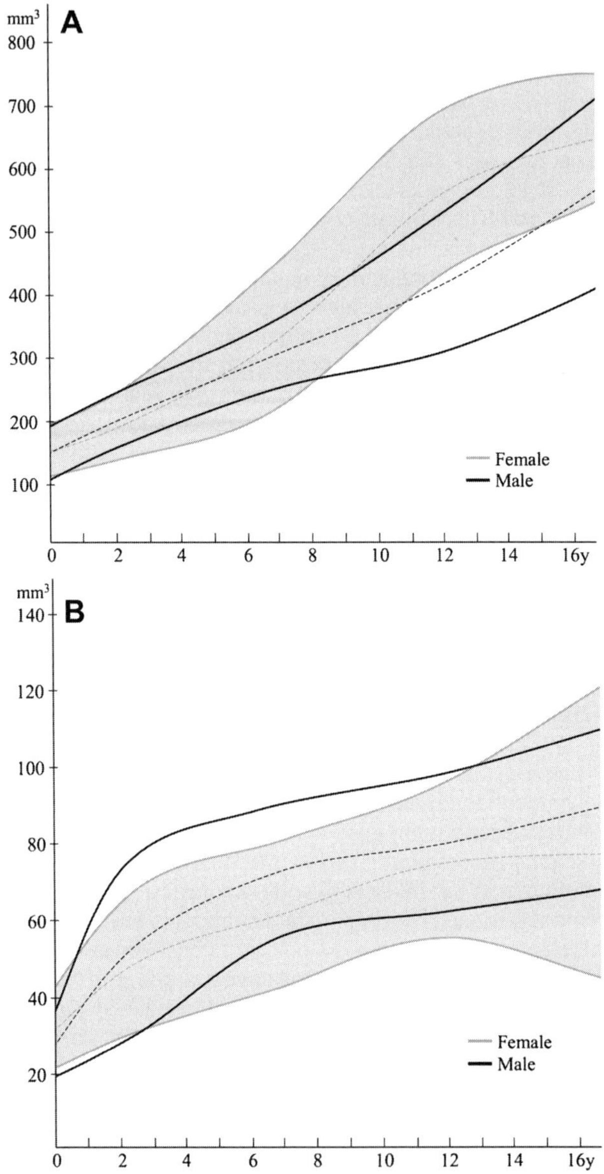


**Fig. 4.** Relative size of the pituitary gland in the first 16 years and contribution of posterior lobe (*Data from* figures *adapted from* Takano K, Utsunomiya H, Ono H et-al. Normal development of the pituitary gland: assessment with three-dimensional MR volumetry. AJNR Am J Neuroradiol 1999;20(2):312–5). (*A*) Diagram illustrating relative growth of the total pituitary. Dashed lines indicating approximate means, with solid lines representing +1 and −1 standard deviation. Black lines indicate boys; gray lines and gray background indicate girls. Boys exhibit a relatively linear growth of the pituitary from birth to the mid-second decade, perhaps exhibiting a slight increase in slope at and beyond puberty. Girls have similar rate of growth in the first half decade, but from that point through puberty the rate increases at a faster rate compared with boys. (*B*) Relative growth of posterior lobe. Line and background shades parallel (*A*). In boys the rate of growth of the posterior gland is most rapid in the first half decade, before resuming a shallower slope through the mid-second decade. In girls the slopes and total volumes tend to be slightly lower, but the total posterior lobe volume shows greater variability after 16 years.

increases in gland width and depth, and the rate of gland growth is similar in boys and girls.

Gender-associated differences in rate of gland growth tend to manifest themselves after 5 years of age, with boys and girls experiencing similar linear growth of their glands up to that point.[17] Boys continue the relatively linear rate of growth into puberty, with slight increase in growth rate beyond this into the late second decade. After the first half decade, overall growth rate in girls is greater than that in boys, until about puberty when the growth slope declines to a rate similar to that seen in the first half decade. A significant portion of gland growth in the first half decade in boys is related to enlargement of the posterior gland, with more balanced gland growth beyond this. Posterior gland growth is less prominent in girls in the first half decade, and anterior lobe growth becomes even more dominant into puberty. By adulthood, female glands are slightly larger than male glands and remain so into old age.

The characteristic neurohypophyseal bright spot on T1-weighted imaging may be absent even in normal patients, but such a pattern is more common in adult populations than in children. When pathologic, absence of this posterior pituitary hyperintensity reflects either a central secretory deficit, disruption of the integrity of axons projecting from hypothalamus to neurohypophysis, or hypoplasia of the gland (**Figs. 5–7**). Fujisawa[16] has defined 4 typical scenarios in which posterior gland intensity is abnormally low:

1. A subset of the normal population does not accumulate significant neurophysin-vasopressin (NP-VP) complex, but these patients are asymptomatic and clinically normal. These patients likely secrete VP soon after it is formed, and therefore do not accumulate enough to confer high signal to the posterior gland.
2. Mass effect within the sella from tumor or even granulomatous disease may, by virtue of its bulk, functionally prevent normal axonal transport of vesicles, resulting in their accumulation just superior to the mass. This is referred to as the "damming phenomenon."
3. When the stalk is transected, either on a congenital basis or from prior trauma, a high signal focus of variable size may be identified along the stalk trajectory

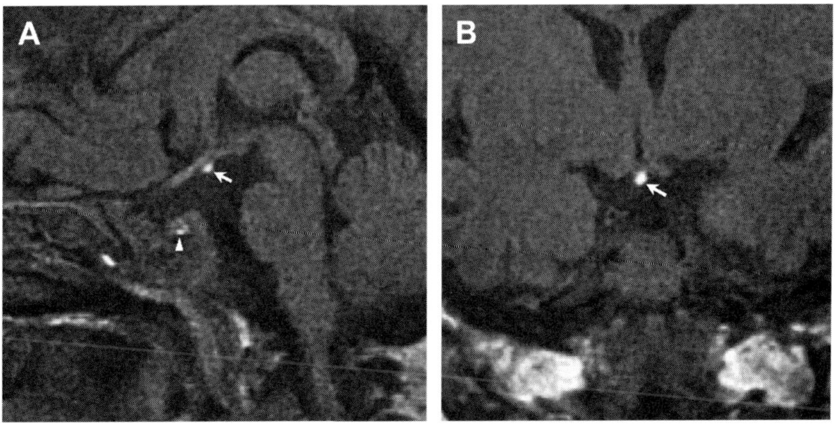


**Fig. 5.** Ectopic posterior pituitary gland. (*A*) Sagittal T1-weighted noncontrast image showing a focal hyperintensity along the inferior hypothalamic margin (*arrow*). No stalk is seen and the pituitary gland is hypoplastic (*arrowhead*). (*B*) Coronal T1-weighted noncontrast image revealing the focal hyperintensity representing nontransported neurophysin-vasopressin vesicles stalled at the inferior hypothalamic margin.

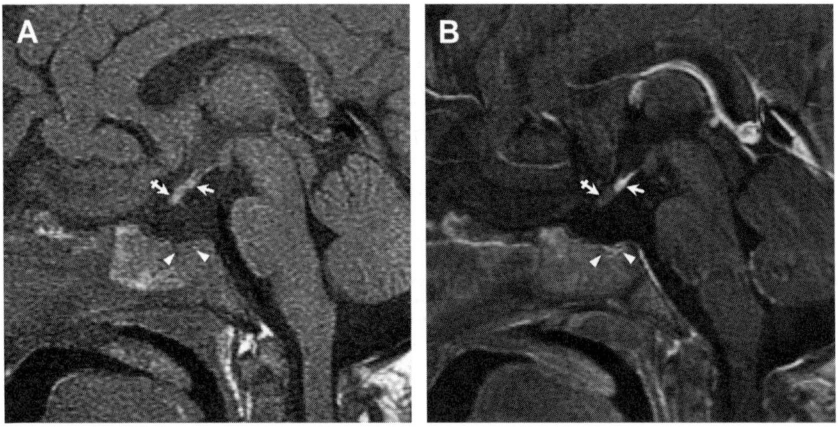

**Fig. 6.** Markedly hypoplastic pituitary with absent bright spot. (*A*) Sagittal noncontrast T1-weighted and (*B*) contrast-enhanced T1-weighted imaging shows almost complete absence of the gland with an associated shallow sella (*arrowheads*). The upper infundibulum is present but the characteristic high T1-weighted signal is not seen on noncontrast imaging. After contrast administration (*B*) the location of the infundibulum and the faint band of sellar pituitary (*arrowheads*) are defined. The chiasm appears thin but is present (*hatched arrow*).

but ectopically (ie, above the level of the normal neurohypophysis). Thus, even though vesicles containing NP-VP may form normally in the hypothalamus, they will not be completely transported into the gland.

4. Patients with central diabetes insipidus may not show any hyperintensity from hypothalamus to pituitary, reflecting an inability to manufacture or package any appreciable NP-VP.

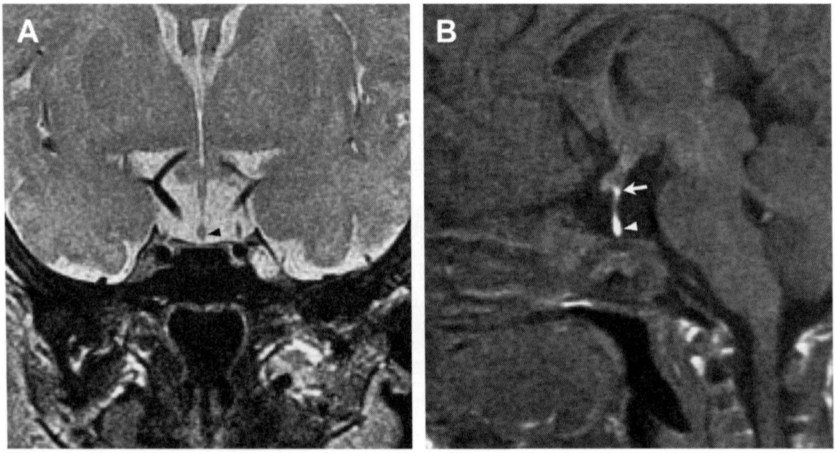

**Fig. 7.** Anterior pituitary aplasia and posterior pituitary ectopia. (*A*) Coronal T2-weighted image reveals a thin stalk terminating in the bulbous, incompletely formed posterior pituitary tissue (*arrowhead*). (*B*) Sagittal T1-weighted noncontrast image showing hypothalamic hypoplasia, a thin infundibulum, and the bulbous neurohypophysis (*arrowhead*) dipping into a shallow, malformed sella. No anterior pituitary was identified.

In the past, anecdotal evidence had suggested that a breech delivery was associated with an ectopic neurohypophysis. Breech delivery was believed to predispose to extreme shearing influences on the stalk, possibly in part related to a consequence of the sharp edge of the diaphragm sella against the stalk. Research has shown that birth trauma may explain only perhaps a third of the cases of pituitary dwarfism, indicating that abnormal mediobasal brain induction may underlie both a pituitary axis abnormality and breech positioning.[21] However, postnatal trauma has more clearly been associated with pituitary dysfunction, with clinically detected endocrine dysfunction in 10% of pediatric patients subject to mild to severe traumatic brain injury. Deficiency of growth hormone is the most prevalent feature.[22] Additional consequences from head trauma include precocious puberty relating to the inability of damaged extrahypothalamic loci to inhibit gonadotropin secretion.

## PITUITARY ADENOMAS

Adenomas arise almost exclusively in the anterior lobe. These tumors seem to behave differently in children than in adults.[23] In adults, tumors that are functional tend to present when small (microadenomas, measuring <10 mm); tumors that are larger (macroadenomas) tend to present because of consequences of mass effect (such as the classic bitemporal hemianopsia seen with chiasmatic compression). In children many of the secreting tumors are quite large at diagnosis. In one pediatric series, at least 70% of tumors had suprasellar extension at diagnosis, and almost 10% were further characterized as giant tumors measuring more than 4 cm.[23]

Pituitary adenomas are rare in childhood, accounting for less than 3% of all supratentorial tumors. Approximately 4% of pituitary adenomas are found in children.[23] However, adenomas are more likely to be functioning in children than in adults.[7] Indeed, some investigators report that up to 95% of pediatric adenomas are hormone-secreting, compared with perhaps one-third in the adult population.[23] Multiple series have shown that prolactinomas are the most common adenoma in the pediatric age group overall, accounting for 48%–52% of tumors. However, prolactinomas are not uniformly prominent throughout the pediatric age range, because the relative proportion of prolactinomas increases steadily through the first decade. In fact, ACTH-releasing tumors with Cushing disease and Nelson syndrome are much more common in the first decade than prolactinomas (71% vs 16%).[24] There is subsequent decrease in ACTH-secreting tumors after the age of 11 years, with these tumors representing 18% to 29% of adenomas for the rest of the second decade. Growth hormone-secreting tumors represent about 8% of lesions, with the proportion slightly higher into later pediatric years.

Detection and conspicuity of microadenomas on imaging depends on lesion size, scan technique, and scan timing. Lesions larger than 3 to 4 mm are usually well seen, regardless of technique employed; resolution of smaller lesions may rely on a higher signal technique to generate thinner sections, higher in-plane resolution, and less imaging noise overall. Typical adenoma signal on routine imaging can vary even within adenoma subtypes, but in general adenomas are isointense or slightly hypointense relative to gray matter on T1-weighted imaging, and isointense to slightly hyperintense on T2-weighted imaging. Hemorrhage may confer susceptibility within the lesion, often seen as diminished T2 signal (and possibly increased T1 signal). Lesions larger than 3 to 4 mm are usually easily seen as areas of diminished signal on postgadolinium imaging, with sensitivity diminishing in smaller lesions (**Fig. 8**). Contrast-enhanced images must be compared with nonenhanced images to confirm parenchymal enhancement, lest an area of high signal be interpreted as enhancement

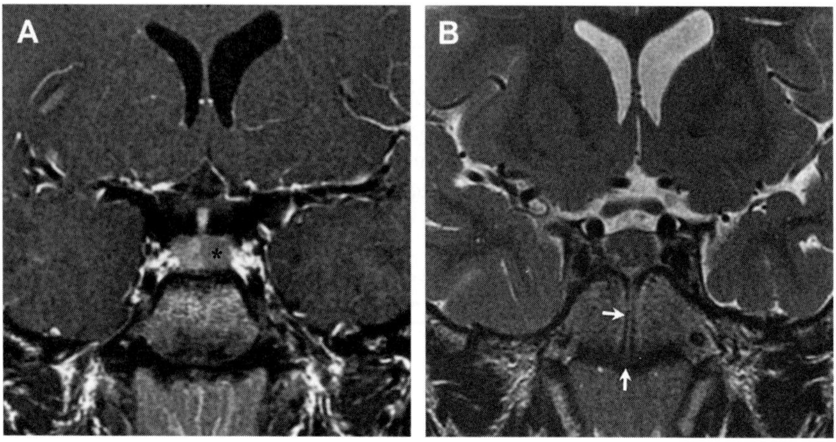


**Fig. 8.** Pituitary adenoma with incidental residual craniopharyngeal canal. (*A*) Coronal T1-weighted contrast-enhanced image reveals an area of diminished enhancement in the left side of the gland (*asterisk*), compatible with a microadenoma. There is only slight right-ward deviation of the stalk in this instance. (*B*) Coronal T2-weighted image fails to show the adenoma, but does show the residual craniopharyngeal canal (*arrows*).

when in fact it was hyperintense on noncontrast imaging to start with (**Fig. 9**). Cystic change may appear hyperintense on T2-weighted imaging, although hemorrhage into a cyst may also be associated with a contradicting reduction in signal.

Because signal in adenomas tends to appear similar to adjacent parenchyma, contrast-enhanced sequences are ordinarily obtained to improve adenoma detection. Although adenomas enhance, they typically do so less strongly than normal pituitary parenchyma, and their peak enhancement lags behind that of the normal gland.

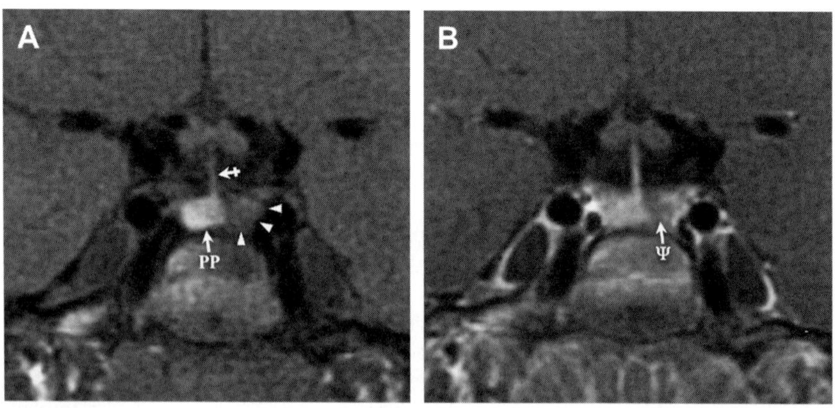


**Fig. 9.** Pseudo-mass in the pituitary. (*A*) Congenitally asymmetric appearance of the bright posterior pituitary (PP) on coronal noncontrast T1-weighted imaging, with perhaps 80% of the posterior lobe sitting to the right of midline. The lower signal in the left side of the gland represents asymmetric positioning of the anterior lobe (*arrowheads*). The stalk (*hatched arrow*) still inserts near the midline. (*B*) After contrast is given the anterior lobe on the left side enhances, but does not become as bright as the posterior lobe on the right, causing a pseudo-mass (ψ).

Ordinarily scanning is begun immediately after contrast administration to capture the maximal difference between gland and adenoma. For each minute that scanning is delayed, one would expect to detect approximately 10% to 15% fewer lesions, so that if scanning is delayed for 7 to 10 minutes after gadolinium injection almost all adenomas would be nearly unresolvable. For this reason the dynamic contrast technique, described earlier, may increase sensitivity further in cases in which a lesion is strongly suspected but not detected on preliminary scanning. In instances where scanning is delayed after contrast administration (eg, mild contrast reaction, nausea, claustrophobia), the examination may still be salvaged by exploiting the differential washout of contrast from the gland (**Fig. 10**). Because contrast clears faster from normal parenchyma than it does from adenomas, on delayed scans adenomas will appear hyperintense relative to the remaining gland, instead of hypointense as they do in the early postinjection period.[25] The crossover point at which enhancement of adenomas begins to surpass normal parenchyma remains poorly defined, but in many cases it may be less than 6 to 8 minutes after contrast injection.

## CYSTIC LESIONS

Rathke cleft cysts (RCCs) are common incidental pituitary cysts that are found in up to 20% of routine autopsies.[26] These cysts arise from the nonobliterated intrasellar lumen of Rathke pouch,[27] and most are so small that they are asymptomatic. When cysts are large (on average 16.3 ± 1.2 mm) they become symptomatic, largely because of their mass effect.[28] Such cysts may exert enough mass effect to

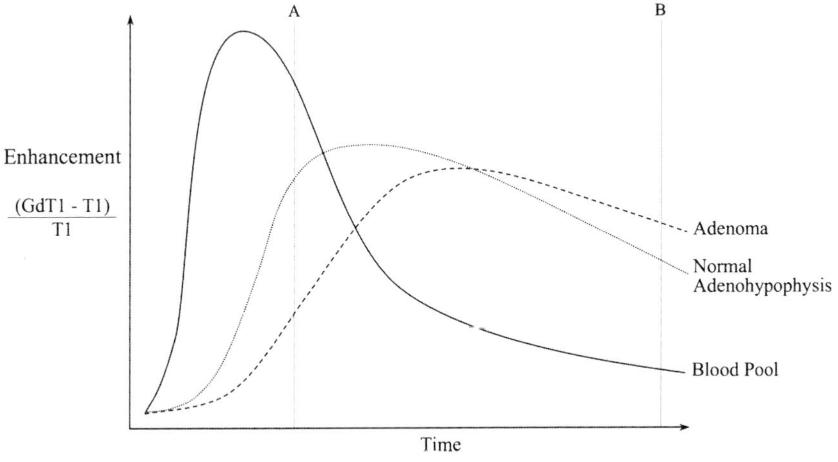


**Fig. 10.** Gadolinium enhancement patterns. The y-axis indicates signal differential between enhanced and baseline images; the x-axis reflects time. The blood pool enhances earliest and strongest, but it also tapers most rapidly with renal clearance of gadolinium. The normal pituitary gland has a shallower increase, somewhat delayed after the blood pool curve, and shows a gradual decrease. Most adenomas have even slower increase and decrease. The greatest difference between parenchyma and adenomas (and therefore greatest conspicuity of adenomas) is in the early gland enhancement period (time point A), when the gland enhances well but the adenoma has only begun to accumulate contrast. If, for some reason, the gland cannot be imaged at that point, the patient may be rescanned, because the adenoma may retain contrast longer and an adenoma will appear as an area of signal that is higher than the gland (time point B).

compromise remaining pituitary tissue, or they may grow superiorly to compress the optic chiasm, resulting in a bitemporal hemianopsia. Larger cysts may also be associated with headaches. On MRI, noncomplicated cysts follow fluid intensity, so they are hypointense on T1-weighted imaging and hyperintense on T2-weighted imaging. RCCs may, over time, develop a higher protein concentration, resulting in an increase in T1 signal and, as protein concentration increases, a reduction in T2 signal (**Fig. 11**). Sludge or intracystic nodules have also been described as areas of layering or nodular signal in the posterior aspect of the gland.[29] RCCs do not enhance centrally and most do not enhance about their periphery unless they have suffered recent hemorrhage or infection; enhancement about a cyst should suggest another diagnosis such as hemorrhagic adenoma or craniopharyngioma.

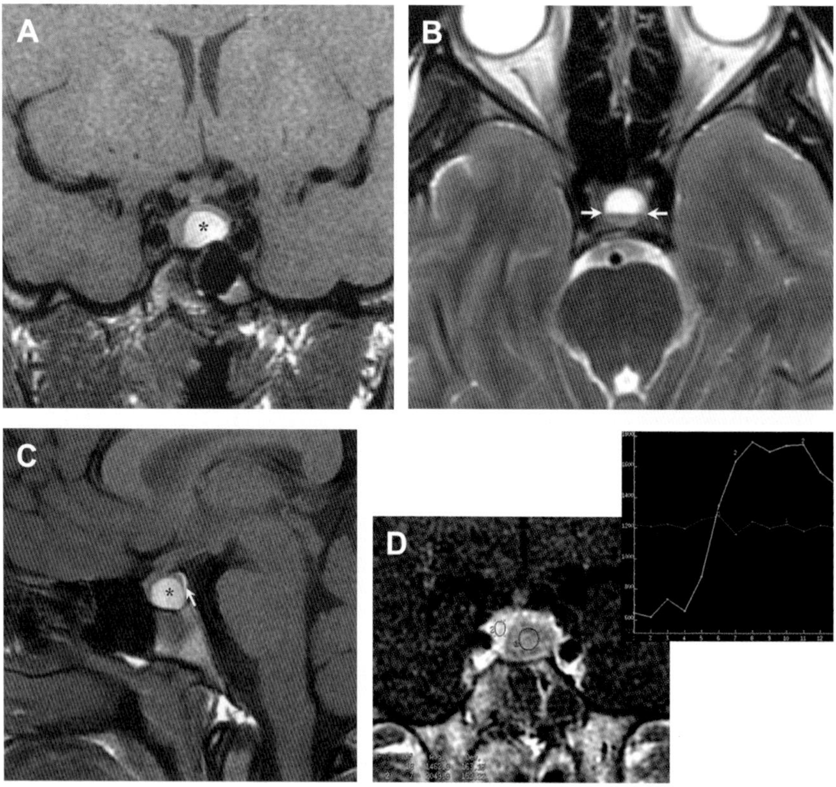


**Fig. 11.** Rathke cleft cyst. (*A*) Coronal T1-weighted noncontrast image shows a rounded focus of high signal (asterisk) situated eccentrically toward the left side of the gland. There is associated bowing of the superior gland margin, presumably related to mass effect from the cyst. (*B*) Axial T2-weighted image, revealing a rounded cavity within the central sella, in which a debris level is present (*between arrows*). Such levels are among the most reliable imaging features confirming a cyst. (*C*) Sagittal T1-weighted noncontrast image reveals the relationship of the cyst (*asterisk*) with the posterior lobe (*arrow*). A thin band of tissue (not labeled) sits between the posterior lobe and the cyst, which presumably reflects the posterior wall of Rathke cleft and makes this cyst more likely to represent a Rathke cleft cyst than a pars intermedia cyst. (*D*) Coronal T1-weighted dynamic sella scan proves the lesion is cystic. The y-axis indicates signal and the x-axis reflects time. Normal pituitary tissue enhances well (curve 2), whereas a cyst will not enhance (curve 1).

Pars intermedia cysts form within the pituitary along the posterior margin of Rathke pouch. These are ordinarily asymptomatic lesions measuring less than 3 mm. Configuration varies, but a flattened cystic cavity broadest in the coronal plane, sitting at the junction of anterior and posterior lobes, suggests this diagnosis (**Fig. 12**). In many instances pars intermedia cysts may be difficult to distinguish from RCCs, which are more common, so many pars intermedia cysts are considered RCCs on imaging.

Craniopharyngiomas (CPs) are benign tumors that, like RCCs, are also derived from embryologic remnants of Rathke pouch. Of the two varieties, the cystic (or adamantinomatous) tumors (ACPs) are more frequent in the pediatric population. These tumors represent about 10% of all childhood brain tumors and account for approximately 90% of pituitary neoplasms in children.[30,31] The squamous-papillary variety, which is most common in the sixth and seventh decades, has more solid configuration. ACPs typically contain one or more large cysts of varying wall thickness, with central proteinaceous fluid typically of "crank-case oil"-like consistency. Because of the proteinaceous nature of the cavities, these lesions may be quite hyperintense on T1-weighted imaging and only mildly elevated on T2-weighted imaging. Enhancement is seen about the rim but not centrally (**Fig. 13**). This peripheral enhancement may be thin or nodular, but with the high T1 signal within the cyst at baseline, any contrast enhancement may be difficult to resolve. ACPs arise within the suprasellar cistern but may grow inferior into the sella; purely intrasellar ACPs are rare. These tumors tend to be large when detected, because they present because of mass effect or local effect of tumor on cranial nerves, and are larger at diagnosis than even symptomatic RCCs (36.2 $\pm$ 4.7 mm vs 16.3 $\pm$ 1.2 mm).[28] If distinction of RCC from ACP proves challenging by MRI, a CT scan that demonstrates calcification around the lesion margin markedly increases the probability of craniopharyngioma. Although these tumors

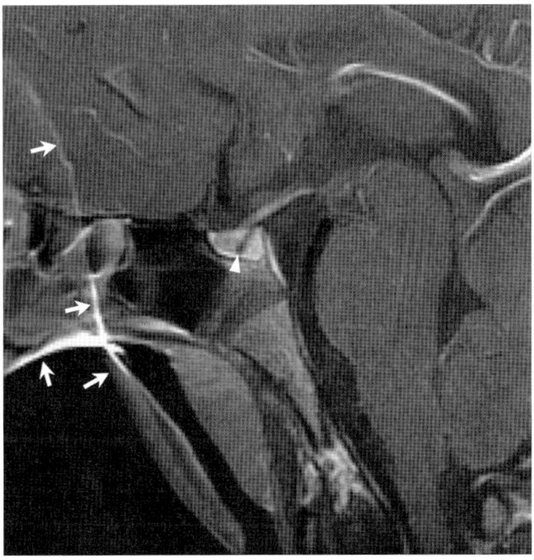

**Fig. 12.** Presumed pars intermedia cyst. Sagittal contrast-enhanced T1-weighted image reveals a thin band of nonenhancement (*arrowhead*) corresponding to the posterior aspect of the anterior lobe. A cyst in this location with thin anterior-posterior diameter relative to height and width is suggestive of a pars intermedia cyst rather than a Rathke cleft cyst. Note the artifact from the patient's dental braces (*arrows*); technologists may be able to modify scanning parameters to eliminate or at least shift the artifacts if they project through structures of interest.

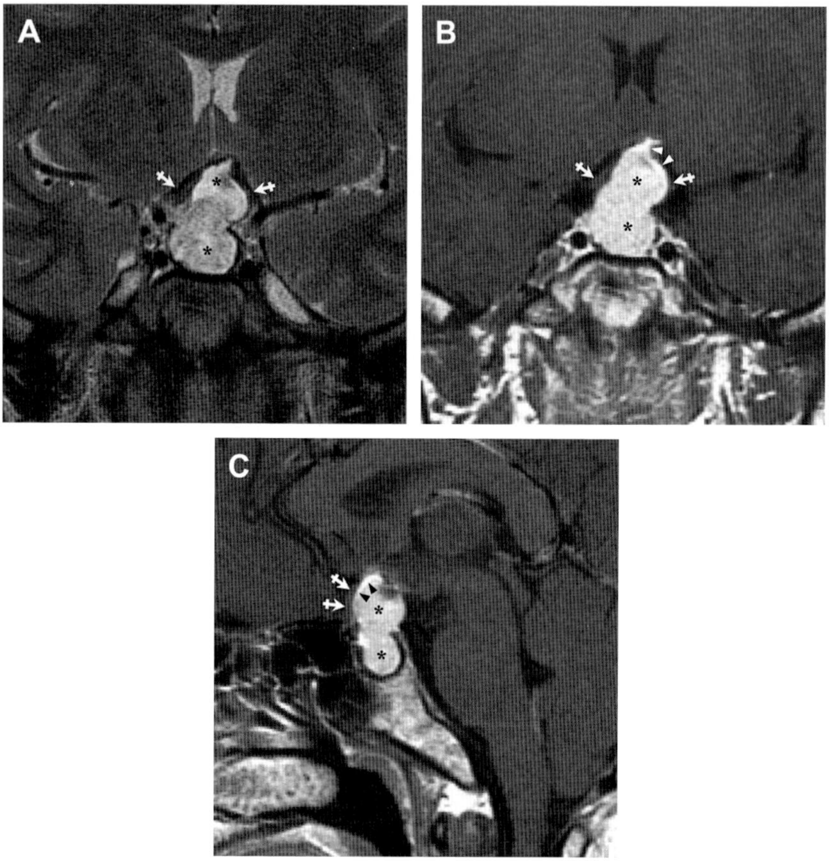


**Fig. 13.** Adamantinomatous (cystic) craniopharyngioma. (*A*) Coronal T2-weighted image reveals a large cyst filling the sella and suprasellar cistern (*asterisks*). Coronal (*B*) and sagittal (*C*) postcontrast T1-weighted imaging reveals the high signal within the cyst (*asterisks*) characteristic of craniopharyngiomas. Enhancement is subtle but can be seen around the superior margin of the cyst (*arrowheads*). In all images the sella is expanded, and mass effect displaces the chiasm superiorly (*hatched arrows*).

are histologically benign, their insinuation into leptomeninges, cranial nerves, and vessels makes surgical eradication difficult if not impossible.

The term "empty sella" is largely a misnomer, as the sella is rarely truly empty. Underlying this phenomenon is atypical transmission of CSF pulsation through the hiatus of the diaphragm sella. This pulsatility may, over time, flatten the pituitary along the floor of the sella. In adults this may be related to an abnormally wide diaphragmatic hiatus, but in children it most commonly results from prior surgery, chemotherapy, or posttraumatic affects. On imaging, the sella appears largely fluid in signal, with hypointense pattern on T1-weighted imaging and hyperintensity on T2-weighted imaging. The gland is typically flattened along the sellar floor and may be most conspicuous after gadolinium administration. In most cases the stalk can be followed to its insertion on the flattened gland along the sellar floor. Little can be inferred from the resulting gland configuration, because gland function may appear clinically normal in many degrees of gland flattening.

Arachnoid cysts are fluid accumulations within the leaves of arachnoid. These are usually congenital, but they may arise after trauma, infection, or hemorrhage.[32] In children, symptomatic arachnoid cysts cause CSF flow disturbances in 95% of patients, and endocrine abnormalities in 5%. Although these are slow-growing cysts, over time they can cause significant mass effect and even bony remodeling. As such, pediatric patients with suprasellar arachnoid cysts may exhibit deficiencies of growth hormone and thyrotropin, excess stimulation of the hypothalamic-pituitary axis, and possibly hyperinsulinism-related tall stature or overweight status.[32,33]

## SUPRASELLAR TUMORS

Gliomas may arise anywhere along the optic pathway (including optic nerve, chiasm, or tract), or within the adjacent hypothalamus. Hypothalamic gliomas are of particular concern with regard to endocrine function, because these tumors may cause symptoms related to obesity, diabetes insipidus, or other hypothalamic-pituitary dysfunction.[34] Most of these gliomas are graded as juvenile pilocytic astrocytomas. These are particularly common in patients with neurofibromatosis type 1 (NF-1, von Recklinghausen disease), but NF-1 patients tend to fare better with this tumor than patients with sporadic hypothalamic gliomas. These lesions are seen on imaging as thickening of the third ventricular floor and hypothalamus, with margins that are sometimes obscure. On MRI, these tumors tend to show an isointense or perhaps slightly hypointense T1 signal and slightly hyperintense T2 signal. However, unlike other low-grade gliomas, these lesions tend to enhance well. Larger tumors may grow directly into the pituitary stalk.

Tuber cinereum hamartomas are nonneoplastic heterotopias that are comprised of an atypical proliferation of normal cellular elements. Two different clinical scenarios may be seen: smaller pedunculated tumors (<1 cm) tend to be associated with precocious puberty, whereas larger sessile tumors (>1 cm) tend to be associated with gelastic seizures. Because these lesions are comprised of neuronal elements, they tend to resemble brain parenchyma on all modes of imaging (**Fig. 14**). Some may show a modestly increased T2 signal.[35] The blood-brain barrier is intact, so they do not enhance appreciably.

Among germ cell tumors, germinomas represent just over half; other less frequent germ cell tumors include teratomas, choriocarcinomas, and embryonal cell carcinomas. More than 90% of germinomas are found in males. They most commonly grow in the pineal region but up to one-third are seen in the suprasellar region, and involvement of both sites simultaneously (bifocal disease) is increasingly recognized.[36] A suprasellar germinoma may present as a consequence of its mass effect, for example, through compression of the optic chiasm (producing a bitemporal hemianopsia), or by disruption of the hypothalamic-infundibular-pituitary axis.[37] These tumors tend to be isointense or slightly hyperintense, with strong enhancement of solid portions after gadolinium administration (**Fig. 15**). Up to half of germinomas contain areas of cystic degeneration, which do not enhance but may appear considerably hyperintense on T2-weighted imaging. Because of the propensity for germinomas to spread within the subarachnoid space, if an intracranial germinoma is suspected additional imaging of the spine is often performed to exclude drop-metastases.

## SYSTEMIC CONDITIONS

Sarcoidosis is a systemic disease in which the primary feature is formation of noncaseating epithelioid granulomas.[38] The lungs and hilar nodes are most frequently

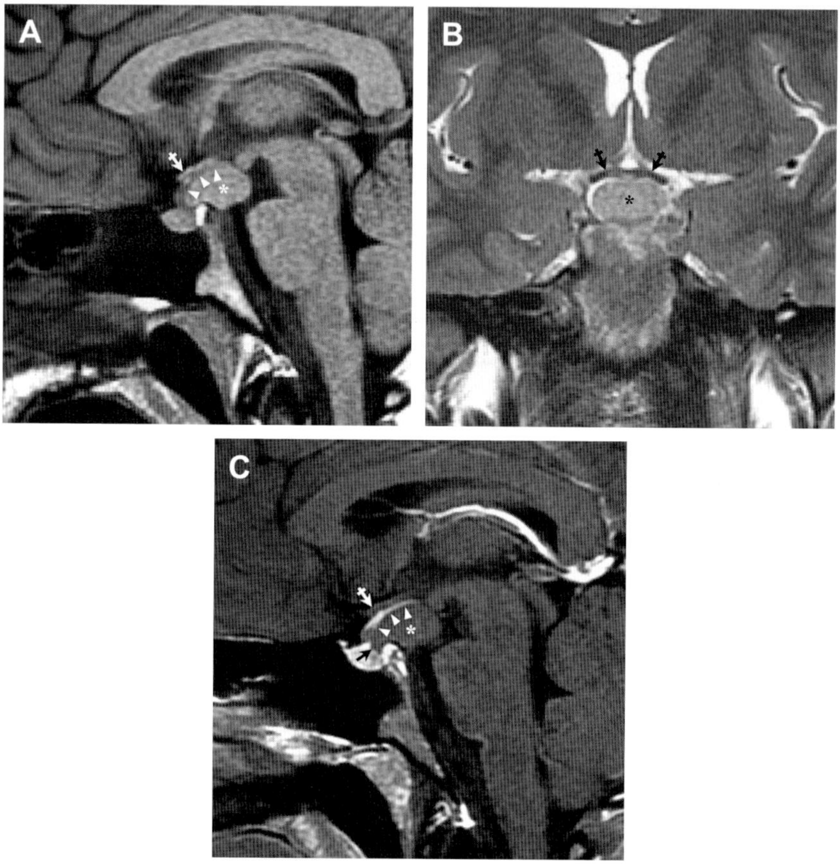


**Fig. 14.** Hypothalamic hamartoma. (*A*) Sagittal T1-weighted image revealing nodular isointense fullness about the hypothalamus (*asterisk*), with displacement of the infundibulum superiorly and the stalk anterosuperiorly (*arrowheads*). The optic chiasm is flattened by the mass (*hatched arrow*). (*B*) Coronal T2-weighted image demonstrating a rounded slightly hyperintense mass in the suprasellar cistern (*asterisk*). The superior displacement and attenuation of the optic chiasm is well seen (*hatched arrows*). (*C*) Sagittal T1-weighted postcontrast image shows no significant enhancement of the tumor (*asterisk*), which actually extends inferiorly into the sella (*arrow*). Contrast does clarify the course of the infundibulum and stalk (*arrowheads*). Again note the flattened optic chiasm (*hatched arrow*).

involved, but sarcoid may also affect the heart, skin, liver, and, infrequently, the central nervous system. When affecting the central nervous system (CNS), sarcoidosis is predominantly extraaxial (ie, it affects brain surfaces rather than brain parenchyma directly). Among extraaxial sites, the sellar and suprasellar regions are preferred, with coarse nodular aggregates typically along the stalk and into the sella that enhance well after contrast. Disease can also involve structures within the subarachnoid spaces, most notably the cranial nerves, in which case they may produce cranial neuropathies. On occasion enhancement from sarcoid may be visualized within parenchyma, deep to the brain surface; in these situations disease is felt to track along perforators from the surface into the parenchyma, mimicking a parenchymal process.

Langerhans cell histiocytosis (LCH) is characterized by pathologic accumulation of Langerhans cells. Typically CNS involvement is seen in patients with systemic disease

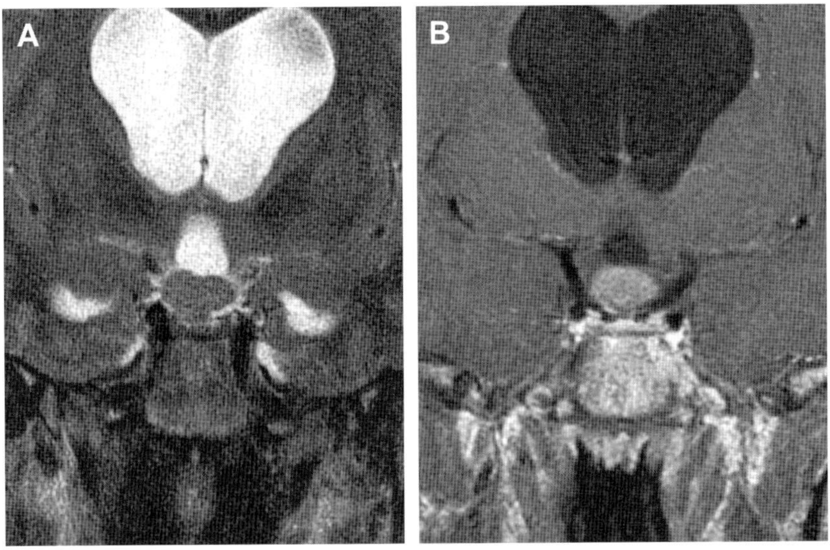


**Fig. 15.** Suprasellar germinoma. Coronal T2-weighted (*A*) and T1-weighted postgadolinium (*B*) scans show a rounded suprasellar mass that enhances moderately well. There is marked dilatation of the lateral ventricles, related to compression of the cerebral aqueduct of Sylvius by simultaneous pineal germinoma (not shown).

or with a skull lesion.[39] It is believed that infiltration into the hypothalamic-pituitary axis causes CNS-associated symptoms; diabetes insipidus is seen in at least 24% of patients with LCH, although some investigators report an even higher incidence.[39,40] Anterior pituitary dysfunction is also reported but is seen less commonly; for example, growth hormone deficiency may be seen in between 10 and 20% of patients with LCH, but these patients usually also have diabetes insipidus. Inflammatory thickening, which is best seen on postcontrast T1 images, may occur anywhere along the infundibulum and stalk. The appearance of this infiltration may mimic other inflammatory disorders such as sarcoid or even a lymphocytic hypophysitis.[41]

McCune-Albright syndrome is a rare sporadic genetic disorder characterized by the classic triad: polyostotic fibrous dysplasia, endocrine hyperfunction, and café-au-lait skin lesions. The best known hormonal association, precocious puberty, is seen more frequently in girls. Additional endocrine manifestations include hypercortisolism, hyperthyroidism, and acromegaly. Occasionally a growth hormone–secreting microadenoma is seen on sellar MRI examination. However, on imaging the most prominent findings relate to fibrous dysplasia. Osseous findings relate to proliferation of fibrous tissue in bone marrow by abnormal preosteoblastic cells.[42] Bone lesions typically extend from medulla to cortex, with either a radiolucent or homogeneous "ground-glass" density. Long bones, ribs, and craniofacial structures are most commonly involved. Radiography exposes patients to a relatively low radiation dose, but CT may be necessary to identify subtle areas of involvement (**Fig. 16**). MRI is a less favorable modality to use for assessment of fibrous dysplasia, although affected areas may occasionally be detected as relatively homogeneous areas of low signal.

## ASSOCIATED MIDLINE LESIONS

Callosal abnormalities range from complete aplasia of the gland (callosal agenesis) to callosal hypoplasia, in which the entire callosum forms but is thin or attenuated.[43]

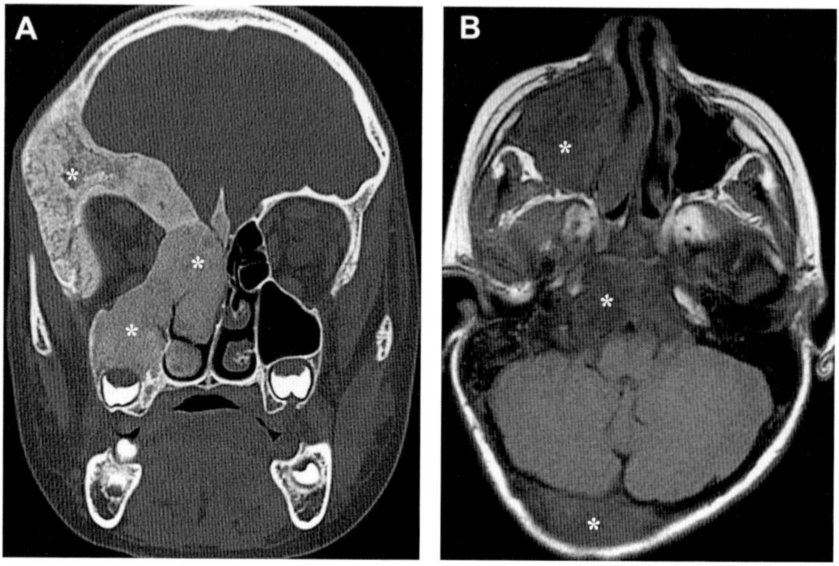


**Fig. 16.** Fibrous dysplasia. (*A*) Coronal CT showing the ground-glass configuration that characterizes fibrous dysplasia through the right maxillary sinus and ethmoid region (*mid and lower asterisk*), with more coarse expansile bone extending along the orbital roof (*upper asterisk*). (*B*) There is a relatively homogeneous and moderately low T1 signal pattern through the nonpneumatized right maxillary sinus, sphenoid bone, and occipital bone (*asterisks*).

*Callosal agenesis.* Complete agenesis is characterized by (1) absent cingulate sulcus; (2) colpocephaly, in which there is a parallel arrangement of the lateral ventricles that have teardrop-shaped posterior horns; (3) superior protrusion of the third ventricle, because its upper margin is not as confined as in normal patients; and (4) abnormal longitudinal fascicles that were meant to cross the midline but instead fold back on themselves, representing disordered bundles of Probst.[44,45] Midline sagittal imaging reveals radiating bands of gyri and sulci from the ventricular margin, in lieu of the cingulum that is normally present.

*Callosal hypogenesis*. The callosum forms in a predictable pattern: genu first, followed by body and splenium, and finally the most anteroinferior rostrum. Segments that fail to form appear the latest embryologically, so hypogenesis almost always involves rostrum, and then may involve splenium, then body, then genu. Thus, in hypogenesis the segments of callosum that do form include G-B-S (genu-body-splenium), G-B, or G (**Fig. 17**). Furthermore, a callosum that possesses an intact rostrum but lacks another segment has likely undergone some destruction of a portion of previously formed segment of the callosum.

*Callosal hypoplasia.* A hypoplastic callosum forms all of its segments, but is somewhat attenuated. As the callosum experiences considerable growth, with thickening over time, assessment of hypoplasia in the first year may prove challenging.

Chiari hindbrain malformations are comprised of a group of 4 developmental cerebellar anomalies. Type I, by far the most common, has been associated with multiple endocrine deficiencies.[46] It is characterized by peglike protrusion of cerebellar tonsils through the foramen magnum. Although numeric thresholds have been used traditionally

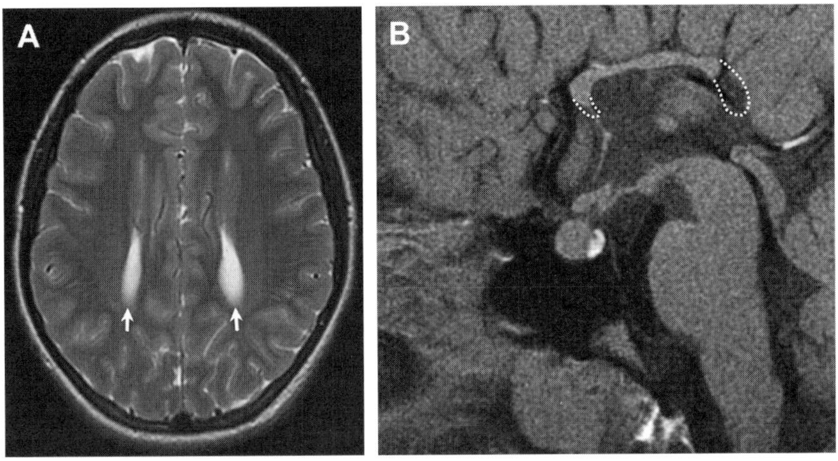


**Fig. 17.** Partial callosal agenesis. (*A*) Axial T2 image through the lateral cerebral ventricles show a parallel (rather than banana-shaped) configuration of the ventricles with colpocephalic tear-drip pattern posteriorly (*arrows*). (*B*) Sagittal T1-weighted image reveals a thin shortened callosum, with absence of the splenium (expected contour margin indicated by posterior dotted line) and rostrum (expected contour margin indicated by anterior dotted line). Note the radiating pattern of gyri and sulci from the callosal margin. The gland is physiologically hypertrophied in this 16-year-old girl.

to confirm this tonsillar ectopia (extension at least 6 mm below the foramen magnum (basion-opisthion line) in the first decade, at least 5 mm in the second and third decades, and so forth[47]) it is becoming clear that what underlies clinically relevant Chiari malformations is actually the alteration in the normal CSF dynamics that result from such a configuration.[48] Thus investigators have used phase-contrast imaging to show where the CSF flow abnormality exists in symptomatic patients, and may ultimately explain why two different patients with the same measured ectopia may exhibit very different symptoms. Additional imaging features may include syringohydromyelia, the abnormal dilatation of the central canal of the cord related to disordered CSF flow patterns. Symptoms from a Chiari I malformation are nonspecific but include suboccipital headaches (28%–63% of patients), cranial nerve palsies or brain stem symptoms (21%), ataxia (6%–25%), and long tract signs.[49]

Septo-optic dysplasia (SOD, de Morsier Syndrome) comprises a spectrum of disorders that affect midline structures.[6,50,51] Although mutations in the HESX1 gene have been implicated, HESX1 causation may be more common in sporadic disease than in familial cases. The most common abnormality is optic nerve hypoplasia (seen in 75%–80% of SOD patients); this is usually bilateral (88%). Microphthalmia or anophthalmia may be seen but is rare. Pituitary symptoms range from isolated growth hormone deficiency to panhypopituitarism; gonadotropin secretion may be preserved in the face of near complete hypopituitarism.[6] Associated brain anomalies include midline forebrain abnormalities such as callosal agenesis, absence of the septum pellucidum and fornix aplasia. Additional features may include schizencephaly and cerebellar hypoplasia. Holoprosencephaly, specifically the lobar variety, may also be seen with SOD.

## SUMMARY

Evaluation of the sella and surrounding structures in pediatric endocrinopathies is best performed with high-resolution MRI scanning. Adequate assessment relies not only on determining the size and shape of the gland but also on confirming normal signal characteristics and homogeneous parenchymal enhancement. Surrounding structures, including the hypothalamus-infundibulum-stalk and the skull base and midline structures about the cerebral hemispheres, warrant careful attention to identify any associated abnormalities. Tumors, whether they arise in the gland or affect gland function through mass effect, are usually well resolved on today's scanners and imaging provides accurate characterization of these lesions.

## REFERENCES


1. Mehta A, Dattani MT. Developmental disorders of the hypothalamus and pituitary gland associated with congenital hypopituitarism. Best Pract Res Clin Endocrinol Metab 2008;22(1):191–206.
2. Ray D, Melmed S. Pituitary cytokine and growth factor expression and action. Endocr Rev 1997;18(2):206–28.
3. Jinkins JR. Atlas of neuroradiologic embryology, anatomy, and variants. Baltimore (MD): Lippincott Williams & Wilkins; 2000.
4. Makulski DD, Taber KH, Chiou-Tan FY. Neuroimaging in posttraumatic hypopituitarism. J Comput Assist Tomogr 2008;32(2):324–8.
5. Rhoton AL Jr. The sellar region. Neurosurgery 2002;51(Suppl 4):S335–74.
6. Kelberman D, Dattani MT. Hypothalamic and pituitary development: novel insights into the aetiology. Eur J Endocrinol 2007;157(Suppl 1):S3–14.
7. Diamond FB Jr. Pituitary adenomas in childhood: development and diagnosis. Fetal Pediatr Pathol 2006;25(6):339–56.
8. Scully KM, Rosenfeld MG. Pituitary development: regulatory codes in mammalian organogenesis. Science 2002;295(5563):2231–5.
9. Kioussi C, O'Connell S, St-Onge L, et al. Pax6 is essential for establishing ventral-dorsal cell boundaries in pituitary gland development. Proc Natl Acad Sci U S A 1999;96(25):14378–82.
10. Mullen RD, Colvin SC, Hunter CS, et al. Roles of the LHX3 and LHX4 LIM-homeodomain factors in pituitary development. Mol Cell Endocrinol 2007;265-266:190–5.
11. Sloop KW, Walvoord EC, Showalter AD, et al. Molecular analysis of LHX3 and PROP-1 in pituitary hormone deficiency patients with posterior pituitary ectopia. J Clin Endocrinol Metab 2000;85(8):2701–8.
12. Cohen LE. Genetic regulation of the embryology of the pituitary gland and somatotrophs. Endocrine 2000;12(2):99–106.
13. Weinmann HJ, Brasch RC, Press WR, et al. Characteristics of gadolinium-DTPA complex: a potential NMR contrast agent. AJR Am J Roentgenol 1984;142(3):619–24.
14. Grobner T, Prischl FC. Patient characteristics and risk factors for nephrogenic systemic fibrosis following gadolinium exposure. Semin Dial 2008;21(2):135–9.
15. Rupp D, Molitch M. Pituitary stalk lesions. Curr Opin Endocrinol Diabetes Obes 2008;15(4):339–45.
16. Fujisawa I. Magnetic resonance imaging of the hypothalamic-neurohypophyseal system. J Neuroendocrinol 2004;16(4):297–302.
17. Takano K, Utsunomiya H, Ono H, et al. Normal development of the pituitary gland: assessment with three-dimensional MR volumetry. AJNR Am J Neuroradiol 1999;20(2):312–5.
18. Kiortsis D, Xydis V, Drougia AG, et al. The height of the pituitary in preterm infants during the first 2 years of life: an MRI study. Neuroradiology 2004;46(3):224–6.

19. Argyropoulou MI, Kiortsis DN. MRI of the hypothalamic-pituitary axis in children. Pediatr Radiol 2005;35(11):1045–55.
20. Dietrich RB, Lis LE, Greensite FS, et al. Normal MR appearance of the pituitary gland in the first 2 years of life. AJNR Am J Neuroradiol 1995;16(7):1413–9.
21. Triulzi F, Scotti G, di Natale B, et al. Evidence of a congenital midline brain anomaly in pituitary dwarfs: a magnetic resonance imaging study in 101 patients. Pediatrics 1994;93(3):409–16.
22. Einaudi S, Bondone C. The effects of head trauma on hypothalamic-pituitary function in children and adolescents. Curr Opin Pediatr 2007;19(4):465–70.
23. Pandey P, Ojha BK, Mahapatra AK. Pediatric pituitary adenoma: a series of 42 patients. J Clin Neurosci 2005;12(2):124–7.
24. Kunwar S, Wilson CB. Pediatric pituitary adenomas. J Clin Endocrinol Metab 1999;84(12):4385–9.
25. Kucharczyk W, Bishop JE, Plewes DB, et al. Detection of pituitary microadenomas: comparison of dynamic keyhole fast spin-echo, unenhanced, and conventional contrast-enhanced MR imaging. AJR Am J Roentgenol 1994; 163(3):671–9.
26. Zada G, Ditty B, McNatt SA, et al. Surgical treatment of Rathke cleft cysts in children. Neurosurgery 2009;64(6):1132–7 [author reply: 1037–8].
27. Takanashi J, Tada H, Barkovich AJ, et al. Pituitary cysts in childhood evaluated by MR imaging. AJNR Am J Neuroradiol 2005;26(8):2144–7.
28. Shin JL, Asa SL, Woodhouse LJ, et al. Cystic lesions of the pituitary: clinicopathological features distinguishing craniopharyngioma, Rathke's cleft cyst, and arachnoid cyst. J Clin Endocrinol Metab 1999;84(11):3972–82.
29. Byun WM, Kim OL, Kim D. MR imaging findings of Rathke's cleft cysts: significance of intracystic nodules. AJNR Am J Neuroradiol 2000;21(3):485–8.
30. Garre ML, Cama A. Craniopharyngioma: modern concepts in pathogenesis and treatment. Curr Opin Pediatr 2007;19(4):471–9.
31. Jagannathan J, Kanter AS, Sheehan JP, et al. Benign brain tumors: sellar/parasellar tumors. Neurol Clin 2007;25(4):1231–49, xi.
32. Mohn A, Schoof E, Fahlbusch R, et al. The endocrine spectrum of arachnoid cysts in childhood. Pediatr Neurosurg 1999;31(6):316–21.
33. Adan L, Bussieres L, Dinand V, et al. Growth, puberty and hypothalamic-pituitary function in children with suprasellar arachnoid cyst. Eur J Pediatr 2000;159(5): 348–55.
34. Koeller KK, Rushing EJ. From the archives of the AFIP. Pilocytic astrocytoma: radiologic-pathologic correlation. Radiographics 2004;24(6):1693–708.
35. Boyko OB, Curnes JT, Oakes WJ, et al. Hamartomas of the tuber cinereum: CT, MR, and pathologic findings. AJNR Am J Neuroradiol 1991;12(2):309–14.
36. Lee L, Saran F, Hargrave D, et al. Germinoma with synchronous lesions in the pineal and suprasellar regions. Childs Nerv Syst 2006;22(12):1513–8.
37. Liang L, Korogi Y, Sugahara T, et al. MRI of intracranial germ-cell tumours. Neuroradiology 2002;44(5):382–8.
38. Tsao CY, Lo WD, Rusin JA, et al. Isolated neurosarcoidosis presenting as headache and multiple brain and spinal cord lesions mimicking central nervous system metastases. Brain Dev 2007;29(8):514–8.
39. Amato MC, Elias LL, Elias J, et al. Endocrine disorders in pediatric-onset Langerhans cell histiocytosis. Horm Metab Res 2006;38(11):746–51.
40. Donadieu J, Rolon MA, Thomas C, et al. Endocrine involvement in pediatric-onset Langerhans' cell histiocytosis: a population-based study. J Pediatr 2004;144(3): 344–50.

41. Gellner V, Kurschel S, Scarpatetti M, et al. Lymphocytic hypophysitis in the pediatric population. Childs Nerv Syst 2008;24(7):785–92.
42. Chapurlat RD, Orcel P. Fibrous dysplasia of bone and McCune-Albright syndrome. Best Pract Res Clin Rheumatol 2008;22(1):55–69.
43. Glenn OA, Barkovich AJ. Magnetic resonance imaging of the fetal brain and spine: an increasingly important tool in prenatal diagnosis, part 1. AJNR Am J Neuroradiol 2006;27(8):1604–11.
44. Lee SK, Kim DI, Kim J, et al. Diffusion-tensor MR imaging and fiber tractography: a new method of describing aberrant fiber connections in developmental CNS anomalies. Radiographics 2005;25(1):53–65 [discussion: 66–8].
45. Lee SK, Mori S, Kim DJ, et al. Diffusion tensor MR imaging visualizes the altered hemispheric fiber connection in callosal dysgenesis. AJNR Am J Neuroradiol 2004;25(1):25–8.
46. Hamilton J, Blaser S, Daneman D. MR imaging in idiopathic growth hormone deficiency. AJNR Am J Neuroradiol 1998;19(9):1609–15.
47. Mikulis DJ, Diaz O, Egglin TK, et al. Variance of the position of the cerebellar tonsils with age: preliminary report. Radiology 1992;183(3):725–8.
48. Quigley MF, Iskandar B, Quigley ME, et al. Cerebrospinal fluid flow in foramen magnum: temporal and spatial patterns at MR imaging in volunteers and in patients with Chiari I malformation. Radiology 2004;232(1):229–36.
49. Hankinson TC, Klimo P Jr, Feldstein NA, et al. Chiari malformations, syringohydromyelia and scoliosis. Neurosurg Clin N Am 2007;18(3):549–68.
50. Kelberman D, Dattani MT. Septo-optic dysplasia – novel insights into the aetiology. Horm Res 2008;69(5):257–65.
51. Mehta A, Hindmarsh PC, Mehta H, et al. Congenital hypopituitarism: clinical, molecular and neuroradiological correlates. Clin Endocrinol (Oxf) 2009;71:376–82.

# Steroid 21 Hydroxylase Deficiency Congenital Adrenal Hyperplasia

Saroj Nimkarn, MD, Karen Lin-Su, MD, Maria I. New, MD*

**KEYWORDS**

- Congenital adrenal hyperplasia • Adrenal steroid
- 21 hydroxylase • 21 OHD

Congenital adrenal hyperplasia (CAH) refers to a group of genetic enzyme deficiencies that impair normal steroid synthesis by the adrenal cortex. The most common form is 21 hydroxylase deficiency (21 OHD), accounting for more than 90% of the cases. Less frequent causes of CAH include deficiencies of 11β-hydroxylase, 3β-hydroxysteroid dehydrogenase, 17α-hydroxylase/17,20-lyase, steroidogenic acute regulatory (StAR) protein (lipoid hyperplasia) and the newly described form of CAH owing to P450 Oxidoreductase defect. In almost all cases, each of these deficiencies results from recessive mutations in the respective genes that encode the enzymes and has distinctive clinical phenotypes. This article focuses on CAH owing to 21 OHD.

## STEROID 21 HYDROXYLASE DEFICIENCY

CAH owing to 21 OHD is divided into classical and nonclassical (NC) CAH. Patients affected with the classical form have more severe symptoms of hyperandrogenism. Beginning in utero, prenatal exposure to potent androgens such as testosterone and $\Delta^4$-androstenedione at critical stages of sexual differentiation virilizes the external genitalia of genetic females, often resulting in genital ambiguity at birth in female patients. The classical form is subdivided into the simple virilizing form (SV) and the salt-wasting form (SW), based on the patient's ability to produce adequate salt-retaining hormone, aldosterone. Salt-wasters account for most of classical 21 OHD CAH patients ($\geq$75%) whereas approximately 25% of individuals are simple virilizers. Newborns who are salt wasters are at risk for life-threatening salt-wasting crises.

Individuals with the NC form of 21 OHD CAH have only mild enzyme deficiency and present postnatally with signs of hyperandrogenism; therefore, females with the NC form are not virilized at birth and do not present with genital ambiguity. Clinical features distinguishing classical and nonclassical forms are shown in **Table 1**. In

Adrenal Steroid Disorders Program, Division of Pediatric Endocrinology, Mount Sinai School of Medicine, 1 Gustave L. Levy Place, Box 1198, New York, NY 10029, USA
* Corresponding author.
*E-mail address:* maria.new@mssm.edu (M.I. New).

Endocrinol Metab Clin N Am 38 (2009) 699–718
doi:10.1016/j.ecl.2009.08.001 

**Table 1**
**Clinical features in individuals with classical and nonclassical 21 OHD CAH**

| Feature | Classical 21 OHD CAH | Nonclassical 21 OHD CAH |
|---|---|---|
| Prenatal virilization | Present in females | Absent |
| Postnatal virilization | Males and females | Variable |
| Salt wasting | ~75% of all individuals | Absent |
| Cortisol deficiency | ~100% | Rare |

males, the clinical distinction between SV and NC-CAH may not be readily apparent, but genetic analysis and adrenocorticotropic hormone (ACTH) stimulation results may clarify the diagnosis.

Screening studies indicate that the worldwide incidence of classical 21 OHD is 1:15,000 to 1:16,000 live births,[1–3] of which approximately 75% are salt wasters. The worldwide incidence of NC-CAH is much higher at 1:1000, with a frequency as high as 1:27 among Ashkenazi Jews.[4,5]

## PATHOPHYSIOLOGY

Adrenal steroid production occurs in three major pathways: glucocorticoids, mineralocorticoids, and sex steroids, as shown in **Fig. 1**. ACTH regulates adrenal steroid production via a rate-limiting step that results in pregnanolone, the principal substrate for the steroidogenic pathway (see **Fig. 1**). It promotes StAR protein function in transporting free cholesterol to the inner mitochondrial membrane, the site where a side chain cleavage occurs and the first step in steroidogenesis takes place. The central nervous system controls the secretion of ACTH, its diurnal variation, and its

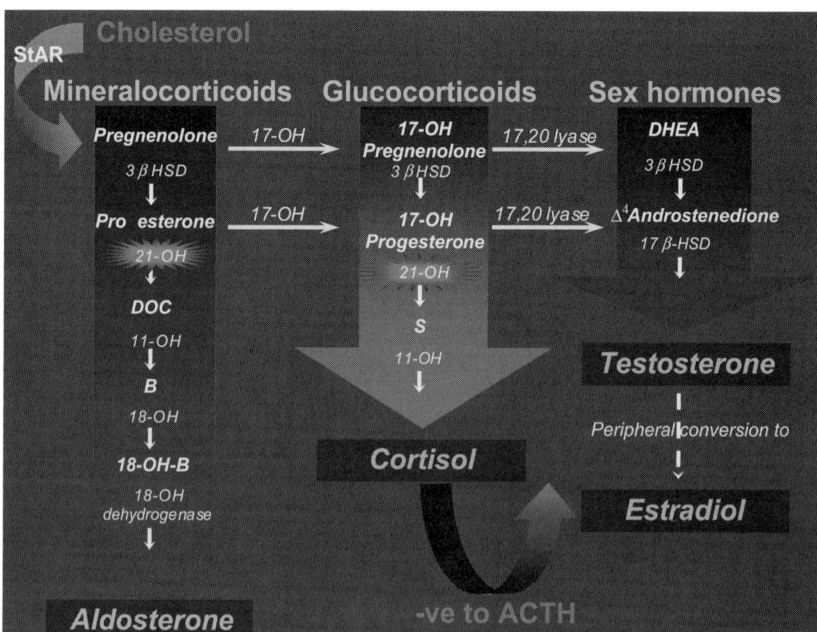


**Fig. 1.** Adrenal steroidogenetic pathways.

increase during periods of physiologic stress via the hypothalamus-produced corticotropin-releasing factor (CRF).[6,7] The hypothalamic-pituitary-adrenal feedback system is mediated through the circulating level of plasma cortisol by its negative feedback on CRF and ACTH secretion. Hence, impeded cortisol secretion in 21 OHD CAH leads to increased ACTH production, which in turn, stimulates (1) excessive synthesis of adrenal products in those pathways unimpaired by the enzyme deficiency and (2) a build-up of precursor molecules, mainly 17 hydroxyprogesterone, in pathways blocked by the enzyme deficiency. The excess 17-OHP is shunted into the intact androgen pathway, where the 17,20-lyase enzyme converts the 17-OHP to $\Delta^4$-androstenedione, which is converted into androgens. Because the mineralocorticoid pathway requires minimal 21 hydroxylase activity, mineralocorticoid deficiency (salt wasting) is a feature of the most severe form of the disease.

## CLINICAL PRESENTATION AND FEATURES

### *External Genitalia*

Adrenocortical function begins around the seventh week of gestation[8]; thus, a female fetus with classical CAH is exposed to adrenal androgens at the critical time of sexual differentiation (approximately 9 to 15 weeks gestational age). In classical CAH patients, the degree of genital virilization may range from mild clitoral enlargement alone to, in rare cases, a penile urethra. Degrees of genital virilization are classified into five Prader stages (**Fig. 2**).[9]

Stage I: clitoromegaly without labial fusion
Stage II: clitoromegaly and posterior labial fusion
Stage III: greater degree of clitoromegaly, single perineal urogenital orifice, and almost complete labial fusion
Stage IV: increasingly phallic clitoris, urethra-like urogenital sinus at base of clitoris, and complete labial fusion
Stage V: penile clitoris, urethral meatus at tip of phallus, and scrotum-like labia (appear like males without palpable gonads)

### *Internal Genitalia*

As the androgens interact with the receptors on genital skin, they induce changes in the developing external female genitalia such as clitoral enlargement, fusion of the labial folds, and rostral migration of the urethral/vaginal perineal orifice. However, internal female genitalia (uterus, fallopian tubes, and ovaries) are normal, as females cannot produce Müllerian-inhibiting hormone because they do not have testicular

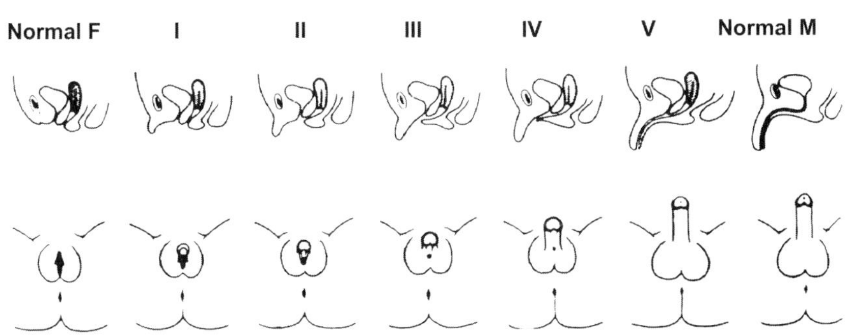


**Fig. 2.** Different degrees of virilization according to the scale developed by Prader.[9]

Sertoli cells. Therefore the Müllerian ducts do not regress, and the internal female internal genitalia develop normally.

### *Postnatal Effects and Growth*

Lack of appropriate postnatal treatment in boys and girls results in continued exposure to excessive androgens, causing progressive penile or clitoral enlargement, the development of premature pubic (pubarche) and axillary hair and acne. Hyperandrogenism during childhood often leads to rapid linear growth accompanied by premature epiphyseal maturation and closure, resulting in a final adult height that is typically below that expected from parental heights (on average −1.1 to −1.5 SD below the midparental target height).[10–13] On the other hand, poor growth can occur in patients with 21 OHD as a result of glucocorticoid treatment when replacement therapy exceeds physiologic requirements.

Final height in classical 21 OHD (as well as NC 21 OHD) is one of the features least amenable to glucocorticoid therapy even among patients with excellent adrenal control. A study of growth hormone therapy alone or in combination with a GnRH analog in CAH patients with compromised height prediction showed improvement in short- and long-term growth to reduce the height deficit.[13,14]

### *Puberty and Secondary Sexual Characteristics*

In most patients treated adequately from early life, the onset of puberty in both girls and boys with classical 21 OHD occurs at the expected chronologic age.[15,16] However, a recent careful study showed that the mean ages at onset of puberty in both males and females were somewhat younger than the general population, but did not differ significantly among the three forms of 21 OHD.[17] Following the onset of puberty, in most successfully treated patients, the milestones of further development of secondary sex characteristics in general appear to be normal.[15–17]

Inadequate treatment leads to an advanced epiphyseal development. This can result in precocious puberty. Also in cases where a significant body maturation at the initial presentation, such as simple virilizing males who were not detected by newborn screening, the exposure to elevated androgens followed by the sudden decreased androgen levels after initiation of glucocorticoid treatment may cause an early activation of the hypothalamic-pituitary-gonadal axis. Studies suggest that excess adrenal androgens (aromatized to estrogens) inhibit the pubertal pattern of gonadotropin secretion by the hypothalamic-pituitary axis.[18] This inhibition, which probably takes place via a negative feedback effect can be reversed by glucocorticoid treatment.

In adolescents and adults, signs of hyperandrogenism in females may include male-pattern alopecia (temporal balding), acne, or infertility, and in females, irregular or absent menses and hirsutism. There is also an association of CAH and polycystic ovarian syndrome (PCOS).[19]

### *Gender Role Behavior*

Prenatal androgen exposure in females with classical forms of 21 OHD CAH has a virilizing effect on the external genitalia and childhood behavior. Prenatal androgen exposure correlates with a decrease in self-reported femininity by adult females, but not an increase in self-reported masculinity by adult females.[20] The rates of bisexual and homosexual orientation were increased in women with all forms of 21 OHD CAH. They were found to correlate with the degree of prenatal androgenization. Of interest, bisexual/homosexual orientation was correlated with global measures of masculinization of nonsexual behavior and predicted independently by the degree of both prenatal androgenization and masculinization of childhood behavior.[21]

Changes in childhood play behavior correlated with reduced female gender satisfaction and reduced heterosexual interest in adulthood. Affected adult females are more likely to have gender dysphoria, and experience less heterosexual interest and reduced satisfaction with the assignment to the female sex. In contrast, males with 21 OHD CAH do not show a general alteration in childhood play behavior, core gender identity, or sexual orientation.[22]

### *Fertility*

Difficulty with fertility in females with CAH may arise for various reasons, including anovulation, secondary polycystic ovarian syndrome, irregular menses, nonsuppressible serum progesterone levels, or an inadequate introitus. Fertility is reduced in SW 21 OHD with rare reports of pregnancy. In a retrospective survey of fertility rates in a large group of females with classical CAH, simple virilizers were shown to be more likely to become pregnant and carry the pregnancy to term.[23] However, more recent data suggest that fertility rates have significantly improved from 60% in SW and 80% in SV patients.[24] Adequate glucocorticoid therapy is probably an important variable with respect to fertility outcome. The development of PCOS in CAH patients is not uncommon and may be related to both prenatal and postnatal excess androgen exposure, which can affect the hypothalamic-pituitary-gonadal axis.

In male patients with classical CAH, several long-term studies indicate that those who have been adequately treated undergo normal pubertal development, have normal testicular function, and normal spermatogenesis and fertility.[17,25–27] However, small testes and reduced sperm count can occur in patients as a result of inadequately controlled disease.[28–32] A complication in postpubertal boys with inadequate control of CAH is hyperplastic nodular testes. Almost all these patients were found to have adenomatous adrenal rests within the testicular tissue, so-called testicular adrenal rest tumor (TART), as indicated by the presence of specific 11β-hydroxylated steroids in the blood from gonadal veins.[33] TART can lead to end-stage damage of testicular perenchyma, most probably as a result of long-standing obstruction of the seminiferous tubules.[34] These tumors have been reported to be ACTH dependent and to regress following adequate steroid therapy.[35–39]

Ironically, some investigators have reported normal testicular maturation as well as normal spermatogenesis and fertility in patients who had never received glucocorticoid treatment.[20,25,27,40]

### *Salt Wasting in 21 OHD*

When the loss of 21 hydroxylase function is severe, adrenal aldosterone secretion is not sufficient for sodium reabsorption by the distal renal tubules, and individuals suffer from salt wasting, in addition to cortisol deficiency and androgen excess. Classical CAH patients who make adequate aldosterone are considered to have SV-CAH. Infants with renal salt wasting have poor feeding, weight loss, failure to thrive, vomiting, dehydration, hypotension, hyponatremia, and hyperkalemic metabolic acidosis progressing to adrenal crisis (azotemia, vascular collapse, shock, and death). Adrenal crisis can occur as early as age 1 to 4 weeks. The salt wasting is presumed to result from inadequate secretion of salt-retaining steroids, primarily aldosterone. In addition, hormonal precursors of the 21 OH enzyme may act as antagonists to mineralocorticoid action in the sodium-conserving mechanism of the immature newborn renal tubule.[41–43] The adrenal medulla may also be incompletely formed in some CAH patients. Merke and colleagues[44] noted that the epinephrine and metanephrine concentrations in CAH patients who manifested salt-wasting crisis was approximately 50% of that of controls, in line with adrenal gland histopathologic studies that showed depleted secretory vesicles.

Affected males who are not detected in a newborn screening program are at high risk for a salt-wasting adrenal crisis because their normal male genitalia do not alert medical professionals to their condition; they are often discharged from the hospital after birth without diagnosis and experience a salt-wasting crisis at home. On the other hand, salt-wasting females are born with ambiguous genitalia that trigger the diagnostic process and appropriate treatment. It is important to recognize that the extent of virilism may not differ among the two classical CAH SV and SW forms. Thus, even a mildly virilized newborn with 21 OHD should be observed carefully for signs of a potentially life-threatening crisis within the first few weeks of life.

It has been observed that an aldosterone biosynthetic defect apparent in infancy may be ameliorated with age.[45,46] Speiser and colleagues[47] reported the spontaneous partial recovery in adulthood of a patient with documented severe salt wasting in infancy. Therefore, it is desirable to follow the sodium and mineralocorticoid requirements carefully by measuring PRA in patients who have been diagnosed in the neonatal period as salt wasters.

Although insufficient aldosterone biosynthesis is clinically apparent only in the SW form of the disease, impaired adrenal capacity to produce aldosterone in response to renin stimulation appeared to be a spectrum in all forms of 21 OHD CAH.[48]

### *Nonclassical Congenital Adrenal Hyperplasia*

Individuals with the NC form of 21 OHD, also known as late-onset 21 OHD, have only mild to moderate enzyme deficiency and present postnatally with signs of hyperandrogenism. NC-CAH may present at any age after birth with a variety of hyperandrogenic symptoms, excluding ambiguous genitalia. This form of CAH results from a mild deficiency of the 21 hydroxylase enzyme. Similar to classical CAH, NC-CAH may cause premature development of pubic hair, advanced bone age, and accelerated linear growth velocity in both males and females. Severe cystic acne has also been attributed to NC-CAH.

Women may present with symptoms of androgen excess, including hirsutism, temporal baldness, and infertility.[49] Menarche in females may be normal or delayed, and secondary amenorrhea is a frequent occurrence. Further virilization may include hirsutism, male habitus, deepening of the voice, or male-pattern alopecia (temporal recession). Clinical course of NC form varies among individuals[50] and it is difficult to predict the appearance of any virilization symptoms.[51]

Polycystic ovarian syndrome may also be seen as a secondary complication in these patients. Possible reasons for the development of PCOS include reprogramming of the hypothalamic-pituitary-gonadal axis from prenatal exposure to androgens, or chronic levels of excess adrenal androgens that disrupt gonadotropin release and have direct effects on the ovary, ultimately leading to the formation of cysts. Because of the overlap of hyperandrogenic symptoms, it is important to consider NC 21 OHD in a patient diagnosed with PCOS. Of note, NC 21 OHD CAH was identified in 2.2% to 10.0% among women who presented with hyperandrogenic symptoms.[50,52,53]

Symptoms in adult males with NC-CAH may include short stature, acne, or oligozoospermia and diminished fertility.[54] Infertility is often caused by TART,[55] although some untreated men have been fertile,[28] as discussed before.

A subset of individuals with NC 21 OHD are completely asymptomatic[56] when detected (usually as part of a family study). Based on longitudinal follow-up of such patients, we observed that symptoms of hyperandrogenism wax and wane with time. The presence of 21 OHD can also be discovered during the evaluation of an incidental adrenal mass.[57] An increased incidence of adrenal incidentalomas has been found, reported as high as 82% in patients with 21 OHD and up to 45% in subjects heterozygous for 21 OHD mutations. This probably arises from hyperplastic tissue areas and does not require surgical intervention.[58]

## DIAGNOSIS OF CONGENITAL ADRENAL HYPERPLASIA

### *Hormonal Diagnosis*

Biochemical diagnosis of 21 OHD can be confirmed by hormonal evaluation. In a randomly timed blood sample, a very high concentration of 17-hydroxyprogesterone (17-OHP), the precursor of the defective enzyme, is diagnostic of classical 21 OHD. The gold standard to establish hormonal diagnosis for NC 21 OHD and for certain enigmatic cases is the corticotropin stimulation test (250 μg cosyntropin intravenously), measuring levels of 17-OHP and $\Delta^4$-androstenedione at baseline and 60 minutes. The 17-OHP values can then be plotted in the published nomogram to ascertain disease severity (**Fig. 3**).[59] The corticotropin stimulation test is crucial in establishing hormonal diagnosis of the NC form of the disease, as even early-morning values of 17-OHP may not be sufficiently elevated to allow accurate diagnosis. For example, an NC patient may have a normal baseline 17-OHP of 100 ng/dL, yet stimulate to greater than 2000 ng/dL, and that would be diagnostic for NC-CAH. Patients with classical CAH typically have stimulated 17-OHP levels of 20,000 to 100,000 ng/dL. The corticotropin stimulation test may also be helpful in males for distinguishing between the NC and SV forms, as males with 21 OHD have normal genitalia.

### *Molecular Genetics*

Hormonally and clinically defined forms of 21 OHD CAH are associated with distinct genotypes characterized by varying enzyme activity demonstrated though in vitro expression studies. The gene encoding 21 hydroxylase is a microsomal cytochrome P450-termed cytochrome P450, family 21, subfamily A, polypeptide 21 (*CYP21A2*) (Online Mendelian Inheritance in Man [OMIM] database number 201,910) located on the short arm of chromosome 6, within the human leukocyte antigen (HLA) complex.[60,61] *CYP21A2* and its homolog, the pseudogene *CYP21A1P* alternate with two genes, *C4B* and *C4A*, that encode the two isoforms of the fourth component of the serum complement system.[62]

More than 100 mutations have been described including point mutations, small deletions, small insertions, and complex rearrangements of the gene.[63] **Table 2** demonstrates the common mutations in *CYP21A2* and their related phenotypes. In recessive disorders, the less severe mutation of the two alleles typically dictates phenotype. Classical 21 OHD is most often caused by two alleles with severe mutations. In contrast to the classical form, patients with NC 21 OHD are predicted to have mild mutations on both alleles or one severe and one mild mutation (compound heterozygosity) of *CYP21A2*. It is not always possible, however, to accurately predict the phenotype on the basis of the genotype—such predictions have been shown to be 79% to 88% accurate[59,76,77] with some nonconcordance. Studies have demonstrated that there is often a divergence in phenotypes within mutation-identical groups, the reason for which requires further investigation.[78,79]

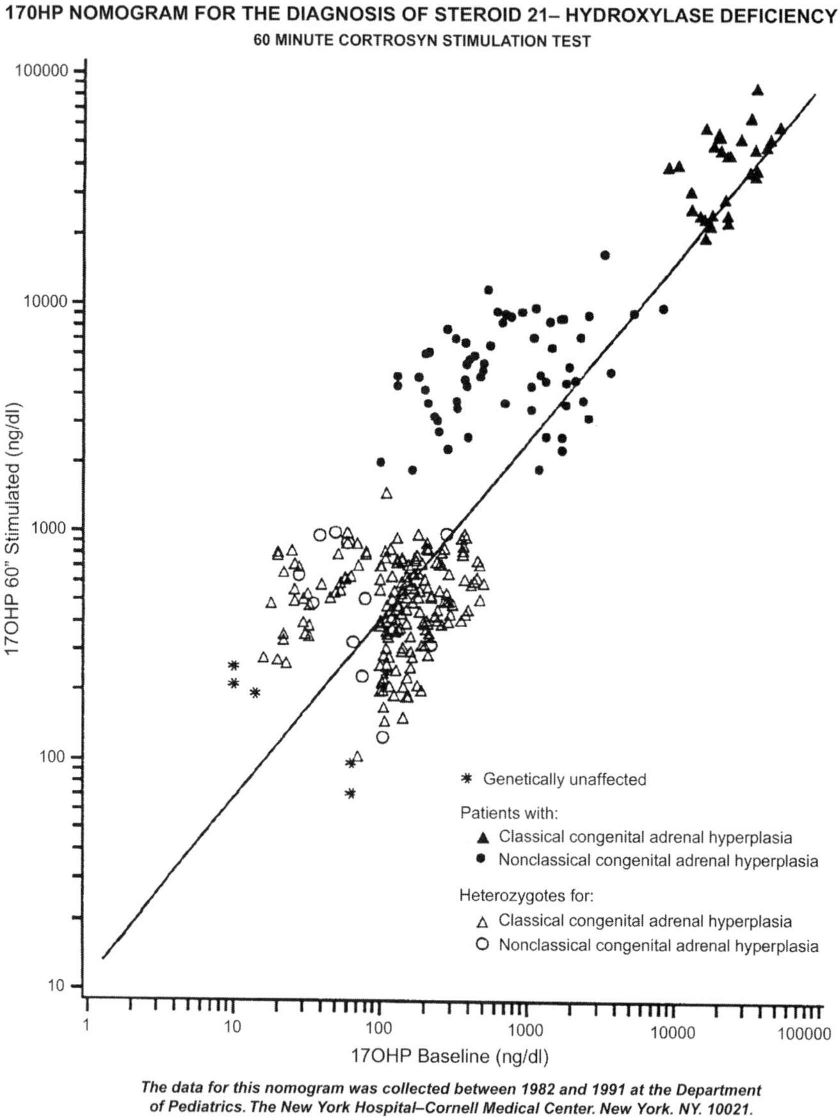


**Fig. 3.** Nomogram of 17 OHP.

## TREATMENT AND MANAGEMENT OF CONGENITAL ADRENAL HYPERPLASIA

### *Hormone Replacement*

The goal of therapy in CAH is to both correct the deficiency in cortisol secretion and suppresses ACTH overproduction. Proper treatment with glucocorticoid reduces stimulation of the androgen pathway, thus preventing further virilization and allowing normal growth and development. The usual requirement of hydrocortisone (or its equivalent) for the treatment of classical CAH is about 10 to 15 mg/m$^2$/day divided into 2 or 3 doses per day. Dosage requirements for patients with NC-CAH may be less. Adults may be treated with the longer-acting dexamethasone or prednisone, alone or in combination with hydrocortisone. A small dose of dexamethasone at

**Table 2**
**Common mutations in CYP21A2 gene and their related phenotypes**

| Study | Exon/Intron | Mutation Type | Mutation | Phenotype | Severity of Enzyme Defect (% enzyme activity) | References |
|---|---|---|---|---|---|---|
| *Nonclassical mutations* | | | | | | |
| Tusie-Luna, 1991 | Exon 1 | Missense mutation | P30L | NC | Mild (30–60) | 64 |
| Speiser, 1988 | Exon 7 | Missense mutation | V281L | NC | Mild (20–50) | 65 |
| Helmberg, 1992 | Exon 8 | Missense mutation | R339H | NC | Mild (20–50) | 66 |
| Helmberg, 1992; Owerbach, 1992 | Exon 10 | Missense mutation | P453S | NC | Mild (20–50) | 66,67 |
| *Classical mutations* | | | | | | |
| White, 1984 | Deletion | 30kb Deletion | — | SW | Severe (0) | 68 |
| Higashi, 1988 | Intron 2 | Aberrant splicing of Intron 2 | 656 A/C-G | SW, SV | Severe (ND) | 69 |
| White, 1994 | Exon 3 | Eight-base deletion | G110 Δ8nt | SW | Severe (0) | 70 |
| Tusie-Luna, 1990; Amor, 1988 | Exon 4 | Missense mutation | I172N | SV | Severe (1) | 71,72 |
| Tusie-Luna, 1990; Amor, 1988 | Exon 6 | Cluster | I236N, V237E, M239K | SW | Severe (0) | 71,72 |
| Globerman, 1988 | Exon 8 | Nonsense mutation | Q318X | SW | Severe (0) | 73 |
| Chiou, 1990 | Exon 8 | Missense mutation | R356W | SW, SV | Severe (0) | 74 |
| Wedell, 1993 | Exon 10 | Missense mutation | R483P[a] | SW | Severe (1–2) | 75 |

*Abbreviations:* NC, nonclassical; ND, not defined; SV, simple virilizing; SW, salt wasting.

bedtime (0.25 to 0.5 mg) is usually adequate for androgen suppression in NC patients. The goal of corticosteroid therapy is to give the lowest dose required for optimal control. Antiandrogen treatment may be useful as adjunctive therapy in adult women who continue to have hyperandrogenic signs despite good adrenal suppression. Females with concomitant PCOS may benefit from an oral contraceptive, although this treatment would not be appropriate for patients trying to get pregnant. Most adult males with NC-CAH are asymptomatic and often remain undiagnosed; therefore, treatment is generally not necessary.[56] For certain cases, however, our group has found that treatment may be helpful in preventing TARTs and preserving fertility. Glucocorticoid treatment may also prevent the development of adrenal adenomas.[80]

Titration of the dose should be aimed at maintaining androgen levels at age and sex-appropriate levels and 17-OHP levels of less than 1000 ng/dL to normalize growth in growing children. Concurrently, overtreatment should be avoided because it can lead to Cushing syndrome and in linear growth suppression in children. Patients with SW-CAH have elevated plasma renin activity (PRA) in response to the sodium-deficient state, and they require treatment with the salt retaining steroid 9$\alpha$-fludrocortisone acetate. It has not been customary to supplement conventional glucocorticoid replacement therapy with the administration of salt-retaining steroids in the SV and NC forms of CAH, although there has been some suggestion that adding fludrocortisone to patients with elevated PRA may improve hormonal control of the disease.[81] The requirement for fludrocortisone appears to diminish with age, and oversuppression of the PRA should be avoided, to prevent complications from hypertension and excessive mineralocorticoid activity.

Monitoring of glucocorticoid/mineralocorticoid replacement therapy is recommended every 3 to 4 months while children are actively growing, and less often thereafter; and monitoring for TART in males every 3 to 5 years after onset of puberty. In adulthood, long-term follow-up in the following areas is recommended: overweight/obesity, bone mineral density, fertility, and cardiovascular risks.

### *Stress Dosing*

In non–life-threatening periods of illness or physiologic stress, the corticosteroid dose should be increased to two or three times the maintenance dose for the duration of that period. We recommend that each family should be given injection kits of hydrocortisone for emergency use (25 mg for infants, 50 mg for children, and 100 mg for adults). In the event of a surgical procedure, our protocol indicated that a total of 5 to 10 times the daily maintenance dose is required during the first 24 to 48 hours. The doses can then be tapered over the following days to the normal preoperative schedule. Stress doses of dexamethasone should not be given because of the delayed onset of action. It is not necessary for increased mineralocorticoid doses during these periods of stress.

It is imperative for all patients who are receiving corticosteroid replacement therapy such as these patients with CAH to wear a Medic-Alert or other identifying bracelets that will enable correct and appropriate therapy in case of emergencies. Additionally, all responsible family members should be trained in the intramuscular administration of hydrocortisone.

### *Surgery*

In the past, it was routine to recommend early corrective surgery for neonates born with ambiguous genitalia. In recent years, the implementation of early corrective surgery has become increasingly controversial because of lack of data on long-term functional outcome.[82] Thus, the role of the parents in sex assignment becomes crucial in all aspects of the decision-making process, and should include full discussion of the controversy and all possible therapeutic options for the intersex child, particularly early versus delayed surgery. Furthermore, a multidisciplinary case-by-case approach, involving pediatric endocrinology, urology, genetics, and psychoendrocrinology, is imperative when considering sex assignment and possible surgical repair.[83,84]

The aim of surgical repair in females with ambiguous genitalia caused by CAH, when the decision is made by parents or patients themselves, is generally to remove the redundant erectile tissue, preserve the sexually sensitive glans clitoris, and provide a normal vaginal orifice that functions adequately for menstruation, intromission, and delivery. A medical indication for early surgery other than for sex assignment is recurrent urinary tract infections as a result of pooling of urine in the vagina or urogenital sinus. The extent of surgery depends on the degree of genital virilization. For female patients with greater degrees of virilization (an enlarged phallus, fused labia, and a single perineal opening), surgical procedures may include reduction of the enlarged clitoris, separation of the labia, and opening of the lower vagina. Further procedures may be required in adolescence and adulthood to provide an adequate introitus for menstruation, tampon use, and coitus. A cross-sectional study of 24 adult women with classical CAH who had undergone genital surgery showed that there was significant impairment to sensitivity in the clitoris compared with unaffected controls and CAH women who had not undergone genital surgery. Sexual function difficulties were also reported, including vaginal penetration, anorgasmia, and intercourse frequency.[85]

A review of sexual and reproductive outcomes in 35 adult women with CAH found that none of the subjects expressed doubts about their gender assignment. Twenty percent had homosexual inclinations; 23% were married; and 37% reported never having had heterosexual intercourse with vaginal penetration. Eighty-one percent of the subjects who had experienced vaginal intercourse reported pain during penetration. Past pregnancy was reported in 8 of the 35 women; 6 of them had children.[86]

Another study of 62 women with CAH demonstrated that they were often less satisfied with their genital function and appearance than controls, regardless of whether or not they had surgery. Half of the CAH women reported that CAH affected their sex life. Clitoral surgery was frequently associated with dissatisfaction with clitoral size and/or sensation. Of the women who had vaginoplasty, 37.5% underwent reoperation because of vaginal stenosis. Painful intercourse was reported in 30% of the subjects. Embarrassment regarding the cosmetic appearance of the external genitalia was also quite common.[87]

### *Bone Mineral Density*

Bone mineral density (BMD) is affected by the competing actions of androgen excess (from undertreatment) and glucocortiocid excess (from overtreatment), which can both occur simulataneously in a patient. To adequately suppress androgen production in patients with CAH, the usual requirement of hydrocortisone is generally higher than the endogenous secretory rate of cortisol. Chronic therapy with glucocorticoids at supraphysiologic levels can result in diminished bone accrual and lead to osteopenia and osteoporosis. Glucocorticoid-induced bone loss is a well-known phenomenon and is the most prevalent form of secondary osteoporosis.[88]

Unlike other diseases treated with chronic glucocorticoid therapy, however, the effect of glucocorticoid replacement in CAH on BMD is unclear. Several studies of patients with 21 OHD have reported decreased BMD,[89,90] whereas other studies have reported increased or normal BMD.[91,92] The discrepancies may be attributable to differences in age and gender, as well as varying treatment regimens. Generally, studies that have included males and older females, particularly postmenopausal women with CAH, have shown a higher incidence of osteopenia and osteoporosis, whereas studies limited to younger patients have not shown such a decrease. It has been postulated that the elevated androgens typically found in young adult women with CAH may have a protective effect on bone integrity, but the precise mechanism is unknown. The increased adrenal androgens, which are converted to estrogens, may counteract the detrimental effects of glucocorticoids on bone mass. This may explain why older CAH women, particularly those who are postmenopausal, are at higher risk for osteoporosis than younger CAH patients. A study is currently under way to examine a potential mechanism by which certain CAH patients are protected against glucocorticoid-induced bone loss.

### *Metabolic Aspects*

Long-term glucocorticoid treatment coupled with increased androgens may lead to undesirable metabolic effects in patients with CAH. Increased body mass index and body fat mass have been described in CAH.[91,93–95] Higher fasting plasma insulin with reduced insulin sensitivity and elevated serum leptin have also been reported in CAH patients,[96–98] as has a higher frequency of gestational diabetes.[99] Other cardiovascular risk factors, such as increased carotid intima-media thickness[98] and hypertension,[95,100] have been described as well.

A decrease in epinephrine reserve with resulting defects in leptin, insulin, and glucose control has been shown during both high- and moderate-intensity exercise in adolescents with classical CAH.[101,102]

### *Fertility and Management during Pregnancy*

#### *Management of congenital adrenal hyperplasia during pregnancy*

As described previously, females with CAH have normal internal female structures and reproductive capability. Although barriers to fertility exist, many CAH females are able to achieve pregnancy with or without medical assistance. Despite genital reconstruction of the external genitalia, many females with classical CAH may have difficulty with a vaginal delivery and will require Caesarean section. Females with NC-CAH should be able to deliver vaginally in the absence of other complications. Because of the physical stress of labor and delivery, particularly if anesthesia is administered, all females with known CAH, who are being treated with glucocorticoid replacement, should receive stress dose hydrocortisone during labor and delivery.

Preferably, the carrier status of the partner should be ascertained before pregnancy. If the partner is found to be genetically unaffected, then the glucocorticoid of choice is hydrocortisone, which does not cross the placenta, as it is inactivated by placental 11β-hydroxysteroid dehydrogenase type 2.[103] Although harm to the fetus from prednisone has not been documented in humans, inactivation of prednisone by the placenta is unpredictable[104]; therefore, prednisone is usually not the preferred treatment for CAH during pregnancy. Our group monitors adrenal hormones, including 17-OHP and androgens, throughout the pregnancy. However, 17-OHP is a necessary hormone for the maintenance of pregnancy, and the serum level of androgens increase during pregnancy owing to increased sex hormone binding globulin (SHBG); therefore, the target levels to maintain during pregnancy should not be as rigid as in the nonpregnant state. For the most part, the prepregnancy dose of hydrocortisone (or the equivalent dose) is adequate to continue throughout pregnancy, although in some instances, dose increases may be necessary.

***Prenatal treatment with dexamethasone***

In pregnancies at risk of the offspring having classical forms of CAH, prenatal diagnosis and treatment can be offered. Conventionally, this occurs in the family where there is a previously affected sibling or first-degree relative with known mutations causing classical CAH, proven by DNA analysis. If the CAH patient's partner is a carrier of a severe mutation, placing the fetus at risk for classical 21 OHD, the patient should be offered prenatal diagnosis and treatment with dexamethasone until chorionic villus sampling or amniocentesis is performed. Prenatal dexamethasone (at a dose of 0.02 mg/kg/day, based on prepregnancy weight, divided into two or three doses), administered at or before 9 weeks of gestation to the mother, has been shown to be effective in reducing virilization in females affected with classical CAH.[105,106] In these studies, no significant or enduring side effects were noted in either the mothers (other than greater weight gain and a higher incidence of striae and edema than untreated mothers) or the fetuses. There was no statistically significant difference between treated and untreated mothers in hypertension or gestational diabetes. All mothers who took partial or full treatment stated they would take dexamethasone again in the event of a future pregnancy. In our report and in others, no cases have been reported of cleft palate, placental degeneration, or fetal death, which have been observed in a rodent model of in utero exposure to high-dose glucocorticoids.[107,108] Another study, in contrast, noted some significant maternal side effects, including excessive weight gain, cushingoid facial features, severe striae resulting in permanent scarring, and hyperglycemic response to oral glucose administration.[109]

A long-term follow-up study of 44 children treated prenatally in Scandinavia demonstrated normal pre- and postnatal growth compared with matched controls.[110] In our study, prenatally treated newborns also did not differ in weight, length, or head circumference from untreated, unaffected newborns.[105,106] Moreover, a survey of 174 prenatally dexamethasone (DEX)-exposed children, ages 1 month to 12 years (including 48 with CAH), compared with 313 unexposed children (including 195 with CAH) found no differences in cognitive or motor development between the two groups.[111] Another report from Sweden suggested that there may be long-term cognitive effects of prenatal treatment with dexamethasone.[112] In their study, DEX-treated CAH children performed less well than unaffected controls on tests measuring verbal processing speed; however, no comparison was made with CAH children who were not DEX-exposed. Full-scale IQ was not different from healthy controls. Another long-term follow-up study of DEX- exposed children did not show any statistically significant differences in measures of psychopathology, behavioral problems, and adaptive functioning. In addition, DEX-exposed children were described by their parents as being more sociable than controls.[113] These studies have prompted Imperative further investigation into the psychological, cognitive, and medical outcome of patients treated prenatally with dexamethasone; more long-term studies are currently under way.

## *Transitioning the Pediatric Patient to Adulthood*

Transitioning the pediatric patient to adulthood is a very important aspect of caring for CAH patients. There are several issues to consider for a smooth transition. During the pediatric period, children with CAH are typically brought to doctor visits by their parents and are monitored very frequently. Once patients reach adulthood, however, they must assume responsibility for understanding their medical condition and for compliance. Medical visits tend to decrease in frequency, and patients are at risk for poor follow-up. Another issue to take into account is that the goals of treatment are different in children compared with adults. Although prevention of Addisonian and salt-wasting crises are critical at any age, the goals in childhood focus on reducing virilization and optimizing growth. Once growth and development are completed, however, the goals of treatment shift toward preventing symptoms of hyperandrogenism in women, preserving fertility, and satisfactory sexual function. The dose and type of glucocorticoid may require adjustment once growth is completed, as growth suppression is no longer a concern. Mineralocorticoid requirements tend to decrease with age.

Although some endocrinologists are trained in both pediatric and adult endocrinology, allowing them to continue caring for their pediatric patients into adulthood, most patients will require some form of transitioning into an adult endocrinology practice. A program of transitioning the pediatric patient into adulthood was developed at the University of Kiel in Germany (the "Kieler Model") as a means for providing a smooth transition.[114] In this program, there is an outpatient clinic staffed by both a pediatric and an adult endocrinologist. The transition usually takes place around 17 to 18 years of age, at which time the CAH patient sees both endocrinologists, and the pediatric endocrinologist provides the adult endocrinologist with an extensive summary of treatment up to that time. Depending on the complexity, the patient is seen several times by both the pediatric and adult endocrinologist in joint appointments until the transition is complete. Similar programs of transitioning may help to optimize the care of CAH patients into adulthood.

## SUMMARY

The pathophysiology of the various types of CAH (the most common being 21 OHD) can be traced to discrete, inherited defects in the genes encoding enzymes for adrenal steroidogenesis. Treatment of CAH is targeted to replace the insufficient adrenal hormones. With proper hormone replacement therapy, normal and healthy development may often be expected. Glucocorticoid and, if necessary, mineralocorticoid replacement, has been the mainstay of treatment for CAH, but new treatment strategies continue to be developed and studied to improve care.

## REFERENCES

1. Pang S, Clark A. Congenital adrenal hyperplasia due to 21-hydroxylase deficiency: newborn screening and its relationship to the diagnosis and treatment of the disorder. Screening 1993;2:105–39.
2. Therrell BJ, Berenbaum S, Manter-Kapanke V, et al. Results of screening 1.9 million Texas newborns for 21-hydroxylase-deficient congenital adrenal hyperplasia. Pediatrics 1998;101:583–90.
3. Balsamo A, Cacciari E, Piazzi S, et al. Congenital adrenal hyperplasia: neonatal mass screening compared with clinical diagnosis only in the Emilia-Romagna region of Italy, 1980–1995. Pediatrics 1996;98:362–7.
4. Speiser PW, Dupont B, Rubinstein P, et al. High frequency of nonclassical steroid 21-hydroxylase deficiency. Am J Hum Genet 1985;37:650–67.
5. Sherman SL, Aston CE, Morton NE, et al. A segregation and linkage study of classical and nonclassical 21-hydroxylase deficiency. Am J Hum Genet 1988; 42:830–8.
6. Ganong W. The central nervous system and the synthesis and release of adrenocorticotrophic hormone. In: Nalbandov A, editor. Advances in neuroendocrinology. Urbana: University of Illinois Press; 1963. p. 92.
7. Guillemin R, Schally A. Recent advances in the chemistry of neuroendocrine mediators originating in the central nervous system. In: Nalbandov A, editor. Advances in neuroendocrinology. Urbana: University of Illinois Press; 1963. p. 314.

8. Goto M, Piper Hanley K, Marcos J, et al. In humans, early cortisol biosynthesis provides a mechanism to safeguard female sexual development. J Clin Invest 2006;116:953–60.
9. Prader A, Gurtner HP. [The syndrome of male pseudohermaphrodism in congenital adrenocortical hyperplasia without overproduction of androgens (adrenal male pseudohermaphrodism)]. Helv Paediatr Acta 1955;10:397–412.
10. Eugster EA, Dimeglio LA, Wright JC, et al. Height outcome in congenital adrenal hyperplasia caused by 21-hydroxylase deficiency: a meta-analysis. J Pediatr. 2001;138:26–32.
11. Muirhead S, Sellers EA, Guyda H. Indicators of adult height outcome in classical 21-hydroxylase deficiency congenital adrenal hyperplasia. J Pediatr 2002;141:247–52.
12. Brunelli V, Russo G, Bertelloni S, et al. Final height in congenital adrenal hyperplasia due to 21-hydroxylase deficiency: the Italian experience. J Pediatr Endocrinol Metab 2003;16(Suppl 2):277–83.
13. Lin-Su K, Vogiatzi MG, Marshall I, et al. Treatment with growth hormone and luteinizing hormone releasing hormone analog improves final adult height in children with congenital adrenal hyperplasia. J Clin Endocrinol Metab 2005; 90:3318–25.
14. Quintos JB, Vogiatzi MG, Harbison MD, et al. Growth hormone therapy alone or in combination with gonadotropin-releasing hormone analog therapy to improve the height deficit in children with congenital adrenal hyperplasia. J Clin Endocrinol Metab 2001;86:1511–7.
15. Jones H, Verkauf B. Congenital adrenal hyperplasia: age at menarche and related events at puberty. Am J Obstet Gynecol 1971;109:292.
16. Ghali I, David M, David L. Linear growth and pubertal development in treated congenital adrenal hyperplasia due to 21-hydroxylase deficiency. Clin Endocrinol (Oxf) 1977;6:425–36.
17. Trinh L, Nimkarn S, Obeid J, et al. Growth and pubertal characteristics in patients with congenital adrenal hyperplasia due to 21-hydroxylase deficiency. ENDO 2006 The Endocrine Society's 88th Annual Meeting. Boston, Massachusetts, June 24–27, 2006. p. 368.
18. Klingensmith G, Garcia S, Jones H, et al. Glucocorticoid treatment of girls with congenital adrenal hyperplasia: effects on height, sexual maturation, and fertility. J Pediatr 1977;90:996–1004.
19. Barnes RB, Rosenfield RL, Ehrmann DA, et al. Ovarian hyperandrogynism as a result of congenital adrenal virilizing disorders: evidence for perinatal masculinization of neuroendocrine function in women. J Clin Endocrinol Metab 1994; 79:1328–33.
20. Long DN, Wisniewski AB, Migeon CJ. Gender role across development in adult women with congenital adrenal hyperplasia due to 21-hydroxylase deficiency. J Pediatr Endocrinol Metab 2004;17:1367–73.
21. Meyer-Bahlburg HF, Dolezal C, Baker SW, et al. Sexual orientation in women with classical or non-classical congenital adrenal hyperplasia as a function of degree of prenatal androgen excess. Arch Sex Behav 2008;37:85–99.
22. Hines M, Brook C, Conway GS. Androgen and psychosexual development: core gender identity, sexual orientation and recalled childhood gender role behavior in women and men with congenital adrenal hyperplasia (CAH). J Sex Res 2004; 41:75–81.
23. Mulaikal RM, Migeon CJ, Rock JA. Fertility rates in female patients with congenital adrenal hyperplasia due to 21-hydroxylase deficiency. N Engl J Med 1987; 316:178–82.

24. Premawardhana L, Hughes I, Read G, et al. Longer term outcome in females with congenital adrenal hyperplasia (CAH): the Cardiff experience. Clin Endocrinol (Oxf) 1997;46:327–32.
25. Prader A, Zachmann M, Illig R. Normal spermatogenesis in adult males with congenital adrenal hyperplasia after discontinuation of therapy. In: Lee P, Platnick L, Kowarski A, et al, editors. Congenital adrenal hyperplasia. Baltimore (MD): University Park Press; 1977. p. 397.
26. Stewart J. A fertile male with untreated congenital adrenal hyperplasia. Acta Endocrinol Suppl 1960;51:661.
27. Urban M, Lee P, Migeon C. Adult height and fertility in men with congenital virilizing adrenal hyperplasia. N Engl J Med 1978;299:1392.
28. Cabrera M, Vogiatzi M, New M. Long term outcome in adult males with classic congenital adrenal hyperplasia. J Clin Endocrinol Metab 2001;86:3070–80.
29. Sugino Y, Usui T, Okubo K, et al. Genotyping of congenital adrenal hyperplasia due to 21-hydroxylase deficiency presenting as male infertility: case report and literature review. J Assist Reprod Genet 2006;23:377–80.
30. Bonaccorsi A, Adler I, Figueiredo J. Male infertility due to congenital adrenal hyperplasia: testicular biopsy findings, hormonal evaluation, and therapeutic results in three patients. Fertil Steril 1987;47:664–70.
31. Claahsen-van der Grinten HL, Sweep FC, Blickman JG, et al. Prevalence of testicular adrenal rest tumours in male children with congenital adrenal hyperplasia due to 21-hydroxylase deficiency. Eur J Endocrinol 2007;157:339–44.
32. Molitor J, Chertow B, Fariss B. Long-term follow-up of a patient with congenital adrenal hyperplasia and failure of testicular development. Fertil Steril 1973;24:319.
33. Blumberg-Tick J, Boudou P, Nahoul K, et al. Testicular tumors in congenital adrenal hyperplasia: steroid measurements from adrenal and spermatic veins. J Clin Endocrinol Metab 1991;73:1129–33.
34. Claahsen-van der Grinten HL, Otten BJ, Hermus AR, et al. Testicular adrenal rest tumors in patients with congenital adrenal hyperplasia can cause severe testicular damage. Fertil Steril 2008;89:597–601.
35. Schoen E, DiRaimondo V, Dominguez O. Bilateral testicular tumors complicating congenital adrenocortical hyperplasia. J Clin Endocrinol Metab 1961;21:518.
36. Miller E, Murray H. Congenital adrenocortical hyperplasia: case previously reported as "bilateral interstitial cell tumor of the testicle". J Clin Endocrinol Metab 1962;22:655.
37. Glenn J, Boyce W. Adrenogenitalism with testicular adrenal rests simulating interstitial cell tumor. J Urol 1963;89:456.
38. Srikanth M, West B, Ishitani M, et al. Benign testicular tumors in children with congenital adrenal hyperplasia. J Pediatr Surg 1992;27:639–41.
39. Rutgers J, Young R, Scully R. The testicular "tumor" of the adrenogenital syndrome. A report of six cases and review of the literature on testicular masses in patients with adrenocortical disorders. Am J Surg Pathol 1988;12:503–13.
40. Wilkins L, Crigler J, Silverman S, et al. Further studies on the treatment of congenital adrenal hyperplasia with cortisone. II. The effects of cortisone on sexual and somatic development, with a hypothesis concerning the mechanism of feminization. J Clin Endocrinol Metab 1952;12:277.
41. Klein R. Evidence for and evidence against the existence of a salt-losing hormone. J Pediatr 1960;57:452.
42. Kowarski A, Finkelstein JW, Spaulding JS, et al. Aldosterone secretion rate in congenital adrenal hyperplasia. A discussion of the theories on the pathogenesis of the salt-losing form of the syndrome. J Clin Invest 1965;44:1505–13.

43. Kuhnle U, Land M, Ulick S. Evidence for the secretion of an antimineralocorticoid in congenital adrenal hyperplasia. J Clin Endocrinol Metab 1986;62:934–40.
44. Merke D, Chrousos G, Eisenhofer G, et al. Adrenomedullary dysplasia and hypofunction in patients with classic 21-hydroxylase deficiency. N Engl J Med 2000;343:1362–8.
45. Stoner E, Dimartino-Nardi J, Kuhnle U, et al. Is salt-wasting in congenital adrenal hyperplasia due to the same gene as the fasciculata defect? Clin Endocrinol (Oxf) 1986;24:9–20.
46. Luetscher JA. Studies of aldosterone in relation to water and electrolyte balance in man. Recent Prog Horm Res 1956;12:175.
47. Speiser PW, Agdere L, Ueshiba H, et al. Aldosterone synthesis in salt-wasting congenital adrenal hyperplasia with complete absence of adrenal 21-hydroxylase. N Engl J Med 1991;324:145–9.
48. Nimkarn S, New MI. Prenatal diagnosis and treatment of congenital adrenal hyperplasia owing to 21-hydroxylase deficiency. Nat Clin Pract Endocrinol Metab 2007;3:405–13.
49. New MI. Nonclassical 21-hydroxylase deficiency. J Clin Endocrinol Metab 2006;91:4205–14.
50. New MI. Extensive clinical experience: nonclassical 21-hydroxylase deficiency. J Clin Endocrinol Metab 2006;91:4205–14.
51. Kashimada K, Ono M, Onishi T, et al. Clinical course of patients with nonclassical 21-hydroxylase deficiency (21-OHD) diagnosed in infancy and childhood. Endocr J 2008;55:397–404.
52. Fanta M, Cibula D, Vrbikova J. Prevalence of nonclassic adrenal hyperplasia (NCAH) in hyperandrogenic women. Gynecol Endocrinol 2008;24:154–7.
53. Escobar-Morreale HF, Sanchon R, San Millan JL. A prospective study of the prevalence of nonclassical congenital adrenal hyperplasia among women presenting with hyperandrogenic symptoms and signs. J Clin Endocrinol Metab 2008;93:527–33.
54. Claahsen-van der Grinten HL, Otten BJ, Sweep FC, et al. Repeated successful induction of fertility after replacing hydrocortisone with dexamethasone in a patient with congenital adrenal hyperplasia and testicular adrenal rest tumors. Fertil Steril 2007;88:705, e5–8.
55. Jaaskelainen J, Tiitinen A, Voutilainen R. Sexual function and fertility in adult females and males with congenital adrenal hyperplasia. Horm Res 2001;56:73–80.
56. Clayton PE, Miller WL, Oberfield SE, et al. Consensus statement on 21-hydroxylase deficiency from the European Society for Paediatric Endocrinology and the Lawson Wilkins Pediatric Endocrine Society. Horm Res 2002;58:188–95.
57. Mokshagundam S, Surks M. Congenital adrenal hyperplasia diagnosed in a man during workup for bilateral adrenal masses. Arch Intern Med 1993;153:1389–91.
58. Jaresch S, Kornely E, Kley H, et al. Adrenal incidentaloma and patients with homozygous or heterozygous congenital adrenal hyperplasia. J Clin Endocrinol Metab 1992;74:685–9.
59. Wilson RC, Mercado AB, Cheng KC, et al. Steroid 21-hydroxylase deficiency: genotype may not predict phenotype. J Clin Endocrinol Metab 1995;80:2322–9.
60. Dupont B, Oberfield SE, Smithwick EM, et al. Close genetic linkage between HLA and congenital adrenal hyperplasia (21-hydroxylase deficiency). Lancet 1977;2:1309–12.

61. Nebert DW, Nelson DR, Coon MJ. The P450 superfamily: update on new sequences, gene mapping, and recommended nomenclature. DNA Cell Biol 1991;10:1–14.
62. White PC, New MI, Dupont B. Structure of the human steroid 21-hydroxylase genes. Proc Natl Acad Sci U S A 1986;83:5111–5.
63. Stenson PD, Ball EV, Mort M, et al. Human Gene Mutation Database (HGMD): 2003 update. Hum Mutat 2003;21:577–81.
64. Tusie-Luna MT, Speiser PW, Dumic M, et al. A mutation (Pro-30 to Leu) in CYP21 represents a potential nonclassic steroid 21-hydroxylase deficiency allele. Mol Endocrinol 1991;5:685–92.
65. Speiser PW, New MI, White PC. Molecular genetic analysis of nonclassic steroid 21-hydroxylase deficiency associated with HLA-B14, DR1. N Engl J Med 1988; 319:19–23.
66. Helmberg A, Tusie-Luna M, Tabarelli M, et al. R339H and P453S: CYP21 mutations associated with nonclassic steroid 21-hydroxylase deficiency that are not apparent gene conversions. Mol Endocrinol 1992;6:1318–22.
67. Owerbach D, Sherman L, Ballard AL, et al. Pro-453 to Ser mutation in CYP21 is associated with nonclassic steroid 21-hydroxylase deficiency. Mol Endocrinol 1992;6:1211–5.
68. White PC, New MI, Dupont B. HLA-linked congenital adrenal hyperplasia results from a defective gene encoding a cytochrome P-450 specific for steroid 21-hydroxylation. Proc Natl Acad Sci U S A 1984;81:7505–9.
69. Higashi Y, Tanae A, Inoue H, et al. Aberrant splicing and missense mutations cause steroid 21-hydroxylase [P-450(C21)] deficiency in humans: possible gene conversion products. Proc Natl Acad Sci U S A 1988;85:7486–90.
70. White PC, Tusie-Luna MT, New MI, et al. Mutations in steroid 21-hydroxylase (CYP21). Hum Mutat 1994;3:373–8.
71. Tusie-Luna M, Traktman P, White PC. Determination of functional effects of mutations in the steroid 21-hydroxylase gene (CYP21) using recombinant vaccinia virus. J Biol Chem 1990;265:20916–22.
72. Amor M, Parker KL, Globerman H, et al. Mutation in the CYP21B gene (Ile-172-Asn) causes steroid 21-hydroxylase deficiency. Proc Natl Acad Sci U S A 1988; 85:1600–7.
73. Globerman H, Amor M, Parker KL, et al. Nonsense mutation causing steroid 21-hydroxylase deficiency. J Clin Invest 1988;82:139–44.
74. Chiou SH, Hu MC, Chung BC. A missense mutation at Ile172–Asn or Arg356–Trp causes steroid 21-hydroxylase deficiency. J Biol Chem 1990;265:3549–52.
75. Wedell A, Luthman H. Steroid 21-hydroxylase (P450c21): a new allele and spread of mutations through the pseudogene. Hum Genet 1993;91:236–40.
76. Speiser PW, Dupont J, Zhu D, et al. Disease expression and molecular genotype in congenital adrenal hyperplasia due to 21-hydroxylase deficiency. J Clin Invest 1992;90:584–95.
77. Wedell A, Ritzen EM, Haglund-Stengler B, et al. Steroid 21-hydroxylase deficiency: three additional mutated alleles and establishment of phenotype-genotype relationships of common mutations. Proc Natl Acad Sci U S A 1992; 89:7232–6.
78. Krone N, Braun A, Roscher A, et al. Predicting phenotype in steroid 21-hydroxylase deficiency? Comprehensive genotyping in 155 unrelated, well defined patients from southern Germany. J Clin Endocrinol Metab 2000;85:p1059–65.
79. Chemaitilly W, Betensky B, Marshal I, et al. Case report: the natural history and genotype-phenotype nonconcordance of HLA identical siblings with the same mutations of the 21-hydroxylase gene. J Pediatr Endocrinol Metab 2005;18:143–54.

80. Rohana AG, Ming W, Norlela S, et al. Functioning adrenal adenoma in association with congenital adrenal hyperplasia. Med J Malaysia 2007;62:158–9.
81. Jansen M, Wit JM, van den Brande JL. Reinstitution of mineralocorticoid therapy in congenital adrenal hyperplasia. Effects on control and growth. Acta Paediatr Scand 1981;70:229–33.
82. Forest MG, Dorr HG. Prenatal therapy in congenital adrenal hyperplasia due to 21-hydroxylase deficiency: retrospective follow-up study of 253 treated pregnancies in 215 families. Endocrinologist 2003;13:252–9.
83. Schachter SC. Handedness in women with intrauterine exposure to diethystilbestrol. Neuropsychologia 1994;32:619–23.
84. Schnitzer J, Donahoe P. Surgical treatment of congenital adrenal hyperplasia. Endocrinol Metab Clin North Am 2001;30:137–54.
85. Crouch NS, Liao LM, Woodhouse CR, et al. Sexual function and genital sensitivity following feminizing genitoplasty for congenital adrenal hyperplasia. J Urol 2008;179:634–8. Epub 2007 Dec 21.
86. Gastaud F, Bouvattier C, Duranteau L, et al. Impaired sexual and reproductive outcomes in women with classical forms of congenital adrenal hyperplasia. Clin Endocrinol Metab 2007;92:1391–6.
87. Nordenskjold A, Holmdahl G, Frisen L, et al. Type of mutation and surgical procedure affect long-term quality of life for women with congenital adrenal hyperplasia. J Clin Endocrinol Metab 2008;93:380–6.
88. Mazziotti G, Giustina A, Canalis E, et al. Glucocorticoid-induced osteoporosis: clinical and therapeutic aspects. Arq Bras Endocrinol Metabol 2007;51:1404–12.
89. Falhammar H, Filipsson H, Holmdahl G, et al. Fractures and bone mineral density in adult women with 21-hydroxylase deficiency. J Clin Endocrinol Metab 2007;92:4643–9.
90. King JA, Wisniewski AB, Bankowski BJ, et al. Long-term corticosteroid replacement and bone mineral density in adult women with classical congenital adrenal hyperplasia. J Clin Endocrinol Metab 2006;91:865–9.
91. Stikkelbroeck N, Oyen W, van der Wilt GJ, et al. Normal bone mineral density and lean body mass, but increased fat mass, in young adult patients with congenital adrenal hyperplasia. J Clin Endocrinol Metab 2003;88:1036–42.
92. Christiansen P, Molgaard C, Muller J. Normal bone mineral content in young adults with congenital adrenal hyperplasia due to 21-hydroxylase deficiency. Horm Res 2004;61:133–6.
93. Cornean RE, Hindmarsh PC, Brook CG. Obesity in 21-hydroxylase deficient patients. Arch Dis Child 1998;78:261–3.
94. Charmandari E, Chrousos GP. Metabolic syndrome manifestations in classic congenital adrenal hyperplasia: do they predispose to atherosclerotic cardiovascular disease and secondary polycystic ovary syndrome? Ann N Y Acad Sci 2006;1083:37–53.
95. Volkl TM, Simm D, Beier C, et al. Obesity among children and adolescents with classic congenital adrenal hyperplasia due to 21-hydroxylase deficiency. Pediatrics 2006;117:e98–105.
96. Speiser PW, Serrat J, New MI, et al. Insulin insensitivity in adrenal hyperplasia due to nonclassical steroid 21-hydroxylase deficiency. J Clin Endocrinol Metab 1992;75:1421–4.
97. Charmandari E, Weise M, Bornstein S, et al. Children with classic congenital adrenal hyperplasia have elevated serum leptin concentrations and insulin resistance: potential clinical implications. J Clin Endocrinol Metab 2002;87:2114–20.

98. Sartorato P, Zulian E, Benedini S, et al. Cardiovascular risk factors and ultrasound evaluation of intima-media thickness at common carotids, carotid bulbs, and femoral and abdominal aorta arteries in patients with classic congenital adrenal hyperplasia due to 21-hydroxylase deficiency. J Clin Endocrinol Metab 2007;92:1015–8.
99. Falhammar H, Filipsson H, Holmdahl G, et al. Metabolic profile and body composition in adult women with congenital adrenal hyperplasia due to 21-hydroxylase deficiency. J Clin Endocrinol Metab 2007;92:110–6.
100. Roche EF, Charmandari E, Dattani MT, et al. Blood pressure in children and adolescents with congenital adrenal hyperplasia (21-hydroxylase deficiency): a preliminary report. Clin Endocrinol (Oxf) 2003;58:589–96.
101. Weise M, Drinkard B, Mehlinger SL, et al. Stress dose of hydrocortisone is not beneficial in patients with classic congenital adrenal hyperplasia undergoing short-term, high-intensity exercise. J Clin Endocrinol Metab 2004;89:3679–84.
102. Green-Golan L, Yates C, Drinkard B, et al. Patients with classic congenital adrenal hyperplasia have decreased epinephrine reserve and defective glycemic control during prolonged moderate-intensity exercise. J Clin Endocrinol Metab 2007;92:3019–24.
103. Burton PJ, Waddell BJ. Dual function of 11beta-hydroxysteroid dehydrogenase in placenta: modulating placental glucocorticoid passage and local steroid action. Biol Reprod 1999;60:234–40.
104. Rennick GJ. Use of systemic glucocorticosteroids in pregnancy: be alert but not alarmed. Australas J Dermatol 2006;47:34–6.
105. Carlson AD, Obeid JS, Kanellopoulou N, et al. Prenatal treatment and diagnosis of congenital adrenal hyperplasia owing to steroid 21-hydroxylase deficiency. In: New MI, editor. Diagnosis and treatment of the unborn child. Reddick (FL): Idelson-Gnocchi Ltd. Publisher; 1999. p. 75–84.
106. New M, Carlson A, Obeid J, et al. Update: Prenatal diagnosis for congenital adrenal hyperplasia in 595 pregnancies. Endocrinologist 2003;13:233–9.
107. Goldman A, Sharpior B, Katsumata M. Human foetal palatal corticoid receptors and teratogens for cleft palate. Nature 1978;272:464–6.
108. Nimkarn S, New MI. Prenatal diagnosis and treatment of congenital adrenal hyperplasia owing to 21-hydroxylase deficiency. Nat Clin Pract Endocrinol Metab 2007;3:405–13.
109. Pang S, Clark AT, Freeman LO, et al. Maternal side-effects of prenatal dexamethasone therapy for fetal congenital adrenal hyperplasia. J Clin Endocrinol Metab 1992;76:249–53.
110. Lajic S, Wedell A, Bui T, et al. Long-term somatic follow-up of prenatally treated children with congenital adrenal hyperplasia. J Clin Endocrinol Metab 1998;83:3872–80.
111. Meyer-Bahlburg HF, Dolezal C, Baker SW, et al. Cognitive and motor development of children with and without congenital adrenal hyperplasia after early-prenatal dexamethasone. J Clin Endocrinol Metab 2004;89:610–4.
112. Hirvikoski T, Nordenstrom A, Lindholm T, et al. Cognitive functions in children at risk for congenital adrenal hyperplasia treated prenatally with dexamethasone. J Clin Endocrinol Metab 2007;92:542–8.
113. Hirvikoski T, Nordenstrom A, Lindholm T, et al. Long-term follow-up of prenatally treated children at risk for congenital adrenal hyperplasia: does dexamethasone cause behavioural problems? Eur J Endocrinol 2008;159:309–16.
114. Kruse B, Riepe FG, Krone N, et al. Congenital adrenal hyperplasia—how to improve the transition from adolescence to adult life. Exp Clin Endocrinol Diabetes 2004;112:343–55.

# Etiology and Treatment of Hypogonadism in Adolescents

Vidhya Viswanathan, MD*, Erica A. Eugster, MD

**KEYWORDS**

- Hypergonadotropic hypogonadism
- Hypogonadotropic hypogonadism
- Adolescents • Delayed puberty • Treatment

Factors that mitigate the onset of puberty have yet to be fully elucidated. Gonadarche refers to the onset of gonadal sex steroid production during puberty. Gonadarche results from pulsatile gonadotropin releasing hormone (GnRH) secretion from the hypothalamus. GnRH secretion occurs every 60 to 90 minutes,[1] and there is subsequent release of the pituitary gonadotropins luteinizing hormone (LH) and follicle stimulating hormone (FSH) initially during sleep,[2] which leads to gonadal stimulation. LH stimulates Leydig cell hyperplasia in males and subsequent testosterone release. FSH has little effect in males until the onset of spermarche (sperm maturation). In females, FSH stimulates the production of estradiol via ovarian follicular development. Testosterone and estradiol secretion lead to the development of secondary sexual characteristics. Adequate functioning at all levels of the hypothalamic-pituitary-gonadal axis is necessary for normal gonadal development and subsequent sex steroid production. Deficiencies at any level of the axis can lead to a hypogonadal state.

In boys, hypogonadism can manifest as a complete lack of secondary sexual development or failure of normal pubertal progression. In girls, it can present with failure of pubertal initiation, failure of pubertal progression, or menstrual irregularities. Abnormalities within the hypothalamus or pituitary lead to *hypogonadotropic hypogonadism* whereas primary gonadal failure is characterized as *hypergonadotropic hypogonadism*.

## HYPOGONADOTROPIC HYPOGONADISM

Hypogonadotropic hypogonadism can be attributed to a variety of congenital origins including single gene mutations, idiopathic forms, and genetic syndromes. Acquired

Section of Pediatric Endocrinology, Department of Pediatrics, Riley Hospital for Children, Indiana University School of Medicine, Room 5960, 702 Barnhill Drive, Indianapolis, IN 46202, USA

* Corresponding author.

*E-mail address:* vviswana@iupui.edu (V. Viswanathan).

Endocrinol Metab Clin N Am 38 (2009) 719–738

doi:10.1016/j.ecl.2009.08.004

0889-8529/09/$ – see front matter. Published by Elsevier Inc.

causes of hypogonadotropic hypogonadism include central nervous system (CNS) insults such as trauma, irradiation, and intracranial tumors. By far the most common cause of hypogonadotropic hypogonadism is transient, and is termed constitutional delay of growth and puberty (CDGP). Each of these causes is briefly discussed here, and the molecular genetic causes of hypogonadotropic hypogonadism are shown in **Table 1**.

### *Constitutional Delay of Growth and Puberty*

CDGP is a variation of normal development that can be difficult to differentiate from pathologic hypogonadotropic hypogonadism. In this condition, puberty and the pubertal growth spurt occur at or later than the extreme upper end of the normal age. The diagnosis is made more often in boys than girls, likely due to referral bias, and has a strongly familial pattern.[3] Skeletal maturation is delayed in comparison with chronologic age. CDGP results in delayed but *normal* puberty; thus puberty progresses through the normal stages but starts at a later time. Children with CDGP achieve their genetic potential for height,[4] and laboratory evaluation is normal. Some patients benefit from short-term treatment to augment secondary sexual development and boost linear growth.[5]

### *Congenital Origins*

#### *Gene defects*

**Nuclear receptor mutations** Nuclear receptors influence gene transcription at multiple levels, and exert their effects in a time- and dosage-specific fashion. An important nuclear receptor involved in gonadotropin secretion is steroidogenic factor-1 (SF-1), a key regulator of genes involved in sexual differentiation, steroidogenesis, and reproduction. SF-1 knockout mice show marked abnormalities in the development of the hypothalamus and impaired development of pituitary gonadotropes, with decreased levels of serum gonadotropins as well as gonadal dysgenesis.[6] Target genes of SF-1 within the hypothalamus and pituitary include the gonadotropin releasing hormone receptor (GnRHR) and the β subunit of LH. Both heterozygous and homozygous mutations in the DNA binding domain of SF-1 result in complete XY sex reversal, testicular dysgenesis, and adrenal failure in genotypic males. A milder phenotype has also been described in which there is impaired gonadal but intact adrenal function.[7] In a genetic female, a heterozygous SF-1 mutation has been associated with primary adrenal failure but normal ovarian development.[8] Thus, SF-1 mutations exist within a broad clinical spectrum that will undoubtedly continue to expand.

DAX-1 is an orphan nuclear receptor that is involved in steroidogenesis and functions as a repressor of SF-1 mediated transcription. Mutations have been identified in *NROB1*, the gene that encodes DAX1, on the Xp21 locus. Males with DAX1 mutations typically present with early-onset adrenal insufficiency and subsequent delayed puberty secondary to hypogonadotropic hypogonadism.[9] However, a delayed presentation of primary adrenal insufficiency has also been reported.[10] DAX1 mutations can lead to both hypothalamic and pituitary dysfunction with decreased GnRH and gonadotropin secretion.[11] DAX1 mutations can also cause defects in spermatogenesis, and in one study affected males also had evidence of azospermia.[12] Therefore, mutations in DAX-1, as in SF-1, can lead to the development of hypogonadism in a multitude of ways.

**Kallman syndrome** Impairment of GnRH secretion can also occur from defects in migration of GnRH producing neurons. Kallman syndrome (KS) refers to the combination of hypogonadotropic hypogonadism and anosmia. The X-linked form results from

**Table 1**
**Molecular genetic causes of hypogonadotropic hypogonadism**

| Gene | Product | Inheritance | Target Sites | Additional Clinical Manifestations |
|---|---|---|---|---|
| *SF-1* | Orphan nuclear receptor | Autosomal recessive | Steroidogenesis in males<br>Hypothalamus<br>Pituitary<br>Adrenals | XY sex reversal, adrenal failure<br>In females: adrenal failure, normal ovarian function |
| *DAX-1* | Orphan nuclear receptor | X-linked recessive | Steroidogenesis<br>Hypothalamus<br>Pituitary<br>Adrenals | In males: spectrum of hypogonadotropic hypogonadism and adrenal insufficiency |
| *KAL-1* | Anosmin | X-linked recessive | Hypothalamic neuronal migration | Anosmia |
| *FGFR1* | FGF receptor | Autosomal dominant | FGF receptor in hypothalamus<br>Pituitary | Cleft palate<br>Agenesis of corpus callosum |
| *GPR54* | G protein coupled receptor | Autosomal recessive | GnRH-secreting neurons<br>Pituitary | Isolated hypogonadotropic hypogonadism |
| *Prop-1* | Transcription factor | Sporadic autosomal recessive | Pituitary gonadotrope development | Growth hormone deficiency<br>Central hypothyroidism |
| *Hesx1* | Transcription factor | Sporadic | Prop-1<br>Pituitary gonadotrope development | Septo-optic dysplasia<br>Central hypothyroidism<br>Central hypocortisolism<br>Diabetes insipidus |
| *LEP* | Leptin | Autosomal dominant | Hypothalamus | Obesity<br>Hyperphagia<br>T-cell immune dysfunction |
| *LEPR* | Leptin receptor | Autosomal dominant | Hypothalamus | Obesity<br>Hyperphagia<br>T-cell immune dysfunction |

a defect in the migration of GnRH and olfactory neurons due to a mutation in the *KAL1* gene. This gene encodes for anosmin-1, a glycoprotein essential for neuronal migration and growth.[13] Individuals with KS also have aplasia of the olfactory bulb as noted on magnetic resonance imaging (MRI).[14] Although *KAL1* gene defects have been the prototype of KS, there is emerging evidence that autosomal forms may be more prevalent than previously thought. In one study, *KAL1* gene defects accounted for only 14% of cases with familial KS. Mutations in unidentified autosomal genes were postulated to cause the remainder. Subjects with presumed autosomal gene defects had some response to GnRH pulses, indicating partial preservation of hypothalamic GnRH-secreting neurons, though still with phenotypic similarity to the X-linked version of the syndrome.[15] Fibroblast growth receptor 1 (FGFR1) mutations may account for as many as 10% of cases,[16] and mutations in the prokineticin 2 (PROK2) gene have also been identified in individuals with KS and normosmic hypogonadotropic hypogonadism.[17] No matter what the underlying molecular genetic cause, lack of adequate GnRH secretion leads to decreased circulating gonadotropins in both autosomal and X-linked cases.

**Isolated hypogonadotropic hypogonadism** Isolated hypogonadotropic hypogonadism (IHH) refers to cases in which anosmia is absent. One potential cause is loss of function mutations of the GnRHR, a G-protein coupled receptor. At least 8 mutations of the GnRHR in 7 families have been identified. Notable genotype-phenotype variation exists even within members of the same kindred due to incomplete activation of GnRHR function.[18] Males with these mutations display signs of hypogonadism and small testes. Females typically present with primary amenorrhea.[19] Another important cause of IHH has been traced to mutations in GPR54, which has a critical role in hypothalamic GnRH signaling and release.[20] Of note, both KS and IHH may be found in the same kindred. IHH has also been noted to be reversible in some patients.[21]

**Transcription factor mutations** Even with intact GnRH production and signal transduction, pituitary gonadotropin synthesis may still be deficient due to mutations in a variety of transcription factors. An important transcription factor involved in the developmental cascade of pituitary gonadotrope cells is Prop-1. Prop-1 is the prophet of the pituitary transcription factor Pit 1, a paired-like homeodomain transcription factor that is responsible for early embryonic pituitary development. Prop-1 gene mutations can result in familial combined pituitary hormone deficiency including growth hormone deficiency, central hypothyroidism, and hypogonadotropic hypogonadism.[22] In one analysis of 8 members of a consanguineous family with Prop-1 gene mutations, all 8 family members had gonadotropin deficiency and failure of spontaneous sexual maturation.[23] There is also a variable pattern of phenotypic expressivity associated with Prop-1 mutations, with different deficiencies appearing at different time periods within the same family.

Like Prop-1, the transcription factor HESX1 is needed for normal pituitary development.[24] Deficiencies in HESX1, initially identified in 1998, are a rare cause of septo-optic dysplasia[25] which may be associated with hypogonadotropic hypogonadism.[26] Other transcription factors implicated in rare cases of hypogonadotropic hypogonadism include LHX4[27] and SOX 2.[28] All patients with hypopituitarism, including idiopathic forms, are at risk for hypogonadotropic hypogonadism.

**Leptin and leptin receptor defects** Congenital leptin deficiency results from loss of function mutations of the *LEP* gene, which encodes for the leptin protein. Leptin interacts with the leptin receptor, a member of the interleukin-6 family of receptors. This interaction stimulates the Jak-Stat pathway and leads to activation of downstream target genes. Leptin deficiency acts as a sign of nutritional deprivation and results in the suppression of the reproductive axis. Classic findings in individuals with leptin deficiency include hyperphagia, obesity, and hypogonadotropic hypogonadism. Administration of leptin seemingly rectifies these abnormalities.[29] Leptin receptor (LEPR) abnormalities have a similar phenotype to congenital leptin deficiency. Females with this mutation have hypogonadotropic hypogonadism. These girls present with delayed puberty, lack of a pubertal growth spurt, and reduced expression of secondary sexual characteristics. Some may have irregular menses due to aromatization of subcutaneous fat to estrogen, which then stimulates uterine hyperplasia. Males with leptin receptor mutations have hypogonadotropic hypogonadism and diminished testosterone production.[30]

#### *Syndromes*

Numerous syndromes include neuroendocrine dysfunction as a potential feature. Perhaps the best known is Prader-Willi syndrome (PWS), which is caused by a genetic defect involving paternal chromosome 15, usually in the form of a microdeletion within the long arm or maternal unipaternal disomy.[31] Hypothalamic dysfunction is marked in these patients as evidenced by their hypotonia, hyperphagia, and intermittent temperature instability. The hypothalamic dysfunction also leads to hypogonadism and may be attributed to an absence of or abnormal location of GnRH neurons. Early studies in individuals with PWS revealed low circulating serum gonadotropins and in males, attenuated testosterone response to human chorionic gonadotropin.[32] Physical findings in boys include micropenis, scrotal hypoplasia, cryptorchidism, and small testes. Either absent or delayed puberty may ensue. In girls, findings may be less remarkable and include hypoplasia of the clitoris or labia minora, primary amenorrhea, and delayed puberty.[33] However, a wide spectrum of hypogonadism exists in PWS, with some women achieving fertility without hormone replacement therapy.[34,35]

### *Acquired Origins*

Any significant CNS insult can result in acquired hypogonadotropic hypogonadism. Two of the most common causes in children are traumatic brain injury and CNS tumors.

#### *Traumatic brain injury*

Traumatic brain injury (TBI) is an insult to the brain that results in neurologic dysfunction. TBI can have significant neurocognitive, neuropsychological, and neuroendocrine sequelae.[36,37] Anterior pituitary insufficiency resulting from TBI has been noted in the past, but is garnering more attention as a high prevalence of pituitary hormone insufficiency has been demonstrated.[38] Some retrospective studies indicate that gonadotropin deficiency may be found in 90% to 95% of those with history of TBI,[39] although prospective studies in adults have noted the prevalence to be far less. In one study, hormonal evaluation was conducted on TBI patients at baseline (acute phase) and at 12 months. In the acute phase, approximately 42% of those evaluated had gonadotropin deficiency. At the 12-month follow-up, many of these patients spontaneously recovered reproductive function. The final prevalence of hypogonadism was 7.7%.[40] It is clear that all patients with a history of TBI require ongoing surveillance for pituitary problems, including hypogonadotropic hypogonadism.

#### *Central nervous system tumors*

Intracranial injury can also occur as a result of CNS tumors. In children, resultant hypogonadotropic hypogonadism can exist as a result of the primary tumor or due to the therapeutic regimen needed to treat the lesion. In a prospective study of 75 children with various CNS tumors, 13% had an abnormality in gonadotropin secretion before initiation of therapy.[41] In a retrospective study focusing on craniopharyngioma, only 1 out of 64 patients had evidence of hypogonadism before treatment. However, after surgical resection and adjuvant radiotherapy, 80% of those evaluated at a pubertal age had evidence of hypogonadism.[42] Gonadotropin deficiency and delayed puberty are most likely in those who receive 40 Gy or more of radiation.[43] Gonadotropin deficiency may continue to evolve for many years after irradiation, with rates of total incidence ranging from 20% to 50%.[44,45] Therefore, all children who have CNS lesions should be monitored for gonadotropin deficiency and signs of pubertal delay.[46]

#### *Hypothalamic amenorrhea*

Hypothalamic amenorrhea is commonly associated with eating disorders such as anorexia nervosa, and also occurs in elite female athletes. Clinical manifestations include absence of menstrual cycles, increased exercise, and weight loss. In these girls, suppression of GnRH secretion results in attenuation of LH and FSH release, and decreased estrogen production.[47] Several theories have been postulated for this hypothalamic dysfunction, including low circulating energy levels due to high energy expenditure and relative deficiency of nutritional intake.[47] Girls with hypothalamic amenorrhea also have low circulating leptin levels. Administration of recombinant leptin to some women with hypothalamic amenorrhea leads to elevated LH and estradiol, resulting in follicular growth and ovulation.[48]

## HYPERGONADOTROPIC HYPOGONADISM

Primary hypogonadism can be due to congenital origins such as chromosomal abnormalities, syndromes, or genetic mutations. Primary hypogonadism can also be acquired later in childhood or adolescence due to autoimmunity or exposure to chemotherapy or radiation. Alterations in gonadotropins, the gonadotropin receptors, or within the gonads themselves can lead to hypogonadism with decreased testosterone and estradiol secretion. The decreased sex steroid secretion causes increased production of gonadotropins manifesting as hypergonadotropic hypogonadism. Congenital causes of primary hypogonadism are outlined in **Table 2**.

### *Congenital Origins*

The most common cause of congenital primary hypogonadism is sex chromosome aneuploidy as is present in Turner syndrome and Klinefelter syndrome. Isolated abnormalities of the X chromosome are also associated with primary ovarian failure.

#### *Turner syndrome*

Turner syndrome (TS) occurs in 1 in 2500 live born females.[49] Diagnosis of the syndrome requires the combination of characteristic physical features, including short stature as well as partial or complete absence of an X chromosome.[50] More than half of girls with TS have chromosomal mosaicism. Approximately 30% will begin puberty spontaneously, but only a small minority will progress to menarche.[51] Spontaneous pregnancy has been reported but is extremely rare in this population.[52] Although initially intrinsically normal, the ovaries in girls with TS undergo accelerated atresia such that ovarian failure is often already present and may be detected at birth. Precisely which genes on the X chromosome are necessary for ovarian maintenance is unknown. FSH levels during early life have been found to be significantly lower in girls with mosaic TS as compared with those who are monosomic.[53]

**Table 2**
**Causes and clinical manifestations of congenital hypergonadotropic hypogonadism**

| Abnormality | Clinical Manifestations | |
|---|---|---|
| Turner syndrome | Short stature, webbed neck, cubitus valgus<br>Streak ovaries | |
| Klinefelter syndrome | Tall stature<br>Eunuchoid body habitus<br>Small, firm testes | |
| X chromosome abnormality | Xq-premature ovarian failure<br>XXX-tall stature<br>GU abnormalities | |
| FSH and LH β subunit mutations | *Males*<br>Delayed puberty<br>Azospermia<br>Infertility | *Females*<br>Primary amenorrhea<br>Menstrual irregularity<br>Polycystic ovary syndrome |
| FSH and LH receptor mutations | *Males*<br>Micropenis<br>Ambiguous genitalia<br>XY sex reversal<br>Infertility | *Females*<br>Primary amenorrhea<br>Gonadal dysgenesis |
| Swyer syndrome (46, XY) | Tall stature<br>Primary amenorrhea<br>Delayed puberty<br>Gonadal tumors | |
| CAIS (46, XY) | Primary amenorrhea<br>Normal breast development<br>Sparse body hair<br>Absent mullerian and wolffian structures | |
| CAH (depending on deficiency) | Hypertension<br>Hypokalemia<br>XY sex reversal<br>Adrenal crisis | |
| Galactosemia | Ovarian failure | |
| Testicular regression sequence | Normal external genitalia | |

### *Klinefelter syndrome*

Klinefelter syndrome is the most common congenital cause of primary hypogonadism and occurs in 1 in 1000 live male births.[54] The most common genotype is XXY, although variants exist with different numbers of X chromosomes. Tall stature, a eunuchoid body habitus, gynecomastia, and small, firm testes are cardinal features. Seminiferous tubule dysgenesis is a classic histologic feature of the testes. Individuals with Klinefelter syndrome exhibit a spectrum of gonadal failure, with many men going undiagnosed until they present with infertility in adulthood. However, a significant number come to attention during adolescence due to delayed puberty or lack of appropriate pubertal progression.

### *X chromosome abnormalities*

Other X chromosome abnormalities, including Xq deletion and Triple X, can cause varying degrees of hypogonadism. Xq deletion can cause a phenotype similar to TS as well as isolated premature ovarian failure.[55] Deletions in the critical region, Xq13-q26, can also lead to premature ovarian failure.[56] Triple X, 47 XXX, is estimated to exist in 1 in 1000 girls and is marked by significant phenotypic variability.[57] Women with this condition can be tall and have normal external genitalia, with preservation of ovarian function.[57] These women can also have ovarian failure as well as significant genitourinary tract anomalies, including cloacal exstrophy and mullerian abnormalities.[58,59]

#### *Abnormalities in gonadotropin production or action*

Mutations within the β subunit of the gonadotropins, the gonadotropin receptors, or forms of resistance to gonadotropins can all result in hypergonadotropic hypogonadism. Females with mutations in the β subunit of FSH present with primary amenorrhea, delayed puberty, and poorly developed secondary sexual characteristics; they have low FSH levels, low estradiol levels, and high LH levels due to lack of feedback inhibition by estradiol.[60,61] Males with the same mutation have normal to delayed puberty and azospermia.[62]

A homozygous mutation within the LH β subunit has resulted in total functional loss in one male.[63] The individual in this case presented with delayed puberty, low serum testosterone, and high LH levels. It was discovered later that several male members in his family were infertile. In further studies, it was noted that females with this defect present with ovarian dysfunction, infertility, menstrual irregularity, or polycystic ovary syndrome.[64]

Inactivating mutations of the G-protein coupled FSH and LH receptors result in a phenotype similar to those with abnormalities in the LH and FSH β subunits. Complete LH resistance results from a loss of function mutation in the LH receptor gene. In males, this causes a phenotype that ranges from micropenis, to ambiguous genitalia, to completely female external genitalia.[65,66] In females, LH resistance results in normal puberty but subsequent amenorrhea, infertility, and elevated LH levels, demonstrating that ovulation requires LH as well as FSH.[67] FSH resistance due to FSH receptor mutations has also been reported, particularly in the Finnish population. Women who are homozygous for this defect have gonadal dysgenesis and primary amenorrhea.[68] In contrast, men from the same kindreds have variable degrees of infertility.

A rare congenital condition associated with gonadotropin resistance is carbohydrate-deficient glycoprotein syndrome, which causes defects in gonadotropin glycosylation. In females with this defect, FSH seems to have less bioactivity and leads to decreased serum estradiol levels. However, exogenous FSH results in an increase in estradiol. Males with this disease advance through puberty but have decreased testicular volume.[69]

Resistance syndromes can also be due to variations in the signal transduction pathway after gonadotropin binding. Pseudohypoparathyroidism is a disease in which the signal transduction pathway of many hormones is altered due to inactivating mutations of the $G_s$ $\alpha$ subunit. The mutation leads to multiple hormone resistance. In a study of 12 patients with pseudohypoparathyroidism, 25% of the pubertal patients had evidence of gonadotropin resistance.[70]

#### *Disorders of sex development*

Disorders of sex development (DSDs) are congenital conditions in which development of chromosomal, gonadal, or anatomic sex is atypical.[71] This broad category includes common entities such as TS and Klinefelter Syndrome, as well as rare disorders such as cloacal exstrophy, mixed gonadal dysgenesis, and congenital aphallia. Many DSDs are associated with ambiguous genitalia, which is beyond the scope of this review. However, a few may present with delayed puberty or primary amenorrhea, and are important to consider in the differential diagnosis of an adolescent with apparent hypogonadism. These DSDs include Swyer syndrome, complete androgen insensitivity syndrome (CAIS), and rare forms of congenital adrenal hyperplasia (CAH), all of which result in female external genitalia.

**Swyer syndrome** Swyer syndrome, also known as XY pure gonadal dysgenesis, is characterized by tall stature, primary amenorrhea, and delayed puberty in a phenotypic female. Laboratory studies reveal elevated gonadotropins, and ultrasonographic examination reveals bilateral streak gonads and a hypoplastic uterus.[72] Fifteen to thirty percent of these individuals have mutations in SRY (sex-determining region of the Y chromosome) or alterations in the Y chromosome.[73] There is also a high risk of gonadal tumors such as dysgerminoma or gonadoblastoma.[73] Therefore, gonadectomy is routinely recommended when this diagnosis is made.

**Complete androgen insensitivity syndrome** CAIS is caused by mutations of the androgen receptor that result in loss of testosterone and dihydrotestosterone mediated action. Androgen receptor mutations are X-linked recessive in 70% of cases, and are found in 1 in 20,000 to 1 in 90,000 genetic males.[74] The most common phenotype is that of an adolescent girl who has normal breast development, but absent or scant body hair and primary amenorrhea. Examination of the external genitalia reveals a normal female phenotype with a blind ending vagina. Eighty percent to 90% of girls with CAIS will also eventually develop inguinal hernias,[75] with some presenting in infancy with this diagnosis.

**Congenital adrenal hyperplasia** Rare forms of CAH can present with hypogonadism due to lack of production of testosterone and estrogen. These conditions include deficiencies of 17α-hydroxylase, side chain cleavage enzyme (SCC), and steroid acute regulatory protein (StAR). Girls with 17α-hydroxylase deficiency can present with primary amenorrhea and absent secondary sexual characteristics. Boys have female external genitalia, a blind vagina, and intra-abdominal testes.[76] Hypertension and hypokalemia may also be present.[77] SCC is the first step in the steroidogenic pathway and converts cholesterol to pregnenolone. SCC deficiency leads to deficiencies in all steroid hormones. SCC deficiency in genetic males leads to XY sex reversal and adrenal insufficiency.[78] StAR, a protein expressed in the adrenal cortex and gonads, increases cholesterol transport in response to steroidogenic stimuli. Affected genetic males present in early infancy with adrenal crisis, and appear phenotypically female.[79] Affected genetic females are normally developed at birth and may have intact ovarian function.[80]

**Galactosemia** Another congenital cause of primary hypogonadism is galactosemia. Galactosemia results from a deficiency in galactose-1-phosphate uridyltransferase (GALT) and presents with clinical manifestations of cataracts, *Escherichia coli* sepsis, poor growth, and feeding dysfunction if undiagnosed in the newborn. In an initial study conducted in 1981, gonadal function was evaluated in 12 women and 8 men with galactosemia. Although gonadal function was normal in men with the disease, the women in this study had evidence of hypergonadotropic hypogonadism, with varying degrees of primary and secondary amenorrhea and oligomenorrhea.[81] Ultrasound studies of the ovaries in those affected demonstrated streak gonads in several women.[81] The cause of the hypogonadism is most likely premature ovarian failure, although the exact pathophysiology is not well understood. Numerous theories exist, including the hypothesis that galactose-1-phosphate is toxic and perhaps competitively inhibits UDP-Galactose transferase and alters FSH and FSH receptors, with subsequent failure of ovarian follicles to develop.[82] This process manifests as an elevated FSH in 85% of girls younger than 10 years who have galactosemia and premature ovarian failure.[82]

**Testicular regression sequence** Testicular regression sequence (TRS), or vanishing testis syndrome, occurs when an initially normal testicle that existed in fetal life subsequently atrophies. Most individuals with TRS have normal male external genitalia, reflecting that normal testicular function existed during prenatal life. The most likely cause of this syndrome is fetal or antenatal testicular torsion, or trauma to scrotal contents in utero.[83] This view is supported by the finding of hemosiderin laden macrophages and dystrophic calcifications under histopatholgic examination.[84] There has also been an association noted between testicular regression and persistence of mullerian duct structures.[85] Thus far, a search for a molecular genetic cause of TRS has been negative.[86]

### *Acquired Origins*

The acquired forms of primary hypogonadism are as varied as the congenital forms. Important acquired origins include treatment for pediatric cancer (radiation and chemotherapy) and autoimmune conditions.

#### *Chemotherapy and radiation*

Both chemotherapy and radiation have been noted to cause primary hypogonadism. In girls, the dose of intra-abdominal radiation needed to destroy more than 50% of developing oocytes is less than 2 Gy.[87] In the 70% of patients who survive pediatric cancer, 1 in 6 female survivors develops primary ovarian failure. Those who do undergo spontaneous menarche have decreased ovarian reserve.[88] In boys, depressed spermatogenesis can be seen after a testicular radiation dose as low as 0.15 Gy, with temporary azoospermia occurring after doses of 0.3 Gy.[89] The effect of radiation on testicular function is age dependent, with prepubertal radiation exposure causing significantly more damage to Leydig cells than postpubertal radiation.[90] Cumulative doses of alkylating agents are also correlated with altered function.[89]

A high prevalence of hypogonadism was noted in young adult survivors of childhood cancer who participated in a study comparing 3 treatment arms for non-Hodgkin lymphoma (NHL) and acute lymphoblastic leukemia (ALL). The study compared treatment with chemotherapy alone (vincristine, prednisolone, l-asparaginase, methotrexate, 6-mercaptopurine), combined chemotherapy and prophylactic cranial radiation, and chemotherapy with total body radiation and bone marrow transplant. All women in the third category had premature ovarian failure. Women in the other 2 categories, however, had intact ovarian function. Among men in the third category, 83% had primary hypogonadism, with a low serum testosterone and elevated FSH and LH. Forty percent of men in all 3 treatment arms had alterations in spermatogenesis, with the greatest dysfunction appearing in those who had received total body radiation.[91]

Despite these findings, there have been reports of spontaneous recovery of testicular or ovarian function in childhood cancer survivors. Although more common in older children and adults, recovery of ovarian function has occurred as long as 12 years post exposure to radiation and alkylating chemotherapy in a young girl.[92] Due to the increased risk of gonadal dysfunction in pediatric cancer patients and also due to the chance of spontaneous recovery, recommendations for surveillance include yearly monitoring of pubertal status with Tanner staging and assessment of growth velocity. Laboratory measurements of FSH and LH as well as estradiol or testosterone are recommended for those with signs of pubertal delay.[93]

***Autoimmune gonadal failure***

Autoimmunity can lead to both testicular and ovarian failure, specifically in those who have other types of autoimmune endocrinopathies. Several autoimmune polyglandular syndromes (APS) have been identified. Of these, APS I and APS II have been associated with premature ovarian failure at prevalence rates of 30% to 50%.[94] APS I consists of a triad of hypoparathyroidism, mucocutaneous candidiasis, and adrenal insufficiency. The mutation is within the *AIRE* gene, the autoimmune regulator. In a Finnish cohort, approximately 50% of the females identified with APS I had premature ovarian failure. Two-thirds of these individuals had autoantibodies to side-chain cleavage enzyme (anti-SCC),[95] one of the enzymes identified in steroid production that is specific to the ovary and is noted in autoimmune ovarian failure. In those who have been diagnosed with APS I and who initially have signs of ovarian failure, the presence of steroid cell antibodies may signal progression of the disease process.[96] APS II consists of autoimmune adrenocortical failure along with thyroid disease or diabetes. Positive antibodies to the P450 enzymes, specifically ovary-specific antibodies, in the steroid production pathway are thought to mediate autoimmune ovarian failure in this syndrome as well.[97] Autoimmunity can also cause isolated premature ovarian failure,[98] and has also been reported in conditions such as systemic lupus erythematous and myasthenia gravis.

Testicular failure occurs at a lower rate than ovarian failure in APS.[99] Autoimmunity to the Leydig cells in APS may be mediated by P450 autoantibodies that are testis specific.[100] Antisperm antibodies have also been noted in prepubertal boys treated with chemotherapy and in those with urogenital tract abnormalities such as cryptorchidism, testicular torsion, or hypospadias.[101]

## EVALUATION

Evaluation of a child with delayed puberty begins with a careful history and physical examination. Important elements on history include the parents' pubertal timing, because late menarche in the mother or delayed completion of adult height in the father is strongly suggestive of CDGP. Eliciting a family history of hypogonadism, autoimmune syndromes, DSDs, or consanguinity is also essential. History in the child should include attention to any CNS insult or symptoms of chronic disease. In the review of systems, lack of sense of smell can be an important clue to the presence of KS.

Physical examination should include height and weight measurements. Neurologic assessment should include evaluation of visual fields. Assessment of secondary sexual characteristics includes Tanner staging and recognition of evidence of androgen exposure. Testicular enlargement, which can sometimes go unnoticed by boys, indicates the onset of central puberty. Stigmata of TS or Klinefelter Syndrome should be noted. The external genitalia should be visually inspected for any signs of anatomic abnormality.

Laboratory evaluation including plasma gonadotropin levels, estradiol, or testosterone may be helpful. Low gonadotropin levels suggest CDGP or pathologic hypogonadotropic hypogonadism, and can be further evaluated with a GnRH stimulation test.[102] In contrast, elevated gonadotropins indicate primary gonadal failure. A bone age radiograph is an essential component of the evaluation. Other tests that may be indicated, depending on the individual situation, include a head MRI, karyotype, autoimmune panel, or molecular genetic analysis. In patients with suspected CDGP, a "wait and see" approach is typically employed to determine whether spontaneous puberty will ensue.

## TREATMENT

Although there are many causes of hypogonadism in children, the treatment is primarily focused on hormone replacement with sex steroids. The overarching goal is to simulate a normal progression of pubertal development that also allows for the attainment of genetic potential for height.

### *Estrogen Replacement*

Estrogen therapy is initially started for pubertal induction and breast development in girls with hypogonadism. Studies regarding estrogen therapy in children have focused primarily on girls with TS. Recommended starting doses of estrogen therapy in this population are one-eighth to one-tenth the doses used for adult replacement, and vary depending on the formulation used. Very low doses have been reported to have a salutary effect on linear growth in TS.[103] Multiple different formulations of estrogen are available, and include oral estradiol, oral conjugated estrogen, transdermal estrogen patches, and estrogen gel. The age at which estrogen therapy is initiated is individualized and incorporates factors such as chronologic age, bone age, absolute height, and psychosocial issues. The starting dose is low and is gradually increased over several years. Equivalent adult doses of oral therapy are micronized estradiol, 2 mg, esterified estrogen, 1.25 mg, ethinyl estradiol, 8 to 10 μg, and conjugated estrogens, 1.25 mg.[104] Addition of progesterone 1 week per month, usually in the form of medroxyprogesterone, after 1 to 2 years of estrogen therapy or post breakthrough bleeding, allows for adequate breast and uterine development. Formulations and available does of estrogen preparations are shown in **Table 3**.

Limitations of oral estrogen therapy include variable bioavailability due to first-pass metabolism within the liver, which subsequently affects liver function and clotting factors.[105,106] As a result, transdermal estrogen formulations are gaining in popularity. Estrogen patches are widely used in adult women, and doses of 0.625 and 1.25 mg of oral conjugated estrogens have been reported to be similar those of 50 and 100 μg of transdermal estradiol per 24 hours.[107] Pubertal induction can be accomplished with transdermal estradiol at a dose as low as 3.1 to 6.2 μg/24 hours.[106] Puberty can then be mimicked with subsequent doubling of the dose after a median duration of 8 months and addition of progesterone 2 years after estrogen initiation. A transdermal estrogen dose of 0.1 mg/d is equivalent to an adult regimen. When comparing transdermal estrogen to oral estrogen, significantly higher levels of 17β-estradiol were noted with oral estrogen. However, no differences in metabolic effects including

**Table 3**
**Estrogen formulations**

| Type of Estrogen | Trade Name | Available Doses |
|---|---|---|
| Oral estradiol | Estrace | 0.5, 1, 2 mg |
| | Gynodiol | 0.5, 1, 2 mg |
| Oral esterified estrogen | Menest | 0.3, 0.625, 1.25, 2.5 mg |
| | Ogen | Equivalent to 0.625 mg and above |
| | Ortho-Est | Equivalent to 0.625 mg and above |
| Oral conjugated equine estrogen | Premarin | 0.3, 0.45, 0.625, 0.9, 1.25 mg |
| Estradiol patches | Vivelle | 0.025, 0.0375, 0.05, 0.075, 0.1 mg/d |
| | Menostar | 0.014 mg/d |
| Estradiol gel | Divigel | 0.5 mg estradiol/5 g gel |

lipolysis, lipid, and carbohydrate oxidation, and resting energy expenditure from short-term transdermal versus oral estrogen therapy have been noted.[105] In contrast, a pilot study of transdermal versus oral conjugated estrogen in girls with TS found better bone mineral accrual and uterine development in the transdermal group.[108]

Percutaneous estradiol gel has also been investigated for pubertal induction in girls with TS at a starting dose of 0.1 mg nightly with increases of 0.1 mg for each additional year up to 5 years. Side effects of percutaneous gel therapy include local skin irritation, and this modality is not currently in use in the clinical setting.[109] For hypogonadal women, estrogen replacement is needed throughout reproductive life.

### *Testosterone Replacement*

In boys, studies involving testosterone for pubertal induction have primarily focused on CDGP and KS. Testosterone therapy is usually initiated at 15% to 25% of adult doses. Approximately 50 to 100 mg of a testosterone ester formulation is given intramuscularly every 2 to 4 weeks for 4 to 6 months with gradual increases to adult doses.[110,111] In boys with CDGP, a 4- to 6-month course of 50 to 100 mg testosterone per month may be offered to bring about initial secondary sexual characteristics and boost linear growth.[110] In boys who have permanent hypogonadism, the need for therapy is lifelong. Even at the initial doses used for pubertal induction, there is a decrease in total fat mass, percent body fat, and whole body proteolysis once testosterone is initiated.[112]

Intramuscular, transdermal, and oral formulations of testosterone exist. The preparations testosterone enanthate and testosterone cypionate are the most often used formulations in children, due to the difficulty in delivering the small doses needed initially for pubertal induction with alternate forms.[113] Intramuscular injections of testosterone, however, can be painful for the adolescent patient population, and studies investigating other formulations are ongoing.

Formal guidelines regarding the use of oral preparations have yet to be delineated, and experience with this form of testosterone is far less than with the intramuscular form. Transdermal testosterone, in the form of testosterone gel, at doses of 50 mg/m$^2$/d has been used in children short-term to treat poor growth secondary to renal failure.[114] In a study of transdermal testosterone delivered via a 5-mg patch, overnight use in boys with delayed puberty resulted in pubertal testosterone concentrations as well

**Table 4**
**Testosterone formulations**

| Formulation | Trade Name | Dose (Adult) |
|---|---|---|
| IM testosterone enanthate | Delatestryl | 250 mg every 2–4 wk |
| IM testosterone cypionate | Depo-Testosterone | 250 mg every 2–4 wk |
| Oral testosterone undecanoate | Andriol (40 mg capsules) | 2 capsules (2–3 times per day) |
| Testosterone patch | Androderm | 5 mg/patch changed twice weekly |
| Testosterone gel | Androgel (25 mg testosterone/2.5 g gel) (50 mg testosterone/5 g gel) | 50–100 mg/d |
| Buccal testosterone | Striant 30 mg tablet | 1 tablet twice a day |
| Testosterone implants | Testopel 75 mg per pellet | 3–4 pellets every 4–6 mo |

short-term growth.[115] Side effects of transdermal testosterone include local skin irritation. As in oral testosterone therapy, there are limited studies regarding the use of transdermal preparations of testosterone, and intramuscular testosterone therapy remains the mainstay of therapy for pediatric patients. Testosterone preparations and adult doses are shown in **Table 4**.

Adjunctive treatment in the form of human chorionic gonadotropin has been suggested in boys with PWS in whom beneficial effects on body composition and endogenous testosterone secretion have been observed.[116]

## SUMMARY

In conclusion, causes of hypogonadism are heterogeneous and may involve any level of the reproductive system. Whereas some conditions are clearly delineated, the exact etiology and underlying pathogenesis of many disorders is unknown. Regardless of the form of hypogonadism, the crux of therapy in children revolves around sex steroid replacement. Continued molecular genetic investigation and prospective clinical trials will enhance knowledge and improve management of hypogonadism in pediatric patients.

## REFERENCES

1. Boyar R, Finkelstein J, Roffwarg H, et al. Synchronization of augmented luteinizing hormone secretion with sleep during puberty. N Engl J Med 1972;287(12): 582–6.
2. Apter D, Butzow TL, Laughlin GA, et al. Gonadotropin-releasing hormone pulse generator activity during pubertal transition in girls: pulsatile and diurnal patterns of circulating gonadotropins. J Clin Endocrinol Metab 1993;76(4):940–9.
3. Sedlmeyer IL, Palmert MR. Delayed puberty: analysis of a large case series from an academic center. J Clin Endocrinol Metab 2002;87(4):1613–20.
4. von Kalckreuth G, Haverkamp F, Kessler M, et al. Constitutional delay of growth and puberty: do they really reach their target height? Horm Res 1991;35(6): 222–5.
5. Bergada I, Bergada C. Long term treatment with low dose testosterone in constitutional delay of growth and puberty: effect on bone age maturation and pubertal progression. J Pediatr Endocrinol Metab 1995;8(2):117–22.
6. Achermann JC, Weiss J, Lee EJ, et al. Inherited disorders of the gonadotropin hormones. Mol Cell Endocrinol 2001;179(1–2):89–96.
7. Kohler B, Lin L, Ferraz-de-Souza B, et al. Five novel mutations in steroidogenic factor 1 (SF1, NR5A1) in 46, XY patients with severe underandrogenization but without adrenal insufficiency. Hum Mutat 2008;29(1):59–64.
8. Biason-Lauber A, Schoenle EJ. Apparently normal ovarian differentiation in a prepubertal girl with transcriptionally inactive steroidogenic factor 1 (NR5A1/SF-1) and adrenocortical insufficiency. Am J Hum Genet 2000;67(6):1563–8.
9. Muscatelli F, Strom TM, Walker AP, et al. Mutations in the DAX-1 gene give rise to both X-linked adrenal hypoplasia congenita and hypogonadotropic hypogonadism. Nature 1994;372(6507):672–6.
10. Yang F, Hanaki K, Kinoshita T, et al. Late-onset adrenal hypoplasia congenita caused by a novel mutation of the DAX-1 gene. Eur J Pediatr 2009;168: 329–31.
11. Habiby RL, Boepple P, Nachtigall L, et al. Adrenal hypoplasia congenita with hypogonadotropic hypogonadism: evidence that DAX-1 mutations lead to

combined hypothalamic and pituitary defects in gonadotropin production. J Clin Invest 1996;98(4):1055–62.
12. Mantovani G, De Menis E, Borretta G, et al. DAX1 and X-linked adrenal hypoplasia congenita: clinical and molecular analysis in five patients. Eur J Endocrinol 2006;154(5):685–9.
13. Franco B, Guioli S, Pragliola A, et al. A gene deleted in Kallmann's syndrome shares homology with neural cell adhesion and axonal path-finding molecules. Nature 1991;353(6344):529–36.
14. Vogl TJ, Stemmler J, Heye B, et al. Kallman syndrome versus idiopathic hypogonadotropic hypogonadism at MR imaging. Radiology 1994;191(1):53–7.
15. Oliveira LM, Seminara SB, Beranova M, et al. The importance of autosomal genes in Kallmann syndrome: genotype-phenotype correlations and neuroendocrine characteristics. J Clin Endocrinol Metab 2001;86(4):1532–8.
16. Sato N, Katsumata N, Kagami M, et al. Clinical assessment and mutation analysis of Kallmann syndrome 1 (KAL1) and fibroblast growth factor receptor 1 (FGFR1, or KAL2) in five families and 18 sporadic patients. J Clin Endocrinol Metab 2004;89(3):1079–88.
17. Pitteloud N, Zhang C, Pignatelli D, et al. Loss-of-function mutation in the prokineticin 2 gene causes Kallmann syndrome and normosmic idiopathic hypogonadotropic hypogonadism. Proc Natl Acad Sci U S A 2007;104(44):17447–52.
18. de Roux N, Young J, Misrahi M, et al. A family with hypogonadotropic hypogonadism and mutations in the gonadotropin-releasing hormone receptor. N Engl J Med 1997;337(22):1597–602.
19. de Roux N, Milgrom E. Inherited disorders of GnRH and gonadotropin receptors. Mol Cell Endocrinol 2001;179(1–2):83–7.
20. de Roux N, Genin E, Carel JC, et al. Hypogonadotropic hypogonadism due to loss of function of the KiSS1-derived peptide receptor GPR54. Proc Natl Acad Sci U S A 2003;100(19):10972–6.
21. Raivio T, Falardeau J, Dwyer A, et al. Reversal of idiopathic hypogonadotropic hypogonadism. N Engl J Med 2007;357(9):863–73.
22. Pfaffle RW, Blankenstein O, Wuller S, et al. Combined pituitary hormone deficiency: role of Pit-1 and Prop-1. Acta Paediatr Suppl 1999;88(433):33–41.
23. Lazar L, Gat-Yablonski G, Kornreich L, et al. PROP-1 gene mutation (R120C) causing combined pituitary hormone deficiencies with variable clinical course in eight siblings of one Jewish Moroccan family. Horm Res 2003; 60(5):227–31.
24. Dasen JS, Barbera JP, Herman TS, et al. Temporal regulation of a paired-like homeodomain repressor/TLE corepressor complex and a related activator is required for pituitary organogenesis. Genes Dev 2001;15(23):3193–207.
25. Dattani MT, Martinez-Barbera JP, Thomas PQ, et al. Mutations in the homeobox gene HESX1/Hesx1 associated with septo-optic dysplasia in human and mouse. Nat Genet 1998;19(2):125–33.
26. Haddad NG, Eugster EA. Hypopituitarism and neurodevelopmental abnormalities in relation to central nervous system structural defects in children with optic nerve hypoplasia. J Pediatr Endocrinol Metab 2005;18(9):853–8.
27. Pfaeffle RW, Hunter CS, Savage JJ, et al. Three novel missense mutations within the LHX4 gene are associated with variable pituitary hormone deficiencies. J Clin Endocrinol Metab 2008;93(3):1062–71.
28. Kelberman D, Rizzoti K, Avilion A, et al. Mutations within Sox2/SOX2 are associated with abnormalities in the hypothalamo-pituitary-gonadal axis in mice and humans. J Clin Invest 2006;116(9):2442–55.

29. Farooqi IS, Matarese G, Lord GM, et al. Beneficial effects of leptin on obesity, T cell hyporesponsiveness, and neuroendocrine/metabolic dysfunction of human congenital leptin deficiency. J Clin Invest 2002;110(8):1093–103.
30. Farooqi IS, Wangensteen T, Collins S, et al. Clinical and molecular genetic spectrum of congenital deficiency of the leptin receptor. N Engl J Med 2007;356(3):237–47.
31. Wharton RH, Loechner KJ. Genetic and clinical advances in Prader-Willi syndrome. Curr Opin Pediatr 1996;8(6):618–24.
32. Jeffcoate WJ, Laurance BM, Edwards CR, et al. Endocrine function in the Prader-Willi syndrome. Clin Endocrinol (Oxf) 1980;12(1):81–9.
33. Crino A, Schiaffini R, Ciampalini P, et al. Hypogonadism and pubertal development in Prader-Willi syndrome. Eur J Pediatr 2003;162(5):327–33.
34. Schulze A, Mogensen H, Hamborg-Petersen B, et al. Fertility in Prader-Willi syndrome: a case report with Angelman syndrome in the offspring. Acta Paediatr 2001;90(4):455–9.
35. Akefeldt A, Tornhage CJ, Gillberg C. A woman with Prader-Willi syndrome gives birth to a healthy baby girl. Dev Med Child Neurol 1999;41(11):789–90.
36. Morton MV, Wehman P. Psychosocial and emotional sequelae of individuals with traumatic brain injury: a literature review and recommendations. Brain Inj 1995;9(1):81–92.
37. Kelly DF, Gonzalo IT, Cohan P, et al. Hypopituitarism following traumatic brain injury and aneurysmal subarachnoid hemorrhage: a preliminary report. J Neurosurg 2000;93(5):743–52.
38. Lieberman SA, Oberoi AL, Gilkison CR, et al. Prevalence of neuroendocrine dysfunction in patients recovering from traumatic brain injury. J Clin Endocrinol Metab 2001;86(6):2752–6.
39. Benvenga S, Campenni A, Ruggeri RM, et al. Clinical review 113: hypopituitarism secondary to head trauma. J Clin Endocrinol Metab 2000;85(4):1353–61.
40. Tanriverdi F, Senyurek H, Unluhizarci K, et al. High risk of hypopituitarism after traumatic brain injury: a prospective investigation of anterior pituitary function in the acute phase and 12 months after trauma. J Clin Endocrinol Metab 2006;91(6):2105–11.
41. Merchant TE, Williams T, Smith JM, et al. Preirradiation endocrinopathies in pediatric brain tumor patients determined by dynamic tests of endocrine function. Int J Radiat Oncol Biol Phys 2002;54(1):45–50.
42. Gonc EN, Yordam N, Ozon A, et al. Endocrinological outcome of different treatment options in children with craniopharyngioma: a retrospective analysis of 66 cases. Pediatr Neurosurg 2004;40(3):112–9.
43. Mills JL, Fears TR, Robison LL, et al. Menarche in a cohort of 188 long-term survivors of acute lymphoblastic leukemia. J Pediatr 1997;131(4):598–602.
44. Constine LS, Woolf PD, Cann D, et al. Hypothalamic-pituitary dysfunction after radiation for brain tumors. N Engl J Med 1993;328(2):87–94.
45. Rappaport R, Brauner R, Czernichow P, et al. Effect of hypothalamic and pituitary irradiation on pubertal development in children with cranial tumors. J Clin Endocrinol Metab 1982;54(6):1164–8.
46. Nandagopal R, Laverdiere C, Mulrooney D, et al. Endocrine late effects of childhood cancer therapy: a report from the Children's Oncology Group. Horm Res 2008;69(2):65–74.
47. Chan JL, Mantzoros CS. Role of leptin in energy-deprivation states: normal human physiology and clinical implications for hypothalamic amenorrhoea and anorexia nervosa. Lancet 2005;366(9479):74–85.

48. Welt CK, Chan JL, Bullen J, et al. Recombinant human leptin in women with hypothalamic amenorrhea. N Engl J Med 2004;351(10):987–97.
49. Nielsen J, Wohlert M. Chromosome abnormalities found among 34,910 newborn children: results from a 13-year incidence study in Arhus, Denmark. Hum Genet 1991;87(1):81–3.
50. Bondy CA. Care of girls and women with Turner syndrome: a guideline of the Turner Syndrome Study Group. J Clin Endocrinol Metab 2007;92(1):10–25.
51. Pasquino AM, Passeri F, Pucarelli I, et al. Spontaneous pubertal development in Turner's syndrome. Italian Study Group for Turner's Syndrome. J Clin Endocrinol Metab 1997;82(6):1810–3.
52. Hovatta O. Pregnancies in women with Turner's syndrome. Ann Med 1999;31(2): 106–10.
53. Fechner PY, Davenport ML, Qualy RL, et al. Differences in follicle-stimulating hormone secretion between 45, X monosomy Turner syndrome and 45, X/46, XX mosaicism are evident at an early age. J Clin Endocrinol Metab 2006; 91(12):4896–902.
54. Bojesen A, Juul S, Gravholt CH. Prenatal and postnatal prevalence of Klinefelter syndrome: a national registry study. J Clin Endocrinol Metab 2003; 88(2):622–6.
55. Abulhasan SJ, Tayel SM, al-Awadi SA. Mosaic Turner syndrome: cytogenetics versus FISH. Ann Hum Genet 1999;63(Pt 3):199–206.
56. Rizzolio F, Bione S, Sala C, et al. Chromosomal rearrangements in Xq and premature ovarian failure: mapping of 25 new cases and review of the literature. Hum Reprod 2006;21(6):1477–83.
57. Linden MG, Bender BG, Harmon RJ, et al. 47, XXX: what is the prognosis? Pediatrics 1988;82(4):619–30.
58. Lin HJ, Ndiforchu F, Patell S. Exstrophy of the cloaca in a 47, XXX child: review of genitourinary malformations in triple-X patients. Am J Med Genet 1993;45(6): 761–3.
59. Holland CM. 47, XXX in an adolescent with premature ovarian failure and autoimmune disease. J Pediatr Adolesc Gynecol 2001;14(2):77–80.
60. Matthews CH, Borgato S, Beck-Peccoz P, et al. Primary amenorrhoea and infertility due to a mutation in the beta-subunit of follicle-stimulating hormone. Nat Genet 1993;5(1):83–6.
61. Layman LC, Lee EJ, Peak DB, et al. Delayed puberty and hypogonadism caused by mutations in the follicle-stimulating hormone beta-subunit gene. N Engl J Med 1997;337(9):607–11.
62. Lindstedt G, Nystrom E, Matthews C, et al. Follitropin (FSH) deficiency in an infertile male due to FSHbeta gene mutation. A syndrome of normal puberty and virilization but underdeveloped testicles with azoospermia, low FSH but high lutropin and normal serum testosterone concentrations. Clin Chem Lab Med 1998;36(8):663–5.
63. Weiss J, Axelrod L, Whitcomb RW, et al. Hypogonadism caused by a single amino acid substitution in the beta subunit of luteinizing hormone. N Engl J Med 1992;326(3):179–83.
64. Furui K, Suganuma N, Tsukahara S, et al. Identification of two point mutations in the gene coding luteinizing hormone (LH) beta-subunit, associated with immunologically anomalous LH variants. J Clin Endocrinol Metab 1994;78(1):107–13.
65. Kremer H, Kraaij R, Toledo SP, et al. Male pseudohermaphroditism due to a homozygous missense mutation of the luteinizing hormone receptor gene. Nat Genet 1995;9(2):160–4.

66. Latronico AC, Anasti J, Arnhold IJ, et al. Brief report: testicular and ovarian resistance to luteinizing hormone caused by inactivating mutations of the luteinizing hormone-receptor gene. N Engl J Med 1996;334(8):507–12.
67. Arnhold IJ, Latronico AC, Batista MC, et al. Clinical features of women with resistance to luteinizing hormone. Clin Endocrinol (Oxf) 1999;51(6):701–7.
68. Aittomaki K. The genetics of XX gonadal dysgenesis. Am J Hum Genet 1994; 54(5):844–51.
69. de Zegher F, Jaeken J. Endocrinology of the carbohydrate-deficient glycoprotein syndrome type 1 from birth through adolescence. Pediatr Res 1995; 37(4 Pt 1):395–401.
70. Gelfand IM, Eugster EA, DiMeglio LA. Presentation and clinical progression of pseudohypoparathyroidism with multi-hormone resistance and Albright hereditary osteodystrophy: a case series. J Pediatr 2006;149(6):877–80.
71. Lee PA, Houk CP, Ahmed SF, et al. Consensus statement on management of intersex disorders. International Consensus Conference on Intersex. Pediatrics 2006;118(2):e488–500.
72. Michala L, Goswami D, Creighton SM, et al. Swyer syndrome: presentation and outcomes. BJOG May 2008;115(6):737–41.
73. Zielinska D, Zajaczek S, Rzepka-Gorska I. Tumors of dysgenetic gonads in Swyer syndrome. J Pediatr Surg 2007;42(10):1721–4.
74. Oakes MB, Eyvazzadeh AD, Quint E, et al. Complete androgen insensitivity syndrome—a review. J Pediatr Adolesc Gynecol 2008;21(6):305–10.
75. Sarpel U, Palmer SK, Dolgin SE. The incidence of complete androgen insensitivity in girls with inguinal hernias and assessment of screening by vaginal length measurement. J Pediatr Surg 2005;40(1):133–6 [discussion: 136–7].
76. Costa-Santos M, Kater CE, Auchus RJ. Two prevalent CYP17 mutations and genotype-phenotype correlations in 24 Brazilian patients with 17-hydroxylase deficiency. J Clin Endocrinol Metab 2004;89(1):49–60.
77. Yang J, Cui B, Sun S, et al. Phenotype-genotype correlation in eight Chinese 17alpha-hydroxylase/17,20 lyase-deficiency patients with five novel mutations of CYP17A1 gene. J Clin Endocrinol Metab 2006;91(9):3619–25.
78. al Kandari H, Katsumata N, Alexander S, et al. Homozygous mutation of P450 side-chain cleavage enzyme gene (CYP11A1) in 46, XY patient with adrenal insufficiency, complete sex reversal, and agenesis of corpus callosum. J Clin Endocrinol Metab 2006;91(8):2821–6.
79. Baker BY, Lin L, Kim CJ, et al. Nonclassic congenital lipoid adrenal hyperplasia: a new disorder of the steroidogenic acute regulatory protein with very late presentation and normal male genitalia. J Clin Endocrinol Metab 2006;91(12): 4781–5.
80. Fujieda K, Tajima T, Nakae J, et al. Spontaneous puberty in 46, XX subjects with congenital lipoid adrenal hyperplasia. Ovarian steroidogenesis is spared to some extent despite inactivating mutations in the steroidogenic acute regulatory protein (StAR) gene. J Clin Invest 1997;99(6):1265–71.
81. Kaufman FR, Kogut MD, Donnell GN, et al. Hypergonadotropic hypogonadism in female patients with galactosemia. N Engl J Med 1981;304(17):994–8.
82. Prestoz LL, Couto AS, Shin YS, et al. Altered follicle stimulating hormone isoforms in female galactosaemia patients. Eur J Pediatr 1997;156(2):116–20.
83. Smith NM, Byard RW, Bourne AJ. Testicular regression syndrome—a pathological study of 77 cases. Histopathology 1991;19(3):269–72.

84. Law H, Mushtaq I, Wingrove K, et al. Histopathological features of testicular regression syndrome: relation to patient age and implications for management. Fetal Pediatr Pathol 2006;25(2):119–29.
85. Imbeaud S, Rey R, Berta P, et al. Testicular degeneration in three patients with the persistent mullerian duct syndrome. Eur J Pediatr 1995;154(3):187–90.
86. Vinci G, Anjot MN, Trivin C, et al. An analysis of the genetic factors involved in testicular descent in a cohort of 14 male patients with anorchia. J Clin Endocrinol Metab 2004;89(12):6282–5.
87. Wallace WH, Thomson AB, Kelsey TW. The radiosensitivity of the human oocyte. Hum Reprod 2003;18(1):117–21.
88. Larsen EC, Muller J, Schmiegelow K, et al. Reduced ovarian function in long-term survivors of radiation- and chemotherapy-treated childhood cancer. J Clin Endocrinol Metab 2003;88(11):5307–14.
89. Lopez Andreu JA, Fernandez PJ, Ferris i Tortajada J, et al. Persistent altered spermatogenesis in long-term childhood cancer survivors. Pediatr Hematol Oncol 2000;17(1):21–30.
90. Shalet SM, Tsatsoulis A, Whitehead E, et al. Vulnerability of the human Leydig cell to radiation damage is dependent upon age. J Endocrinol 1989;120(1): 161–5.
91. Steffens M, Beauloye V, Brichard B, et al. Endocrine and metabolic disorders in young adult survivors of childhood acute lymphoblastic leukaemia (ALL) or non-Hodgkin lymphoma (NHL). Clin Endocrinol (Oxf) 2008;69(5):819–27.
92. Rahhal SN, Eugster EA. Unexpected recovery of ovarian function many years after bone marrow transplantation. J Pediatr 2008;152(2):289–90.
93. Meacham LR, Ghim TT, Crocker IR, et al. Systematic approach for detection of endocrine disorders in children treated for brain tumors. Med Pediatr Oncol 1997;29(2):86–91.
94. Schatz DA, Winter WE. Autoimmune polyglandular syndrome. II: clinical syndrome and treatment. Endocrinol Metab Clin North Am 2002;31(2): 339–52.
95. Wolff AS, Erichsen MM, Meager A, et al. Autoimmune polyendocrine syndrome type 1 in Norway: phenotypic variation, autoantibodies, and novel mutations in the autoimmune regulator gene. J Clin Endocrinol Metab 2007;92(2):595–603.
96. Ahonen P, Miettinen A, Perheentupa J. Adrenal and steroidal cell antibodies in patients with autoimmune polyglandular disease type I and risk of adrenocortical and ovarian failure. J Clin Endocrinol Metab 1987;64(3):494–500.
97. Uibo R, Aavik E, Peterson P, et al. Autoantibodies to cytochrome P450 enzymes P450scc, P450c17, and P450c21 in autoimmune polyglandular disease types I and II and in isolated Addison's disease. J Clin Endocrinol Metab 1994;78(2): 323–8.
98. Hoek A, Schoemaker J, Drexhage HA. Premature ovarian failure and ovarian autoimmunity. Endocr Rev 1997;18(1):107–34.
99. Buzi F, Badolato R, Mazza C, et al. Autoimmune polyendocrinopathy-candidiasis-ectodermal dystrophy syndrome: time to review diagnostic criteria? J Clin Endocrinol Metab 2003;88(7):3146–8.
100. Perniola R, Falorni A, Clemente MG, et al. Organ-specific and non-organ-specific autoantibodies in children and young adults with autoimmune polyendocrinopathy-candidiasis-ectodermal dystrophy (APECED). Eur J Endocrinol 2000;143(4):497–503.

101. Sinisi AA, D'Apuzzo A, Pasquali D, et al. Antisperm antibodies in prepubertal boys treated with chemotherapy for malignant or non-malignant diseases and in boys with genital tract abnormalities. Int J Androl 1997;20(1):23–8.
102. Goodpasture JC, Ghai K, Cara JF, et al. Potential of gonadotropin-releasing hormone agonists in the diagnosis of pubertal disorders in girls. Clin Obstet Gynecol 1993;36(3):773–85.
103. Rosenfield RL, Perovic N, Devine N, et al. Optimizing estrogen replacement treatment in Turner syndrome. Pediatrics 1998;102(2 Pt 3):486–8.
104. Donaldson MD, Gault EJ, Tan KW, et al. Optimising management in Turner syndrome: from infancy to adult transfer. Arch Dis Child 2006;91(6):513–20.
105. Mauras N, Shulman D, Hsiang HY, et al. Metabolic effects of oral versus transdermal estrogen in growth hormone-treated girls with turner syndrome. J Clin Endocrinol Metab 2007;92(11):4154–60.
106. Ankarberg-Lindgren C, Elfving M, Wikland KA, et al. Nocturnal application of transdermal estradiol patches produces levels of estradiol that mimic those seen at the onset of spontaneous puberty in girls. J Clin Endocrinol Metab 2001;86(7):3039–44.
107. Chetkowski RJ, Meldrum DR, Steingold KA, et al. Biologic effects of transdermal estradiol. N Engl J Med 1986;314(25):1615–20.
108. Nabhan ZM, DiMeglio LA, Qi R, et al. Oral versus transdermal estrogen replacement in girls with Turner syndrome: a pilot comparative study. J Clin Endocrinol Metab 2009;94(6):2009–14.
109. Piippo S, Lenko H, Kainulainen P, et al. Use of percutaneous estrogen gel for induction of puberty in girls with Turner syndrome. J Clin Endocrinol Metab 2004;89(7):3241–7.
110. Richman RA, Kirsch LR. Testosterone treatment in adolescent boys with constitutional delay in growth and development. N Engl J Med 1988;319(24):1563–7.
111. Soliman AT, Khadir MM, Asfour M. Testosterone treatment in adolescent boys with constitutional delay of growth and development. Metabolism 1995;44(8):1013–5.
112. Arslanian S, Suprasongsin C. Testosterone treatment in adolescents with delayed puberty: changes in body composition, protein, fat, and glucose metabolism. J Clin Endocrinol Metab 1997;82(10):3213–20.
113. Rogol AD. Pubertal androgen therapy in boys. Pediatr Endocrinol Rev 2005;2(3):383–90.
114. Kassmann K, Rappaport R, Broyer M. The short-term effect of testosterone on growth in boys on hemodialysis. Clin Nephrol 1992;37(3):148–54.
115. Mayo A, Macintyre H, Wallace AM, et al. Transdermal testosterone application: pharmacokinetics and effects on pubertal status, short-term growth, and bone turnover. J Clin Endocrinol Metab 2004;89(2):681–7.
116. Eiholzer U, Grieser J, Schlumpf M, et al. Clinical effects of treatment for hypogonadism in male adolescents with Prader-Labhart-Willi syndrome. Horm Res 2007;68(4):178–84.

# Sonography of the Pelvis in Patients with Primary Amenorrhea

Henrietta Kotlus Rosenberg, MD, FACR, FAAP

**KEYWORDS**

- Sonography • Duplex/color Doppler sonography
- Primary amenorrhea • Pelvic sonography

Duplex/color Doppler sonography (US) is the modality of choice for evaluation of the patient who presents with primary amenorrhea.[1–9] Without the use of ionizing radiation, intravenous contrast material, or sedation/anesthesia, an enormous amount of information can be obtained that helps to narrow the differential diagnosis. Familiarity with the normal sonographic appearance of the uterus and ovaries during different phases of growth and development is essential for correlation of the anatomic findings with the clinical history, physical examination, and laboratory information. This article discusses the wide gamut of etiologies of primary amenorrhea, the US appearance of pathologic processes that result in primary amenorrhea, and helps the reader understand when additional higher tech imaging is indicated.

## DEFINITIONS

Amenorrhea is defined as absence of menstruation.[10–12] It is a symptom, not a disease entity, that may be caused by a variety of physiologic and pathologic processes. Primary amenorrhea is defined as a lack of menses by 16 years and secondary amenorrhea is defined by cessation of menstruation any time after menarche and before menopause.

## IMPORTANCE OF MEDICAL HISTORY, FAMILY HISTORY, AND LABORATORY EVALUATION

Medical history plays an important role in the assessment of patients with primary amenorrhea. In the perinatal period, maternal hormone ingestion and maternal androgen-producing tumor may be significant. In addition, a neonatal history of

Department of Radiology, The Mount Sinai Medical Center, The Mount Sinai School of Medicine, One Gustave L. Levy Place, New York, NY 10029, USA
*E-mail address:* Henrietta.Rosenberg@mountsinai.org

Endocrinol Metab Clin N Am 38 (2009) 739–760
doi:10.1016/j.ecl.2009.09.002
endo.theclinics.com

hypoglycemia may have been associated with hypopituitarism. Beyond the neonatal period, childhood growth data must be carefully assessed as well as any history of prior surgery, irradiation, chemotherapy, eating disorders, and psychological difficulties. The age at which the patient's mother achieved menarche should be considered, as well as any endocrine-related abnormalities in the patient including those secondary to congenital adrenocortical hyperplasia, ovarian tumors, and thyroiditis. Laboratory evaluation of gonadotrophic releasing hormone (GnRH), luteinizing hormone (LH), and follicle-stimulating hormone (FSH) are essential as well.[12]

## ETIOLOGIES OF PRIMARY AMENORRHEA

All the components necessary for menstruation can be found in the normal female at the time of birth. There are, however, many congenital and acquired conditions that can interfere with that process ranging from disorders affecting the hypothalamus, pituitary gland, adrenal glands, and ovaries, as well as uterine and vaginal structural abnormalities.[10–14] Conditions affecting the hypothalamus include systemic illness, chronic disease (cystic fibrosis, sickle cell disease, Crohn's disease), stress (child abuse), competitive athletics, eating disorders, obesity, medications (chemotherapy, steroids), and pelvic irradiation. Pituitary etiologies include idiopathic hypopituitarism, trauma (child abuse), tumor, infection (brain abscess, tuberculosis), cranial irradiation, and hemochromatosis. Thyroid conditions including both hypothyroidism and hyperthyroidism may cause primary amenorrhea. Adrenal abnormalities that may cause primary amenorrhea include congenital adrenal hyperplasia, Cushing syndrome, and adrenal tumor. Ovarian etiologies include gonadal dysgenesis, ovarian failure, polycystic ovary syndrome, and ovarian tumor. Structural anomalies that do not allow for the menstrual cycle to develop include uterine agenesis or obstruction, vaginal agenesis or obstruction, or ovarian agenesis. In the presence of imperforate hymen, the menstrual cycle is generally well established but the menstrual products cannot be expelled. In addition, it is always important to consider that a patient with primary amenorrhea may be pregnant.

## PUBERTY

Puberty is a 4-year process that begins with the activation of the hypothalamic-pituitary-ovarian-uterine axis. During this time, the gonads mature, there is increased production of sex hormones, secondary sexual characteristics develop, there is a growth spurt, and the development of reproductive capability ensues. During the course of normal pubertal development, healthy girls pass through four stages, first of which is thelarche (breast development) at approximately 8 to 13 years. Pubic hair develops any time from 8 to 14 years, the growth spurt occurs between 9.5 and 14.5 years, axillary hair becomes apparent from 10 to 16 years, and menarche begins any time between 10 and 16 years. In general, menarche usually occurs 2 to 5 years after breast bud development. If a girl does not have clinical evidence of puberty by 13 years, an evaluation should be done. However, the evaluation may be delayed for 1 year if there is a known debilitating illness or the patient is involved in competitive or endurance sports (eg, ballet, track).

## PHYSICAL EXAMINATION

Patients with primary amenorrhea should have a comprehensive physical examination that includes evaluation for visual field disturbance and neurologic abnormalities that may reflect pituitary or other central nervous system disease.[11] Breast development should be assessed as well as the presence, absence, and quality of axillary and pubic hair. A bulging introital mass should be looked for which could be indicative of hydrometrocolpos. The vaginal mucosa should be examined, as estrogen deficiency may cause the vaginal mucosa to become red and thin, as compared with normal estrogenization, which results in a pink, moist vagina. The patient should also be examined for any signs of pregnancy and a pregnancy test should be performed as part of the evaluation.

## DUPLEX/COLOR DOPPLER SONOGRAPHIC EVALUATION

Duplex/color Doppler high-resolution, real-time sonography has emerged as the modality of choice for the evaluation of the pelvis in infants, children, adolescents, and adults.[3,4,6] Patients should be well hydrated before pelvic sonography so that the bladder is optimally filled. The distended bladder (either from natural distention following drinking an adequate amount of clear liquids or following installation of sterile water via a catheter) lifts the small bowel superiorly and out of pelvis, which allows the bladder to serve as an excellent acoustic window to the gynecologic structures that are posterior/posterolateral to it. In addition, the lower urinary tract, pelvic musculature, and blood vessels can be demonstrated and assessed as well. The use of sterile water as a contrast agent to outline the vagina (hydrosonovaginography [water vaginography]), rectum (water enema),[15] or urogenital sinus may be very helpful in the evaluation of the patient with a pelvic mass or complex congenital anomalies of the genitourinary (GU) tract. Sonography can be performed during real-time imaging of these structures as they are being filled in a retrograde manner. When transabdominal sonography provides suboptimal images in mature, sexually active teenage or young adults, endovaginal US can be performed, which provides higher resolution with more detailed sonograms.[16] With this technique, which is particularly helpful in obese females and in those patients who cannot maintain adequate bladder distention, more refined detail can be obtained of the structures within the field of view than with borderline or unclear transabdominal US of the pelvis. This technique often aids in the demonstration of the gynecologic structures and in determining the origin and characteristics of pelvic masses and complex adnexal lesions. Couplant gel is placed into a probe cover (usually a condom), which is then placed over the probe. Transducer gel is also used on the outside of the probe cover before insertion of the probe into the vagina. As endovaginal sonography is performed following complete bladder emptying, it is quite well tolerated and generally well accepted by sexually active patients. In the virginal patient, transperineal (translabial) sonography may be done by placing the covered probe (endovaginal, curvilinear, or linear) at the introitus. In addition, 3-dimensional (3-D) US has proven to be helpful in the assessment of uterine and vaginal anomalies.[17,18]

Given that the urinary bladder is used as a sonic window, it is important to be familiar with the normal sonographic appearance of this pelvic structure.[19] The wall of the urinary bladder should be smooth in a distended state, with its wall thickness not greater than 3 mm during bladder distention and not greater than 5 mm when the bladder is empty or partially distended. In the nondistended state, the internal aspect of the bladder wall generally appears slightly irregular sonographically. The distal ureters, with the exception of the submucosal intravesical portion, are not ordinarily visualized unless they are abnormally dilated. The trigone, however, is easily demonstrated. The bladder neck and urethra can be demonstrated and when a urethral abnormality is noted on suprapubic imaging, scans through the perineum or transrectally can confirm these findings via a different imaging plane. Hydrosonourethrography may be used to detect urethral abnormalities (strictures, calculi, foreign bodies, bladder neck dyssynergia, diverticuli, and trauma) and to differentiate urethra from other tubular structures such as the vagina. The urethra can be further assessed during real-time observation during voiding or during a retrograde hand injection of saline into the urethra.

CT and MRI provide a more global view of the pelvis and are particularly useful when it is important to assess the musculoskeletal structures, mesentery, and bowel and for confirmation of fat and/or calcium.[20] Although these higher tech imaging modalities can be used for elucidation of unclear sonographic findings, there are disadvantages to both of them. Radiation exposure as well as the need for intravenous and gastrointestinal contrast are disadvantages of CT. In addition, CT is limited in patients with a paucity of adipose tissue. The cost of both CT and MRI outweigh those of US and some patients having MRI will require sedation to avoid intolerable claustrophobia.

## NORMAL ANATOMY

### *The Uterus*

Identification of the uterus and sonographic assessment of its size, configuration, and endometrial stripe provides essential information in the imaging workup of the patient with primary amenorrhea (**Fig. 1**). The uterus and ovaries undergo a series of changes

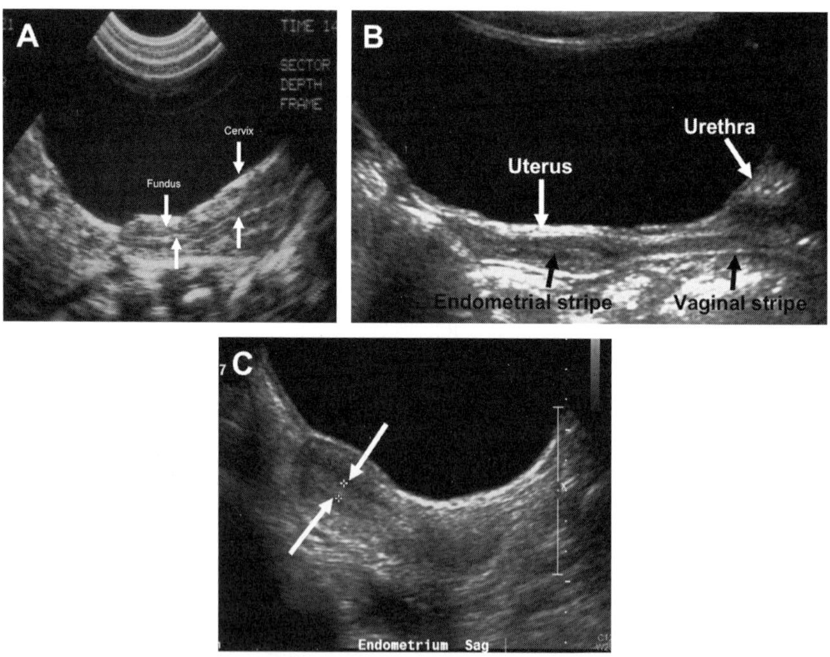


**Fig. 1.** (*A*) Normal newborn uterus. Sagittal sonogram obtained using the bladder as a sonic window demonstrates the spade-shape configuration of the prominent newborn uterus. The fundus to cervix ratio is 1:2 when assessing either the depth or the length of the uterus. Note the prominent echogenic endometrial lining (*arrows*) owing to maternal utero hormonal stimulation. (*B*) Normal prepubertal uterus in a 2-year-old female. Sagittal sonogram shows the tubular configuration of the uterus, which demonstrates a fundus-to-cervix ratio of 1:1. The endometrial stripe is pencil-line thin owing to a lack of hormonal stimulation. (*C*) Normal postpubertal uterus in a 15-year-old female. Sagittal sonogram demonstrates the normal mature configuration of the uterus with a fundus-to-cervix ratio of 3:1. The endometrial stripe (*arrows*) thickness indicates early secretory phase of the menstrual cycle.

in size and configuration during normal growth and development and thus, it is important to be aware of the US characteristics of these structures during various phases of life.[2–4]

The size and shape of the gynecologic structures are strongly influenced during the first few months of life, owing to high circulating gonadotropin levels that develop as the maternal estrogen and progesterone declines after separation of the neonate from the placenta. In the newborn female, the uterus is prominent and thickened with a brightly echogenic endometrial lining caused by the in utero maternal hormonal stimulation. The newborn uterine configuration is spade shaped with the length measuring approximately 3.5 cm. The fundus:cervix ratio based on anterior/posterior (AP) dimensions is 1:2. The neonatal cervix is also longer than the corresponding fundus. It is not uncommon for a hypoechoic halo to be demonstrated around the endometrial stripe or intracavity fluid, both of which findings are far more typical of an adolescent or adult uterus under the cyclical hormonal influences of postmenarchal life.

At 2 to 3 months of age, the uterus regresses to a prepubertal size and develops a somewhat tubular configuration. The uterine length of the prepubertal uterus is 2.5 to 3.0 cm, with the fundus:cervix ratio 1:1. The endometrial stripe when it is seen appears as thin as a pencil line. The uterine length increases gradually between 3 and 8 years of age, measuring up to 4.3 cm at the end of this phase of development. The tubular uterine configuration during this time is maintained until puberty, at which time the uterine length gradually increases to 5 to 7 cm. The uterus then assumes a pear-shaped configuration at puberty with the fundus:cervix AP ratio 3:1. The echogenicity and thickness of the endometrial lining then varies according to the phase of the menstrual cycle. After puberty, the uterus descends deeper into the pelvis and may not maintain the typical prepubertal position, and may appear anteverted or retroverted. The uterus is supplied by bilateral uterine arteries, which are branches of the internal iliac arteries. Color Doppler imaging generally demonstrates flow in the myometrium, with little or no flow in the endometrium.

### The Vagina

Digital and visual examination of the vagina may be difficult in young patients and in those with congenital anomalies resulting in no obvious vaginal introitus. State-of-the-art real-time US most often obviates the need for pelvic examination under sedation or general anesthesia. In the patient with an interlabial mass, sonography can generally determine the cause, although at times MRI may be necessary. The vagina is best visualized on midline longitudinal scans obtained by using the distended bladder as a sonic window. The vagina appears as a long, tubular structure in continuity with the uterine cervix. The apposed mucosal surfaces cause a long, bright, slender central linear echo. Transverse suprapubic images may also be obtained along the course of the vagina. In addition, transperineal (translabial) and hydrosonovaginography can be used as needed for further clarification (**Fig. 2**).

### The Ovary

Sonographic visualization of the ovaries, particularly in children, can be variable, depending on their location, size, and the age of the patient, but when not obscured by bowel gas can generally be easily visualized. The normal ovary has an ovoid configuration and is located within the mesovarium of the broad ligament (**Fig. 3**).[21] Each ovary is generally located posterior or lateral to the uterus, medial and anterior to its ipsilateral iliac vessels, and adjacent to its ipsilateral obturator internus muscle. Contained follicles and lack of peristaltic motion help differentiate an ovary from collapsed bowel. Ovaries may be found anywhere along their embryologic course from the

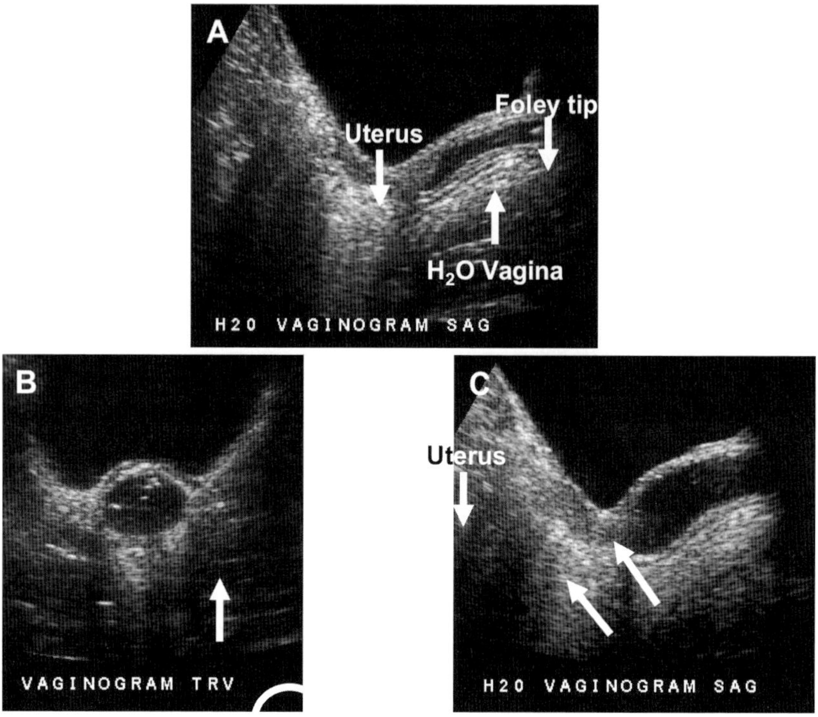


**Fig. 2.** Normal hydrosonovaginography in a prepubertal female. (*A*) Sagittal sonogram demonstrates the tip of the Foley catheter in a partially fluid-distended vagina. A normal prepubertal uterus is seen. (*B*) Transverse sonogram of the bladder following increased fluid distention. The contained artifacts are a result of air bubbles inadvertently introduced at the time the instillation of sterile water. (*C*) Sagittal sonogram with the bladder completely fluid distended.

inferior border of the kidney to the broad ligament. As the true absence of an ovary is rare, the absence of an ovary and its ipsilateral fallopian tube, as may be noted at surgery, suggests antenatal torsion with secondary necrosis. In addition, an ovary may be involved with an indirect hernia and extend as low as the labia majora. Because of a generally long pedicle and a small pelvis in the neonate, the ovaries in this age patient may be found anywhere between the lower pole of the kidneys and the true pelvis.

The appearance and size of the ovaries varies with the degree of hormonal stimulation. Ovarian size is most reproducible and best described by measurement of the ovarian volume, which can be calculated mechanically on the US unit or by a simplified modified equation for determination of the volume of a prolate ellipse: length $\times$ width $\times$ depth $\times$ 0.523 = volume (in mL). The mean ovarian volumes in girls younger than 6 years old is usually less than or equal to 1 mL. Neonatal ovarian volumes, however, may be quite large as a result of maternal hormonal stimulation during intrauterine life, which may take several months to regress. Ovarian volume gradually begins to increase again at approximately 6 years with the mean ovarian volume measurement in premenarchal girls between 6 and 11 years of age ranging between 1.2 mL and 2.5 mL (**Table 1**). There is marked enlargement in ovarian size

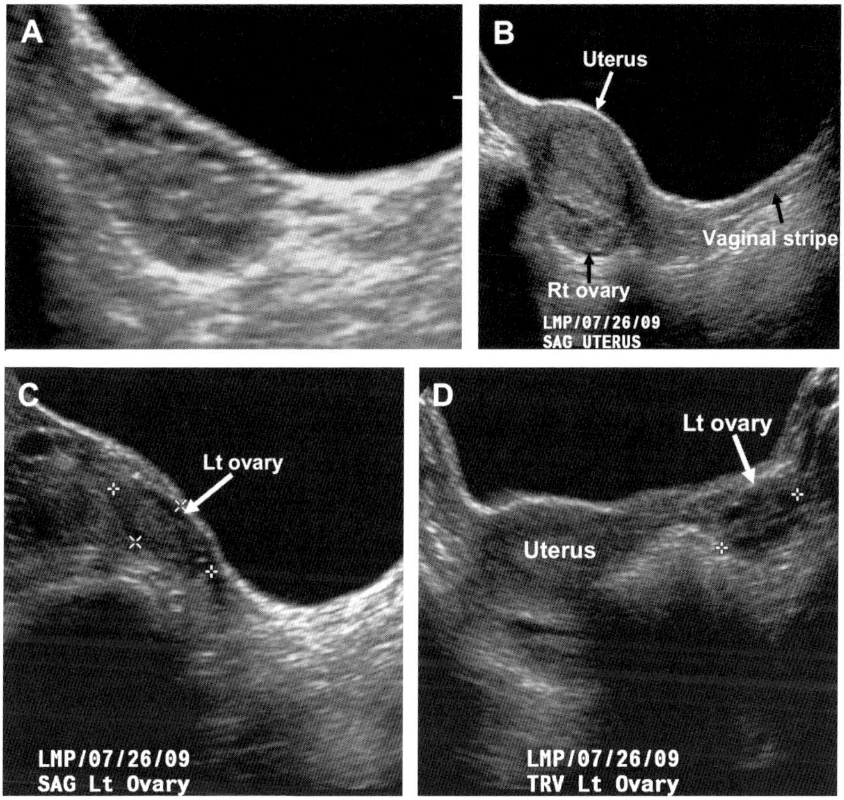


**Fig. 3.** Ovaries. (*A*) Normal ovary in a prepubertal child. The ovary is almond-shaped (ovoid) and appears heterogeneous because of multiple small follicles. (*B*) Normal right ovary in a postpubertal teenager. Sagittal sonogram demonstrates the mature uterine configuration with the ovoid-shaped right ovary located deep in the cul de sac posterior to the uterus. Multiple small follicles are seen throughout the ovary. (*C* and *D*) Normal left ovary in a postpubertal teenager. Sagittal (*C*) and transverse (*D*) sonogram of the normal-appearing left ovary, which contains multiple follicles.

postpuberty; thus, ovarian sizes in menstruating females in late childhood will be larger than in their premenarchal counterparts. Cohen and colleagues[21] reported a mean ovarian volume of 9.8 mL with a 96% confidence interval between 2.5 mL and 21.9 mL in menstruating females.

Multiple cysts are common within the ovaries and are considered physiologic when the largest cross-sectional diameter measures less than 3 cm.[21] In the neonatal period, the typical ovary appears heterogeneous because of the presence of small cysts. The demonstration of follicles within a structure thought to be a gonad is most helpful in establishing that the structure is in fact an ovary and not a testis, which should demonstrate a homogeneous echotexture devoid of follicles. Cohen and colleagues[21] observed ovarian cysts in 84% of children aged 1 day to 2 years and in 68% of children aged 2 to 12 years. Macrocysts (cysts measuring larger than 9 mm) were more frequently seen in the ovaries of girls in their first year of life compared with those in their second year, which probably accounts for the larger mean and top-normal ovarian volume measurements obtained in girls 0 to 3 months of age (mean ovarian volume of 1.06 mL with range of 0.7 to 3.6 mL) versus those

**Table 1**
**Pediatric ovarian volume measurements**

| | Age | Mean Ovarian Volume cm$^3$ (+SD) |
|---|---|---|
| Premenarchal | | |
| | 0–5 y | ≤1 cm$^3$ |
| | 1 d to 3 mo | 1.06 (±0.96) |
| | 4–12 mo | 1.05 (±0.67) |
| | 13–24 mo | 0.67 (±0.35) |
| | 3 y | 0.7 (±0.4) |
| | 4 y | 0.8 (±0.4) |
| | 5 y | 0.9 (±0.02) |
| | 6–8 y | 1.2 cm$^3$ |
| | 6 y | 1.2 (±0.4) |
| | 7 y | 1.3 (±0.6) |
| | 8 y | 1.1 (±0.5) |
| | 9–10 y[a] | 2.1 cm$^3$ |
| | 9 y | 2.0 (±0.8) |
| | 10 y | 2.2 (±0.7) |
| | 11 y[a] | 2.5 cm$^3$ (±1.3) |
| | 12 y[a] | 3.8 cm$^3$ (±1.4) |
| | 13 y[a] | 4.2 cm$^3$ (±2.3) |
| Menstrual | | 9.8 cm$^3$ (±5.8) |

[a] Note that these measurements may differ, depending on degree of maturation and presence of menarche.

*Data from* Cohen HL, Shapiro MA, Mandel FS, et al. Normal ovaries in neonates and infants: a sonographic study of 77 patients 1 day to 24 months old. AJR Am J Roentgenol 1993;160:583–6.

13 to 24 months of age (mean ovarian volume 0.67 mL with a range of 0.1 to 1.7 mL). These findings are probably secondary to the higher residual maternal hormone level in younger infants.

The blood supply of the ovary is dual, arising from the ovarian artery, which originates directly from the aorta, and from the uterine artery, which supplies an adnexal branch to each ovary. Blood flow can be seen in 90% of adolescent ovaries, but Doppler imaging cannot distinguish between the two blood supplies. Typically, on color flow Doppler imaging, the intraovarian arteries appear as short, straight branches located centrally within the normal ovary.

### *Duplex/color Doppler Sonography Findings in Primary Amenorrhea*

US has proven to be an indispensable tool for the evaluation of the pelvis in patients with primary amenorrhea, as it allows for rapid evaluation of the gynecologic structures and serves to confirm or deny their presence, and to characterize them when present.[10,11] If the ovaries are not identified in the expected location, high-resolution linear array technology can be used to examine the inguinal regions and the labia majora. When US cannot provide sufficient information because of a limited field of view, when excess bowel gas obscures an area of interest, or there is a need for assessing the extent of a malignant disease process before surgical resection, CT and/or MRI play a role.[20] With these modalities, a more global view is obtained and there is no difficulty in imaging skeletal structures, muscles, mesentery, and bowel. They assist in the differentiation of fat and calcium, and provide comprehensive information regarding resectability of masses.

### Amenorrhea with Delayed Sexual Development

Amenorrhea with delayed sexual development is suspected when breast budding does not occur by age 13 years.[22,23] The patient will have signs of being hypoestrogenic and assessment of FSH/LH levels is important in narrowing the possible causes of amenorrhea. US will demonstrate an infantile uterus, rather than a adult type (**Fig. 4**).

### Hypogonadotropic Hypogonadism

Hypogonadotropic hypogonadism is suspected when the FSH/LH levels are low, which suggests pituitary or hypothalamic dysfunction. High prolactin also suggests a pituitary cause. Low prolactin suggests hypothalamic suppression of the pituitary gland. Pituitary dysfunction may occur in the presence of child abuse, head trauma, tumors, systemic illness, and anorexia.

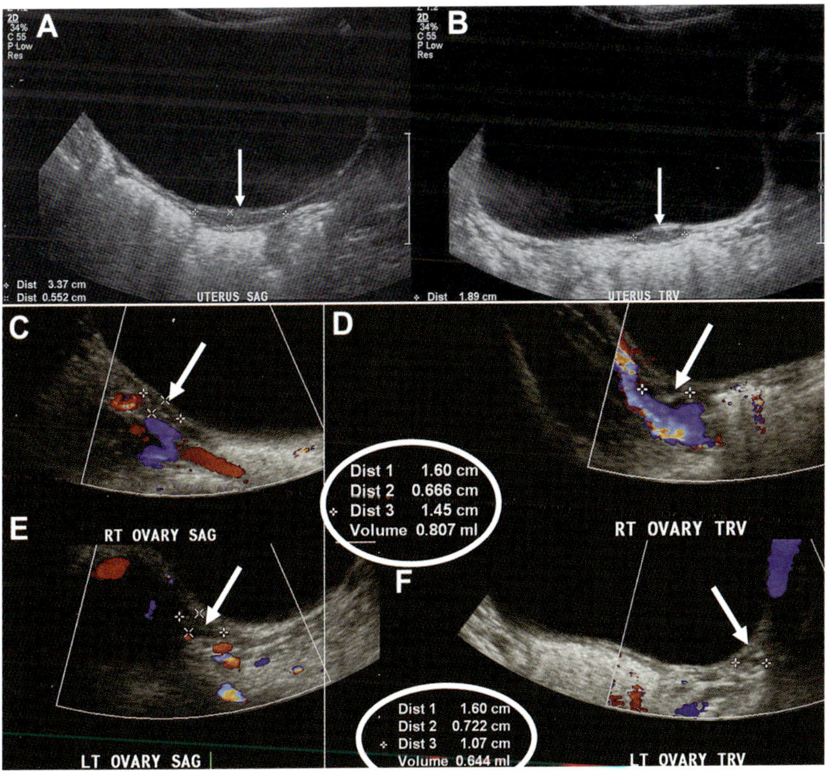


**Fig. 4.** Hypoplasia of the uterus and ovaries in a 16-year-old with primary amenorrhea. Sagittal (*A*) and transverse (*B*) sonograms of the uterus demonstrate a small tubular-shaped prepubertal configuration with the uterus measuring 3.4 cm in length by 0.6 cm in depth by 1.2 cm in width. Sagittal (*C*) and transverse (*D*) images of the right ovary and sagittal (*E*) and transverse (*F*) images of the left ovary demonstrate their diminutive size with the volume of the right ovary measuring 0.8 mL and that of the left ovary measuring 0.6 mL.

### *Hypergonadotropic Hypogonadism*

Hypergonadotropic hypogonadism is suspected when the FSH/LH levels are high. In this condition, the gonadal tissues fail to respond to endogenous gonadotropins. In the pure forms, there are no secondary sexual characteristics. At times, it may be a result of an abnormal karyotype such as Turner's syndrome (45,XO gonadal dysgenesis).[24,25] Turner's syndrome is characterized by sexual infantilism, although there is variability in the size and configuration of the uterus and ovaries in these patients and primary amenorrhea is quite common (**Fig. 5**). In Turner's syndrome, the most common form of gonadal dysgenesis, there is delayed or absent puberty associated with short stature, webbed neck, cubitus valgus deformities, shield chest, and scoliosis. Other anomalies include renal duplication, horseshoe kidney, coarctation of the aorta, bicuspid aortic valve, and lymphatic obstruction. In those girls with pure 45,XO karyotypes, the ovaries may not be visualized sonographically although a prepubertal uterus may be demonstrated. In genetic mosaicism with 45,XO/46,XX karyotype, the ovaries can vary from nonvisualized streak ovaries to normal adult ovaries. The uterine configuration also may be variable, appearing prepubertal in some patients and intermediate length in others measuring less than that of the

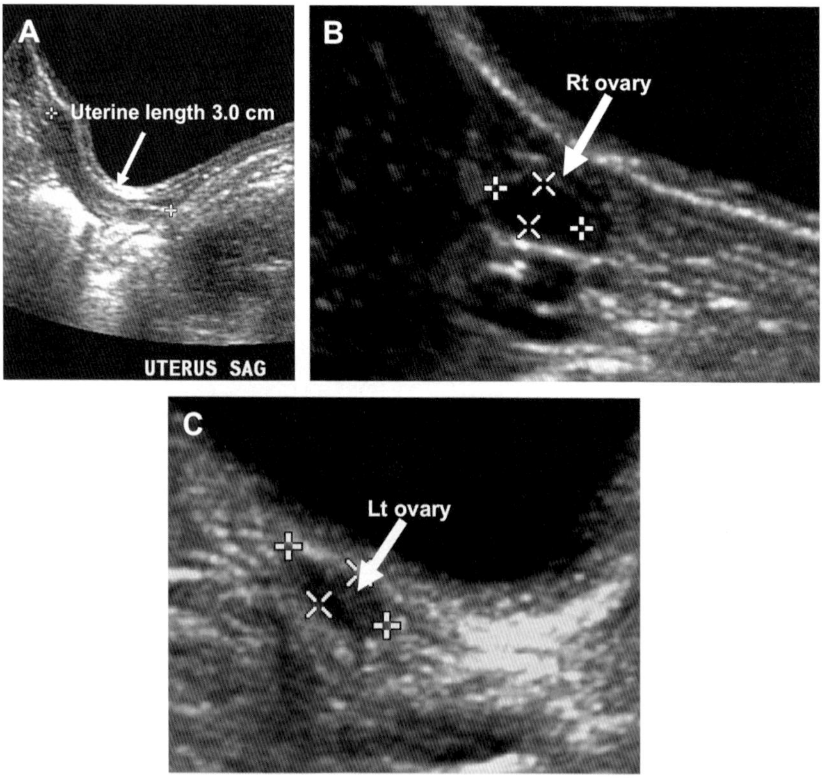


**Fig. 5.** Gonadal dysgenesis: Turner's Syndrome in a teenager with primary amenorrhea. (*A*) The uterus is smaller than normal measuring 3 cm in length with a prepubertal configuration. Right ovary (*B*) and left ovary (*C*) demonstrate diminutive ovaries with a dominant follicle within the right ovary.

healthy adult female. One or both ovaries were detected in 44% of 93 patients with Turner's syndrome. Within the prepubertal group, the mean uterine volume and mean ovarian volume measurements were significantly lower than those of the healthy controls ($P<.001$) (0.5 ± 0.3 mL vs 1.0 ± 0.3 mL and 0.3 ± 0.3 mL vs 0.6 ± 0.4 mL, respectively). In prepubertal girls, no significant relationship was found between age and uterine size or ovarian volume. Both uterine volume and ovarian volume of 19 women with spontaneous puberty increased during breast development, although mean uterine volume and mean ovarian volume were significantly ($P<.01$) lower than those of pubertal control patients.

### *Other Forms of Pure and Mixed Gonadal Dysgenesis*

Other forms of gonadal dysgenesis are also associated with nonvisualization of the ovaries as a result of absent or streak gonads. In pure gonadal dysgenesis (Swyer's syndrome),[26] the patients have 46,XX or 46,XY karyotypes and normal height. Mixed gonadal dysgenesis is a genetic mosaic of karyotypes 45,X/46,XY with a streak ovary and a contralateral intra-abdominal testis. Both of these forms of gonadal dysgenesis have an increased risk of gonadal tumors as a result of the presence of the Y chromosome. Noonan's syndrome (pseudo-Turner's syndrome) is characterized by phenotypic changes of Turner's syndrome, normal ovarian function, and normal ovaries on US.

### *Pseudointersex (Formerly Pseudohermaphrodite)*

Pseudointersex (formally pseudohermaphrodite) is a term that has been applied to patients with discordant karyotype, gonadal anatomy, and genital development.[27] True intersex is rare, whereas pseudointersex, mixed gonadal dysgenesis, and testicular feminization syndrome are more common, although they are also rare conditions. Female intersex is most often as a result of congenital adrenal hyperplasia (CAH). In this condition, the chromosomes are normal (46,XX). CAH is usually diagnosed in the neonatal period as a result of the presence of masculinized external genitalia, which results from excess production of androgens by the adrenal glands. These neonates may exhibit findings that include clitoral hypertrophy, partial fusion of the labia majora simulating the appearance of a scrotum, and a persistent urogenital sinus. Female intersex is rarely attributable to maternal ingestion of androgens during early pregnancy, or to a maternal masculinizing ovarian tumor. Male intersex may present with hypergonadotropic amenorrhea. Lack of production of Müllerian inhibition leads to variable development of the Müllerian elements. Incomplete testosterone production results from early destruction or dysgenesis of the testes. Therefore, the patients are karotypic normal males and phenotypically females, except for partial masculinization of their external genitalia. Secondary sexual development does not occur at puberty.

Testicular feminization is an unusual form of intersex that is another cause of primary amenorrhea.[28–30] It is a sex-linked recessive abnormality, resulting in end-organ insensitivity to androgens. These patients are phenotypic females who demonstrate normal breast development and a peculiar lack of body hair. The Müllerian system is inhibited and thus the uterus, fallopian tubes, and upper two-thirds of the vagina do not develop. These patients develop secondary female sexual characteristics as a result of circulating estrogens from the testes and adrenal glands. There is no turn-off mechanism for testosterone. The vagina ends blindly, and the testes are undescended and located within the abdomen, pelvis, canals, or within the labia majora (**Fig. 6**, **Fig. 7**). Gonadal biopsy reveals a lack of seminiferous tubules and germ cells.

At times, female adolescents with primary amenorrhea present with virilization. These girls develop a constellation of findings that may include deepening of their

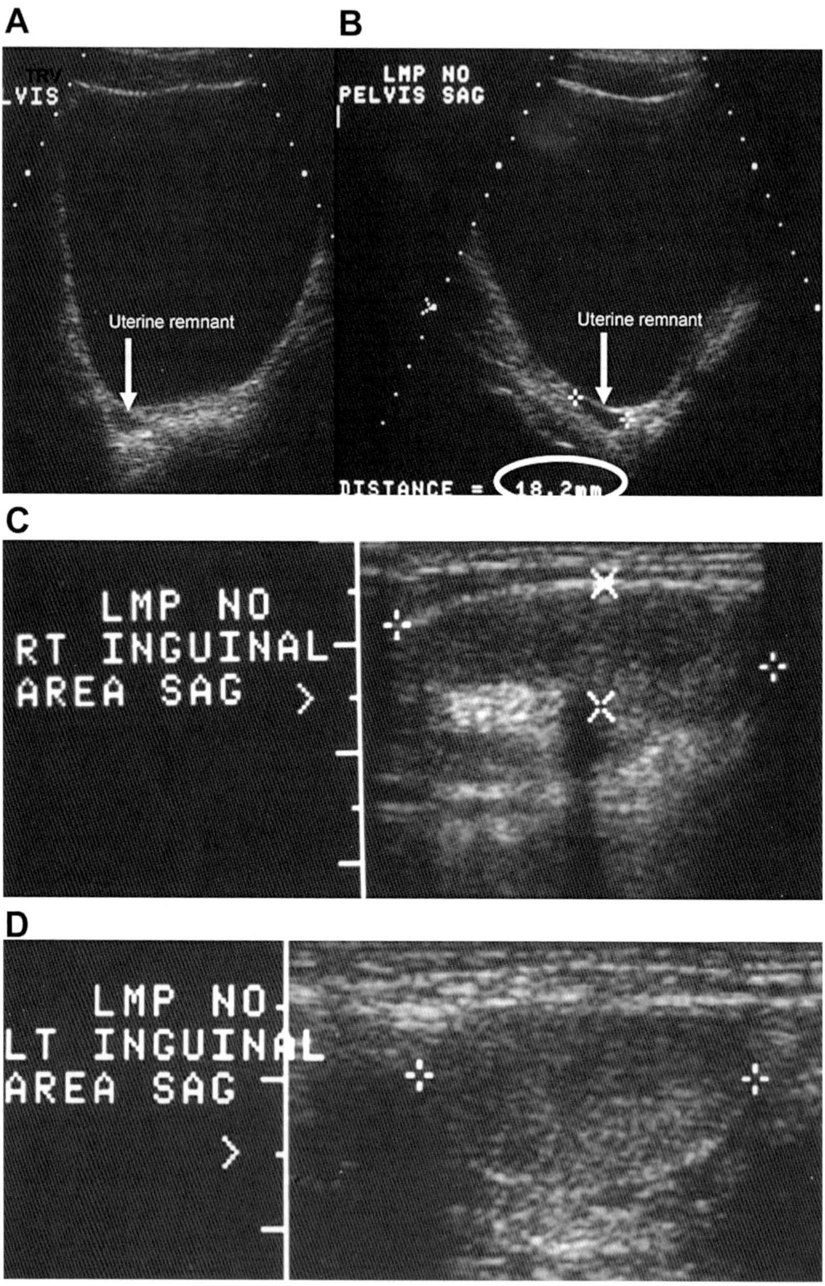


**Fig. 6.** Testicular feminization in a 16-year-old with primary amenorrhea. Transverse (*A*) and sagittal (*B*) sonograms of the markedly small uterine remnant, which measures 1.8 cm in length. Attempt was made to insert a #8 Fr catheter into a tiny opening at the introitus but the catheter advanced no deeper than 1 cm. No gonadal structures were identified within the true pelvis. Right (*C*) and left (*D*) gonads imaged in a sagittal plane when scanning over the ipsilateral inguinal region of each gonad. Note the homogeneous echotexture of these structures which lack ovarian follicles and are consistent with male gonads.

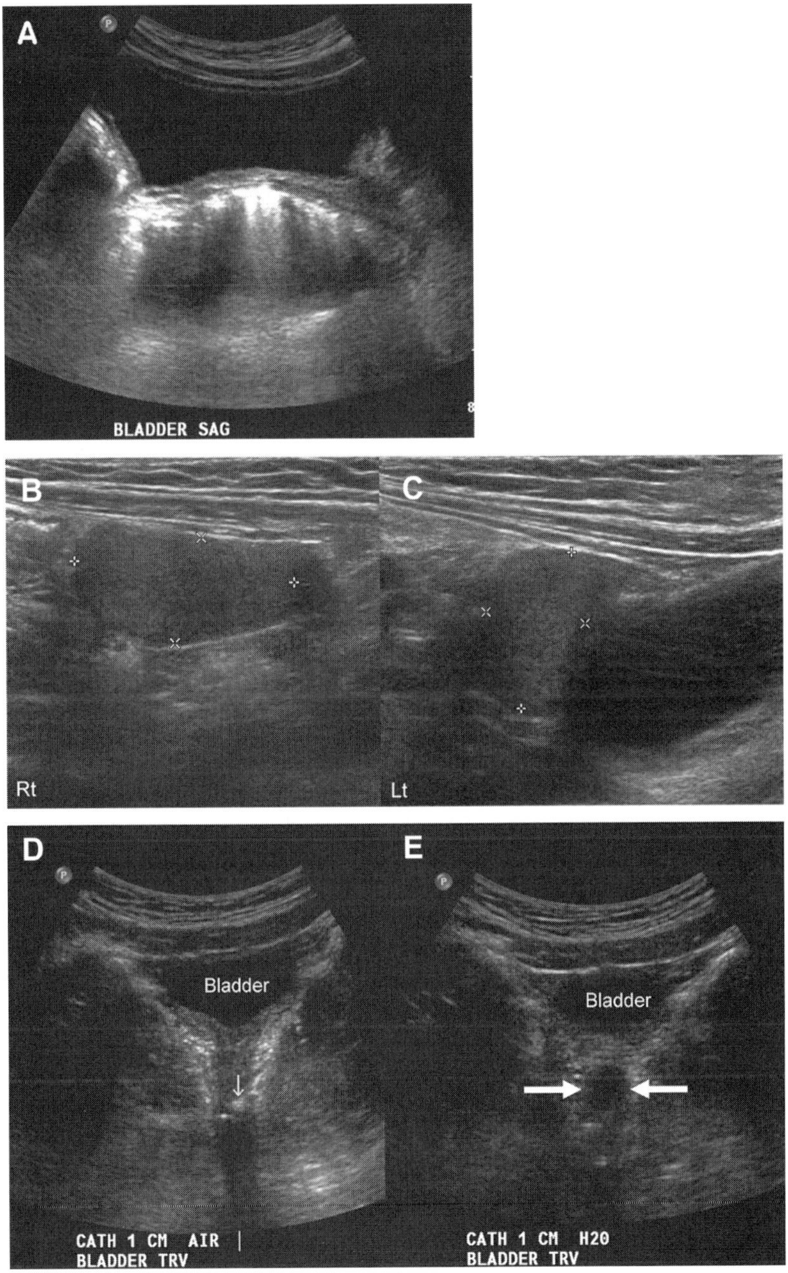


**Fig. 7.** (*A–E*) Testicular feminization in a 6-year-old female who underwent bilateral inguinal herniorrhaphies at which time the surgeon noted atypical gonads in both hernia sacs which on biopsy proved to be testes. (*A*) Sagittal sonogram of the bladder showing the lack of a uterine structure. Right (*B*) and left (*C*) -sided gonads identified in each respective inguinal region bilaterally. Note that the gonads are homogeneous and devoid of follicles. (*D, E*) Transverse scans of the bladder during an attempt to inject air (*D*) and water (*E*) into the 1-cm-long introital opening.

voices, cliteromegaly, increased muscle mass, and temporal balding.[31] Diagnostic etiologies may include virilizing ovarian tumors (eg, gonadal stromal tumors 67% 13–30 years [arrhenoblastoma, gynandroblastoma]), Sertoli-Leydig cell 39% 10–30 years, hilus cell 80% > 40 years, and adrenal rest tumors 45% 11–30 years.

Patients with Polycystic Ovary Syndrome (PCOS) may present with primary amenorrhea, although they most often manifest oligomenorrhea or secondary amenorrhea and come in seeking medical assistance for evaluation of infertility.[32–35] Sixty-two percent of patients with PCOS manifest hirsuitism and 31% are obese. US findings include bilateral ovarian enlargement, rounded ovarian configuration, "string of pearls" distribution of ovarian follicles around the periphery of the ovaries, 5- to 8-mm diameter follicles, more than 5 follicles within each ovary, and a moderate amount of free fluid (**Fig. 8**).

### *Uterine/Vaginal Obstruction*

Congenital anomalies of the uterus and vagina are uncommon and may present as an abdominal or pelvic mass secondary to obstruction, although more mature patients with an anomaly that causes obstruction may present with primary amenorrhea (**Fig. 9**).[35–37] The uterus, cervix, and upper two-thirds of the vagina are formed by the fused caudal ends of the Müllerian (paramesonephric) ducts and the paired fallopian tubes are formed by the unfused upper ends, whereas the lower third of the vagina is derived from the urogenital sinus. Because Müllerian duct development into the uterus is dependent on the formation of the Wolffian (mesonephric) duct, abnormal development of the Müllerian duct results in uterine and vaginal anomalies, and is often associated with renal anomalies. The terminology used to describe the resulting abnormalities is as follows: uterus (metro-) vagina (colpos), hydro- (distended by anechoic secretions), and hemato- (distended by echogenic blood). The uterus and vagina can be differentiated by the expected thicker uterine wall compared with that of the vagina. Scattered echoes are often present proximal to obstruction as a result of cellular debris, mucoid material, and/or blood. Superimposed infection is quite rare.

The most common congenital uterine abnormality is a bicornuate uterus (**Figs. 9** and **10**), which results when the two Müllerian ducts fuse only inferiorly resulting in two uterine horns that are joined at a variable level above the single cervix (see **Fig. 9**). A single vagina is present.[38,39] With complete duplication of the Müllerian ducts, there is duplication of the uterus and cervix and a septated vagina. In either anomaly, obstruction of

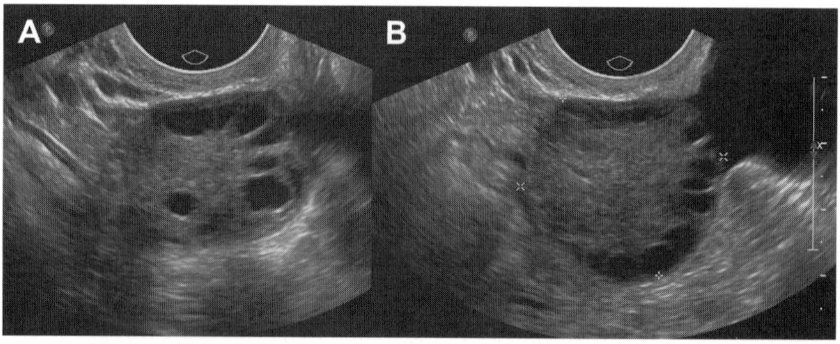


**Fig. 8.** Polycystic ovarian disease in a 16-year-old with amenorrhea, obesity, and hirsuitism. Right (*A*) and left (*B*) ovaries are larger than normal with a rounded configuration, a "string of pearls" distribution of ovarian follicles around the periphery of the ovaries, 5- to 8-mm diameters of each follicle, and more than 5 follicles within each ovary.

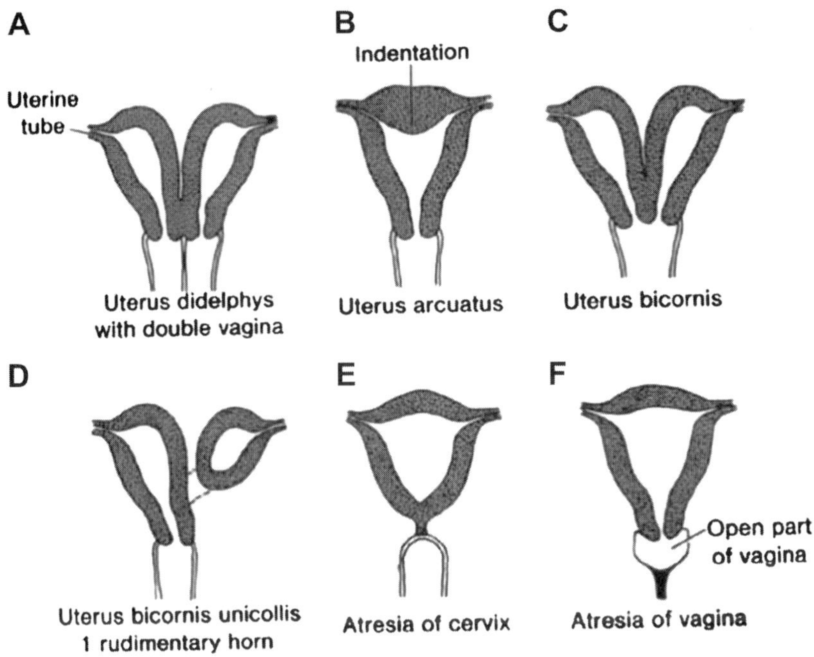


**Fig. 9.** Uterine anomalies (*A–F*). (*From* Sadler TW. Langman's Medical Embryology. 6th edition. Philadelphia: Williams & Wilkins; 1990. p. 282; with permission.)

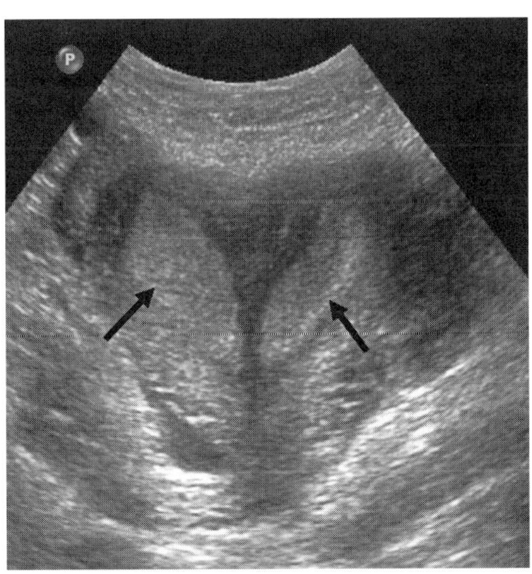

**Fig. 10.** Bicornuate uterus. Transverse sonogram obtained during the secretory phase of the menstrual cycle with each arrow pointing to a uterine horn.

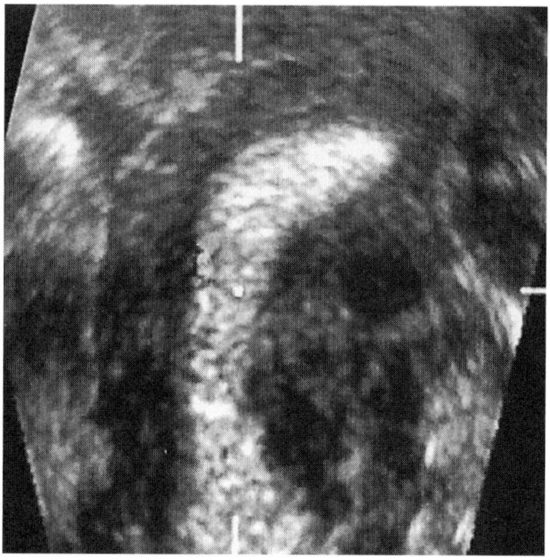

**Fig. 11.** Unicornuate uterus as shown by 3-D ultrasound reconstruction. (*From* Salem S, Wilson SR. Gynecologic ultrasound. In: Rumack CM, Wilson Charboneau JW, editors. Diagnostic ultrasound. 3rd edition. St Louis: Mosby, Inc; 2005. p. 536; with permission.)

one uterine horn can result in a pelvic mass as a result of unilateral hydrometra or hematometra. Agenesis of only one Müllerian duct results in development of a unicornuate uterus (one horn) (**Fig. 11**).[40] Although routine US is often sufficient for demonstration of congenital anomalies of the uterus, 3-D US is an excellent modality for obtaining planar reformatted sections through the uterus, which allows for precise evaluation of the anatomy.[17]

Hydrocolpos or hydrometrocolpos, is secondary to an imperforate hymen, a transverse vaginal septum, or a stenotic or atretic vagina and results in an accumulation of secretions proximal to the obstruction.[41–45] In neonates, the secretions are secondary to intrauterine and postnatal stimulation of uterine and cervical glands by maternal estrogens and accounts for 15% of abdominal masses in newborn girls (**Fig. 12**). In girls who have reached menstrual age, the low-level echoes within the fluid represent blood. These girls do not experience the onset of menarche despite their obvious

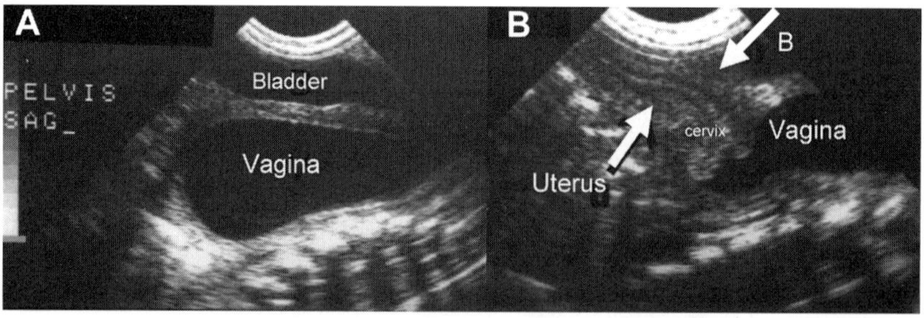


**Fig. 12.** Hydrocolpos in a newborn with history of prenatal hydronephrosis. (*A*) Sagittal scan of pelvis in newborn showing large, conical, fluid-filled mass representing obstructed vagina (V) behind bladder (B). (*B*) Sagittal scan, angled higher than in *A*, shows uterus (*arrows*) with cervix projecting into dilated vagina (V). B, bladder. (*From* Rosenberg HK. Sonography of pediatric urinary tract abnormalities. Pt I. Am Urol Assoc Weekly Update Series 1986;35(5):1–8; with permission.)

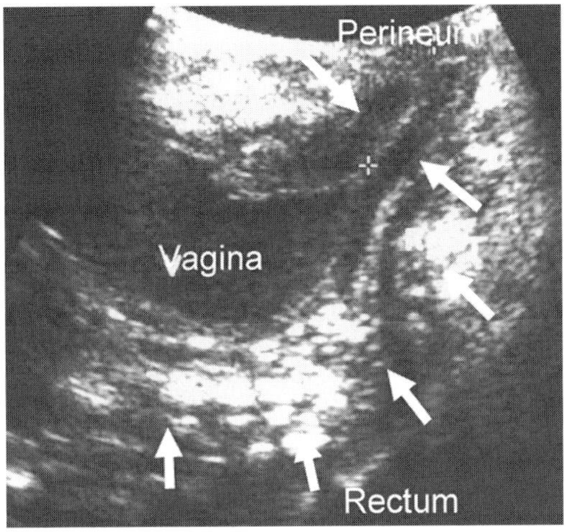


Fig. 13. Hydrocolpos with distal vaginal atresia. There is dilatation of the vagina proximal to the long segment area of distal atresia (*arrows*). The echoes within the dilated vaginal canal are a result of secretions secondary to maternal in utero hormonal stimulation.

postpubertal sexual development. They often present with primary amenorrhea in a setting of intermittent or monthly abdominal or pelvic pain, abdominal mass, and difficulty with micturition. Transabdominal US is useful for determining the extent of uterine and/or vaginal obstruction. Hydrocolpos appears as a large tubular, cystic mass posterior to the bladder, which is distal to the cervix and extends inferior to the pubic symphysis (**Fig. 13**). The blood-filled dilated uterine cavity can be shown in continuity with the dilated vagina. Transperineal US is useful for defining and measuring the distance of an obstructed vaginal compartment from the perineum (**Fig. 14**).[46] A simple imperforate hymen is not usually associated with other congenital anomalies. On the other hand, vaginal atresia or a midtransverse or high-transverse vaginal septum is associated with a high incidence of genitourinary (secondary urinary retention and hydronephrosis, cloacal exstrophy, persistent urogenital sinus), gastrointestinal (imperforate anus), and skeletal anomalies. Rarely, peritoneal calcifications may be seen in very young patients with hydrometrocolpos, as a result of a sterile inflammatory reaction to spillage of accumulated secretions into the peritoneal cavity.[47]

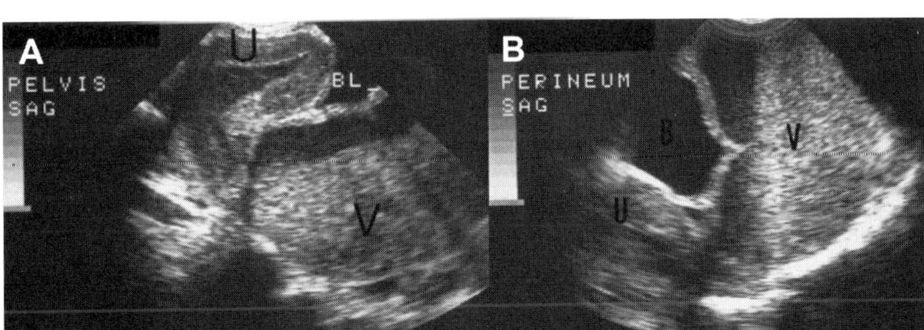


Fig. 14. Hematometrocolpos in a 13-year-old female who presented with cyclic pelvic pain and primary amenorrhea. (*A*) Sagittal transabdominal scan of pelvis shows dilated thicker walled uterine cavity (U) filled with echogenic debris (blood). (*B*) Perineal scan demonstrates fluid-debris level is seen in dilated, obstructed vagina (V).

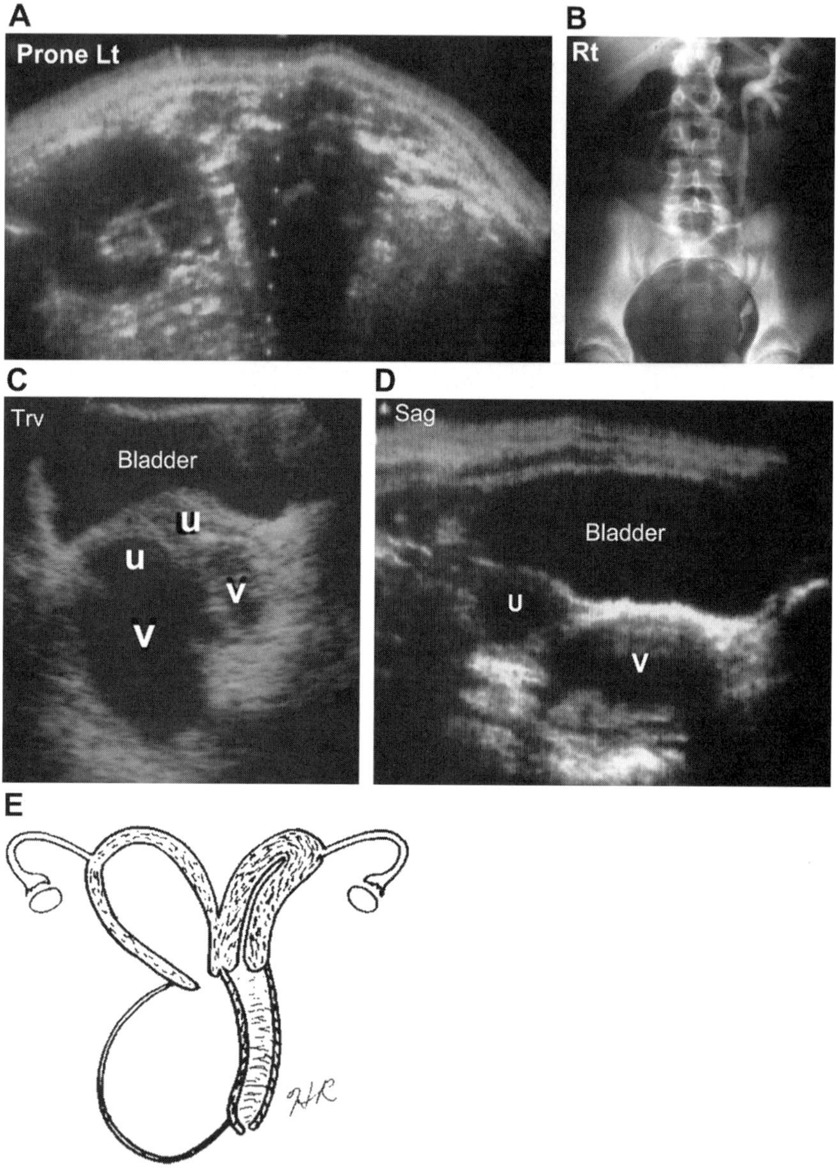


**Fig. 15.** Mayer-Rokitansky Kuster-Hauser syndrome with duplication of the uterus and vagina with an obstructed right uterus and vagina associated with renal agenesis on the side of the hematometrocolpos. (*A*) Prone US transverse scan demonstrates absence of the right kidney. (*B*) Intravenous pyelogram confirms the US findings of right renal agenesis. (*C* and *D*) Transverse US demonstrates duplication of the uterus and vagina with an obstructed right side uterus and vagina (u, uterus; v, vagina). (*E*) Drawing of the duplicated uterus and vagina with right-sided hydrometrocolpos. (*From* Rosenberg HK, Udassin R. Howell C. et al. Duplication of the uterus and vagina, unilateral hydrometrocolpos, and ipsilateral renal agenesis: sonographic aid to diagnosis. J Ultrasound Med 1982;1(7):289–91; with permission.)

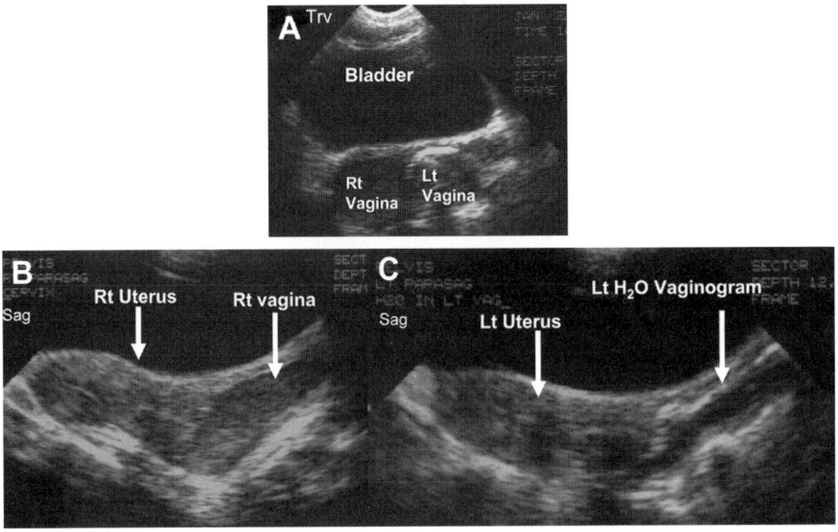


**Fig. 16.** Mayer-Rokitansky-Kuster-Hauser syndrome in a 13-year-old female with duplication of uterus and vagina, obstructed right-sided vagina, and fenestrated vaginal septum with cyclic pelvic pain and normal menstrual periods. (*A*) Transverse image of the pelvis demonstrates both vaginal compartments in cross-sectional view with air/fluid in the left-sided vagina and a miniscule amount of fluid outlining the echogenic blood products within the right-sided vagina. (*B*) The right-sided uterus is normal in size and configuration and the vagina is distended with blood products. (*C*) A left-sided normal-appearing uterus is clearly seen in the sagittal plane and following hand injection of sterile water into the single introitus, the left-sided vagina was demonstrated. During real-time observation, tiny amounts of water could be seen intermittently in the right-sided vagina, suggesting the presence of a fenestrated vaginal septum. (*From* Rosenberg HK, Sherman NH, Tarry WF, et al. Mayer-Rokitansky-Küster-Hauser syndrome: ultrasound aid to diagnosis. Radiology 1986;161:815–9; with permission.)

The Mayer-Rokitansky-Küster-Hauser syndrome is the second most common cause of primary amenorrhea.[48–52] The US findings result from defects in Müllerian development and include findings such as vaginal atresia and a spectrum of uterine anomalies (rudimentary, hypoplasia, duplication, partial lumen, septate or bicornuate uterus, unilateral or bilateral obstruction). The broad and round ligaments, fallopian tubes, and ovaries are normal. These girls have a normal female karyotype, secondary sexual development, and external genitalia. There is a high incidence of unilateral renal (50%) and skeletal (12%) anomalies. Unilateral renal agenesis or ectopia is the most common renal anomaly. The most common sonographic findings are uterine didelphys with unilateral hydrometrocolpos and ipsilateral renal agenesis. Water vaginography can help identify the septated vagina with unilateral vaginal obstruction (**Fig. 15** A,B; **Fig. 16**).

## SUMMARY

US is the imaging modality of choice for the evaluation of patients with primary amenorrhea. Careful correlation with clinical history, physical examination, and laboratory findings significantly narrows the diagnostic possibilities thus allowing for a more precise diagnosis.

## REFERENCES

1. Stranzinger E, Strouse PJ. Ultrasound of the pediatric female pelvis [a review]. Semin Ultrasound CT MR 2008;29(2):98–113.
2. Garel L, Dubois J, Grignon A. US of the pediatric female pelvis: a clinical perspective. Radiographics 2001;21:1393–407.
3. Siegel MJ, editor. Female pelvis. Pediatric sonography. 3rd edition. Philadelphia: Lippincott Williams and Wilkins; 2002. p. 530–77.
4. Cohen HL, Bober SE. Imaging the pediatric pelvis: the normal and abnormal genital tract and simulators of its diseases. Urol Radiol 1992;14:273–83.
5. Arbel-DeRowe Y, Tepper R, Rosen DJ, et al. The contribution of pelvic ultrasonography to the diagnostic process in pediatric and adolescent gynecology. J Pediatr Adolesc Gynecol 1997;10:3–12.
6. Rosenberg HK. The pediatric pelvis. In: Rumack CM, Wilson SR, Charboneau JW, editors. Diagnostic ultrasound. 3rd edition. St Louis (MO): Mosby, Inc; 2005. p. 1977–2033.
7. Teele RL, Share JC. Ultrasonography of the female pelvis in childhood and adolescence. Radiol Clin North Am 1992;30(4):743–58.
8. Comstock CH, Boal DK. Pelvic sonography of the pediatric patient. Semin Ultrasound CT MR 1984;5:54–67.
9. Siegel MJ. Pediatric gynecologic sonography. Radiology 1991;179:593–600.
10. Cohen HL. Evaluation of the adolescent and young adult with amenorrhea: role of US. In: Bluth E, Arger P, Hertzberg B, et al, editors. Syllabus: a special course in ultrasound: clinical questions, practical answers. Oak Brook (IL): RSNA Publications; 1996. p. 171.
11. Reid R. Amenorrhea. In: Copeland L, editor. Textbook of gynecology. Philadelphia: WB Saunders; 1993. p. 367.
12. Mashchak CA, Kletzky OA, Davajan V, et al. Clinical and laboratory evaluation of patients with primary amenorrhea. Obstet Gynecol 1981;57(6):715–21.
13. Falsetti L, Pasinetti E, Mazzani M, et al. Weight loss and menstrual cycle: clinical and endocrinological evaluation. Gynecol Endocrinol 1992;6:49.
14. Lee PA. Physiology of puberty. In: Principles and practice of endocrinology and metabolism. Philadelphia: JB Lippincott; 1990. p. 740.
15. Rubin C, Kurtz AB, Goldberg BB. Water enema: a new ultrasound technique in defining pelvic anatomy. J Clin Ultrasound 1978;6:28–33.
16. Bellah RD, Rosenberg HK. Transvaginal ultrasound in a children's hospital: is it worthwhile? Pediatr Radiol 1991;21:570–4.
17. Benacerraf BR, Shipp TD, Bromley B. Which patients benefit from a 3-D reconstructed coronal view of the uterus added to a standard routine 2D pelvic sonography? AJR Am J Roentgenol 2008;190(3):626–9.
18. Ghate SV, Crockett MM, Boyd BK, et al. Sonohysterography: do 3D reconstructed images provide additional value? AJR Am J Roentgenol 2008;190(4):841–2.
19. Jequier S, Rousseau O. Sonographic measurements of the normal bladder wall in children. AJR Am J Roentgenol 1987;149:563–6.
20. Hamm B, Kubik-Huch RA, Fleige B. MR imaging and CT of the female pelvis: radiologic-pathologic correlation—pictorial review. Eur Radiol 1999;9:3–15.
Lee PA. Neuroendocrinology of puberty. Semin Repord Endocrinol 1988;6:13.
21. Cohen HL, Shapiro MA, Mandel FS, et al. Normal ovaries in neonates and infants: a sonographic study of 77 patients 1 day to 24 months old. AJR Am J Roentgenol 1993;160:583–6.
22. Rosenfeld RL. Clinical review 6: diagnosis and management of delayed puberty. J Clin Endocrinol Metab 1990a;70:559.

23. Mulayim B, Celik NY. Pubertal failure and primary amenorrhea with uterine hypotrophy due to hypogonadotropic hypogonadism. J Pediatr Adolesc Gynecol 2009 Apr;22(2):e1–3.
24. Haber HP, Ranke MB. Pelvic sonography in Turner syndrome: standards for uterine and ovarian volume. J Ultrasound Med 1999;18:271–6.
25. Bakalov VK, Shawker T, Cenbiceros I, et al. Uterine development in Turner syndrome. J Pediatr. 2007;151(5):528–31.
26. Hetu V, Caron E, Francoeur D. Hypoplastic uterus and clitoris enlargement in Swyer syndrome. J Pediatr Adolesc Gynecol 2009. [Epub ahead of print].
27. Dreger AD, Chase C, Sousa A, et al. Changing the nomenclature/taxonomy for intersex: a scientific and clinical rationale. J Pediatr Endocrinol Metab 2005;18:729–33.
28. Norris JR, Ryley TJ, Urbach GI. Testicular feminization syndrome. Can Med Assoc J 1965;93:765–7.
29. Shah R, Woolley M, Costin G. Testicular feminization syndrome: the androgen insensitivity syndrome. J Pediatr Surg 1992;27:757.
30. Goske MJ, Emmens RW, Rabinowitz R. Inguinal ovaries in children demonstrated by high resolution real-time ultrasound. Radiology 1984;151:635–6.
31. Rosenfield RI. Hyperandrogenism in peripubertal girls. Pediatr Clin North Am 1990;37:1333.
32. Hann LE, Hall DA, McArdle CR, et al. Polycystic ovarian disease: sonographic spectrum. Radiology 1984;150:531–4.
33. Dolz M, Osborne NG, Blanes J, et al. Polycystic ovarian syndrome: assessment with color Doppler angiography and three-dimensional sonography. J Ultrasound Med 1999;18:303–13.
34. Jeffrey Chang R, Coffler MS. Polycystic ovary syndrome: early detection in the adolescent. Clin Obstet Gynecol 2007;50(1):178–87.
35. Lakhani K, Seifalian AM, Atiomo WU, et al. Polycystic ovaries. Br J Radiol 2002; 75(889):9–16.
36. Blask ARN, Sanders RC, Rock JA. Obstructed uterovaginal anomalies: demonstration with sonography. Part I: neonates and infants. Radiology 1991;179: 79–83.
37. Blask ARN, Sanders RC, Rock JA. Obstructed uterovaginal anomalies: demonstration with sonography. Part II. Teenagers. Radiology 1991;179:84–8.
38. Sadler TW. Langman's Medical Embryology. 6th edition. Philadelphia: Williams & Wilkins; 1990. p. 282.
39. Tiker F, Yildirim SV, Barutcu O, et al. Familial Müllerian agenesis. Turk J Pediatr 2000;42(4):322 4.
40. Brody JM, Koelliker KL, Frishman GN. Unicornuate uterus: imaging appearance, associated anomalies, and clinical implications. AJR Am J Roentgenol 1998;171: 1341–7.
41. Sanders RM, Nakajima ST. An unusual late presentation of imperforate hymen. Obstet Gynecol 1994 May;83(5 Pt 2):896–8.
42. Messina M, Severi FM, Bocchi C, et al. Voluminous perinatal pelvic mass: a case of congenital hydrometrocolpos. J Matern Fetal Neonatal Med 2004;15(2):135–7.
43. Fisher MR, Kricun ME, editors. Imaging of the pelvis. Gaithersburg (Md): Aspen; 1989.
44. Capito C, Echaieb A, Lortat-Jacob S, et al. Pitfalls in the diagnosis and management of obstructive uterovaginal duplication: a series of 32 cases. Pediatrics 2008;122(4):e891–7 [Epub 2008].
45. Mifkovic LJ, Mirkovic D, Boskovic V, et al. Uterus didelphys with obstructed hemivagina and ipsilateral renal agenesis. Acta Chir Iugosl 2007;54:137–9.

46. Scanlan KA, Pozniak MA, Fagerholm M, et al. Value of transperineal sonography in the assessment of vaginal atresia. AJR Am J Roentgenol 1990;54:545–8.
47. Hu MX, Methratta S. An unusual case of neonatal peritoneal calcifications associated with hydrometrocolpos. Pediatr Radiol 2001;31:742–4.
48. Meglin AJ, Balotin RJ, Jelinek JS, et al. Cloacal exstrophy: radiologic findings in 13 patients. AJR Am J Roentgenol 1990;155:1267–72.
49. Warne SA, Wilcox DT, Creighton S, et al. Long-term gynecological outcome of patients with persistent cloaca. J Urol 2003;170(4 Pt 2):1493–6.
50. Rosenberg HK, Sherman NH, Tarry WF, et al. Mayer-Rokitansky-Küster-Hauser syndrome: ultrasound aid to diagnosis. Radiology 1986;161:815–9.
51. Pittock ST, Babovic-Vuksanovic D, Lteif A. Mayer-Rokitansky-Küster-Hauser anomaly and its associated malformations. Am J Med Genet A 2005;135(3):314–6.
52. Rosenberg HK, Udassin R, Howell C, et al. Duplication of the uterus and vagina, unilateral hydrometrocolpos, and ipsilateral renal agenesis: sonographic aid to diagnosis. J Ultrasound Med 1982;1(7):289–91.

# Optimizing Potential for Fertility: Fertility Preservation Considerations for the Pediatric Endocrinologist

Peter A. Lee, MD, PhD[a,b,*], Alan Rogol, MD[b,c], Christopher P. Houk, MD[d]

**KEYWORDS**

- Cryopreservation • Sperm retrieval • Oocyte retrieval
- Infertility • Assisted fertility • Fertility preservation

Modern medicine now offers hope for many patients who would have been infertile in the past. Fertility preservation and assisted reproduction in adults has received considerable attention. In women, discussion of fertility preservation typically arises in patients with malignancies or nononcologic conditions that either require treatment with gonadotoxic drugs, ovariectomy,[1] or pelvic radiation. Among adult men, fertility preservation should be considered whenever testicular damage may result from medical/surgical therapy or from trauma. Fertility preservation is a consideration that should be discussed in those undergoing treatment for malignancy as well as those with genetic or other congenital conditions.

The dramatic success noted in the treatment for childhood cancers has resulted in a marked increase in survival rates creating many long-term cancer survivors with unique medical challenges. Preservation of fertility is one such challenge that has mandated the need to assess future reproduction among these individuals.[2] Topics related to fertility preservation in pediatric and adolescent patients being treated for

[a] Department of Pediatrics, Penn State College of Medicine, MC-H085, The Milton S. Hershey Medical Center, PO Box 850, 500 University Drive, Hershey, PA 17033-0850, USA
[b] Department of Pediatrics, Indiana University School of Medicine, Riley Hospital for Children, Indianapolis, IN 46202, USA
[c] Department of Pediatrics, University of Virginia, Charlottesville, VA 22908, USA
[d] Department of Pediatrics, Medical College of Georgia, Augusta, GA 31403, USA
* Corresponding author. Department of Pediatrics, MC-H085, The Milton S. Hershey Medical Center, PO Box 850, 500 University Drive, Hershey, PA 17033-0850.
*E-mail address:* plee@psu.edu (P. Lee).

Endocrinol Metab Clin N Am 38 (2009) 761–775
doi:10.1016/j.ecl.2009.08.003
endo.theclinics.com
0889-8529/09/$ – see front matter 

cancers, including ethical considerations, have recently been summarized.[3] Given the recent improvements in fertility preservation, this issue must now become part of an overall care plan for such children and adolescents.

Awareness of current and developing techniques is appropriate for the pediatric endocrinologist because of the improved potential for fertility in children with malignancy who have undergone chemotherapy or radiation therapy as well as children and adolescents with other diagnoses, including endocrinopathy, who have long been considered to be infertile.

Efforts to address fertility preservation should be considered as soon as the risk is realized. This applies to those with gonadal failure previously considered to be incompatible with biologic parenthood such as Turner or Klinefelter syndromes. Parenthood may also be possible, albeit at considerable expense, for patients with hypogonadotropic hypogonadism, polycystic ovarian disease, or other ovulatory dysfunction. The potential for such therapies should be assessed at an early age.

## ATTAINMENT OF FERTILITY POTENTIAL IN THE HUMAN

Although fertility potential is not normally attained until early or midpuberty, a low level of gonadal activity is present during childhood with limited follicular development and early stages of spermatogenesis. Even though mature sperm are not present until a mean age of 14 years, meiosis results in development of spermatids in the prepubertal testis.[4] Semen cryopreservation has been reported to be feasible in roughly two-thirds of boys aged 13.7 to 18.9 years.[5] Although sperm counts cannot accurately be predicted by hormone measurements, it is likely that an adequate sample for preservation could be obtained around midpuberty in those without chronic debilitating illness. Similar findings have also been noted in 14- to 17-year-old boys with malignancies.[6] Among females, there is no conclusive evidence of further oocyte production after birth and meiosis occurs during follicular maturation. There is potential for in vitro maturation of primordial oocytes into oogonia. Before ovarian failure, all females will produce mature follicles in response to gonadotropin stimulation. In fact most females are capable of ovulation by midpuberty.

## ETHICAL CONSIDERATIONS FOR THE CHILD

Ethical and legal issues including risk-benefit determination, must be considered[7] before implementing fertility preservation procedures. These must be proposed to parents, and, in an age-appropriate way, to the patient. Investigational review boards require a pediatric counselor to discuss the proposed preservation with the child. Such discussion may be awkward for families who have recently been given a diagnosis of malignancy. In addition, the importance of future fertility may be difficult for the prepubertal child to assess; therefore, parents can and should play a role in decision making in this arena. Consent must be obtained from parents with appropriate assent from the child before attempting to obtain and cryopreserve germ cells or gonadal tissue. Any procedures should be presented to an appropriate ethical review board as experimental, as protocols to preserve fertility in children are only now being developed.

## DIAGNOSES IN CHILDREN AND ADOLESCENTS FOR FERTILITY PRESERVATION CONSIDERATIONS

Procedures for adolescent women and prepubertal boys and girls being investigated[8] are listed in **Box 1**. Efficacy of these procedures must be verified in adults before they are used in children. Procedures applicable to children include oocyte banking,

**Box 1**
**Potential methods to preserve or stimulate fertility in children and adolescents**

A. Among prepubertal individuals being treated with gonadotoxic agents or radiation or those with endocrinological diagnoses of primary hypogonadism
   a. Girls
      i. Cryopreservation of immature oocytes and in vitro follicular maturation
      ii. Ovarian tissue cryopreservation
      iii. Ovarian transposition out of radiation field
   b. Boys
      i. Testicular tissue cryopreservation
      ii. Spermatogonial stem cell transplantation
      iii. Shielding testes from radiation
B. Pubertal and postpubertal adolescents
   a. Girls
      i. Oocyte cryopreservation
      ii. GnRH analog
      iii. Ovarian tissue cryopreservation
   b. Boys
      i. Semen cryopreservation
C. Among those with hypogonadotropic hypogonadism
   a. Gonadotropin or gonadotropin-releasing hormone (intermittent stimulation)

ovarian tissue cryopreservation, in vitro follicular maturation for females, and testicular tissue cryopreservation and spermatogonial stem cell transplantation in males.[9]

Fertility preservation in children (**Box 2**) who face therapy that may preclude fertility or have congenital or early-onset gonadal dysfunction will focus on preserving remaining germ cells. Examples of children and adolescents in this category include those whose gonads have been damaged as a result of therapy for malignant or autoimmune diseases, those with incomplete primary hypogonadism, including patients with Klinefelter syndrome, Turner syndrome, some types of DSD (disorders of sex development) such as ovotesticular DSD and those with gonadal damage following trauma, torsion, inflammatory process, or surgery. For those with congenital or acquired hypogonadotropic hypogonadism, the focus of therapy involves the pulsatile administration of GnRH (currently unavailable in the United States), or intermittent gonadotropin stimulation.

## FERTILITY PRESERVATION IN MALIGNANT DISEASES OF CHILDHOOD AND ADOLESCENCE

Consequences of therapy for childhood cancers may interfere with the ability to produce mature germ cells and achieve future fertilization. Accordingly, survivors of childhood cancer may have difficulty becoming pregnant, have increased spontaneous abortions as a consequence of altered uterine anatomy, and suffer higher rates of neonatal death and low-birth-weight infants.[10] An increased risk of congenital malformations or childhood cancer in the offspring of patients who received cancer treatment in childhood has not been reported.

**Box 2**
**Fertility preservation or stimulation among children and adolescents**

1. To preserve germ cells among those who
   - face therapy for malignant or autoimmune diseases that may preclude fertility
   - have congenital or early-onset gonadal dysfunction
     - males with incomplete primary hypogonadism, including most boys with Klinefelter syndrome, those with gonadal damage after torsion, orchitis, or partial removal of the testes
     - females with Turner syndrome whose ovaries contain follicles, and some patients with potentially functional ovaries having disorders of sex development (DSD), such as the female with ovotesticular DSD.
2. Stimulate germ cell maturation via pulsatile administration of GnRH or intermittent gonadotropin stimulation
   - Males and females have congenital or acquired hypogonadotropic hypogonadism

Fertility preservation techniques have progressed as survival rates of many cancers have improved, particularly in young adult men and women. These techniques apply to adolescents who have completed puberty who show adult-type spermatogenesis or ovulation. For adolescent males, sperm banking is relatively simple, well tested, and does not delay therapy for the underlying malignancy. In the postmenarchal adolescent female, delay of therapy for the malignancy is usually necessary to permit retrieval of ova.

Although the need for fertility preservation for children and adolescents is clear, there are few outcome studies that examine only those who have not had fertility preservation. Therefore, fertility rates are unknown. A survey of adult cancer survivors indicates that 34 of 260 participants or partners achieved pregnancy, with 30 of these having one or more children[11]; the data do not report what percentage of these patients had attempted pregnancy. Also, the data did not account for the almost 25% of participants who indicated that they did not want children, in part because of a fear that the cancer would return or would develop in their child.

Damage to the gonad from chemotherapy is age-related, varies between the sexes, and is more likely with use of gonadotoxic drugs. Adolescents treated before puberty are at high risk for severe damage to spermatogenetic potential and ovarian follicular dysfunction.[12] Impaired fertility following chemotherapy for malignancy[13] is related to the age at therapy. The prepubertal testicle appears to be more vulnerable to cytotoxic effects of chemotherapy than is the adult testis[14]; in contrast, the prepubertal ovarian reserve is less susceptible to cytotoxic damage than the mature ovary. In fact, most prepubertal girls are expected to retain normal ovarian function. Seventy-five percent of 25 male cancer survivors diagnosed between ages 0.9 and 15.9 years[15] had normal sperm counts. Sperm concentrations correlated positively with testicular volume and inhibin B levels and negatively with follicle stimulating hormone (FSH) concentrations.

In a group of men who had gonadotoxic therapy before puberty,[16] such fertility markers have been found to be indicative of compromised fertility although the utility of these measures in individual patients was less helpful. Differences in inhibin B, testosterone, luteinizing hormone (LH) and FSH levels, testicular volume, and sperm counts were found when men who were long-term cancer survivors were compared with a control group (**Table 1**). Low inhibin B levels but near normal testosterone levels are consistent with the greater vulnerability of sperm-producing elements than the

**Table 1**
**Parameters of fertility among adult male survivors of childhood cancer and control men**

| | Range Survivors | Range Controls | *P* value | % Abnormal Survivors | % Abnormal Controls |
|---|---|---|---|---|---|
| Inhibin B, ng/L | 0–393 | 60–556 | <.0001 | 65 | 25 |
| Testosterone, nmol/L | 2.8–45.1 | 4.7–27.7 | .05 | 8 | 10 |
| FSH, U/L | 0.3–65.8 | 0.6–18.0 | .01 | 32 | 17 |
| LH, U/L | 0.1–16.3 | 0.3–19.2 | <.0001 | 10 | 2 |
| Sperm density, $1 \times 10^6$ mL | 0.0–158.0 | 21.1–234.0 | <.0001 | 76 | 0 |
| Testis vol, mL | 2–35 | 11–30 | .391 | 17 | 14 |

Although the range is of limited usefulness for the individual patient, the overlap among the subjects with controls is pertinent.

*Abbreviations:* FSH, follicle-stimulating hormone; LH, luteinizing hormone.

*Data from* Van Casteren NJ, ver der Linden GHM, Hakvoort-Cammel FGAJ, et al. Effect of childhood cancer treatment on fertility markers in adult male long-term survivors. Pediatr Blood Cancer 2009;52:108–12.

testosterone-producing Leydig cells, both hormone levels being significantly lower in survivors than in control men. Increased LH levels in survivors suggest a component of compensation whereby greater stimulation is required to achieve physiologic testosterone levels. Mean testicular volume did not differ between the two groups, although sperm concentrations were dramatically lower in the survivors where 67% showed oligospermia or azoospermia. Individual assessment of sperm parameters, both concentration and motility, is clearly the best determinant of subfertility or infertility.

## FERTILITY PRESERVATION IN ENDOCRINE DISORDERS IN CHILDREN AND ADOLESCENTS

### *Hypothalamic-pituitary Dysfunction*

Patients with hypothalamic-pituitary dysfunction may also be candidates if the gonads developed or are preserved sufficiently so that gonadotropin-responsive germ cells are present. These conditions may be acquired, such as following high-dosage cranial irradiation, or congenital.

### *Gonadal Dysfunction, Hypoplasia, or Dysplasia*

In patients with gonadal dysgenesis who show arrested gonad development or early gonadal degeneration, there may be sufficient germ cells to permit harvesting. A small portion of Turner syndrome patients have normal puberty and normal gonadotropin secretion and are likely to be spontaneously fertile[17]; such patients do not require fertility preservation.

Conversely, most patients with Turner syndrome have very little peripubertal gonadal function and are therefore not candidates for fertility preservation; only the small portion of patients with persistent oocytes will benefit from fertility preservation. Such patients are likely to have some early, albeit usually limited, pubertal development. Their karyotype is likely mosaic or involves the loss of only a portion of the X chromosome. Moderate elevations of circulating gonadotropin levels may be present as evidence of follicular dysfunction. Because ultrasonography or MRI evaluations do not accurately assess ovarian structure or detect the presence of follicles, it is important to verify the presence of ovarian follicles with a definitive technique such as laparoscopic ovarian biopsy.

Evaluation of prognostic factors for follicular development have been reported for 57 patients with Turner syndrome.[18] The patients were categorized into three groups: (1) 15 found to have follicles after laparoscopic ovarian biopsy, (2) 32 with no follicles seen on biopsy, and (3) ovarian streaks identified and no biopsy done. Results are summarized in **Table 2** and **Fig. 1**. Baseline data are the most compelling in group one (those with follicles), which showed that 12 had mosaic karyotypes or structural abnormalities, 11 had spontaneous puberty, and 8 reached spontaneous menarche. The eight patients reaching menarche had Tanner stage 4 or 5 breast development at the time of evaluation.

In addition to spontaneous pubertal development and karyotype, positive predictive factors for detecting follicles in Turner syndrome patients were a normal serum FSH level (<11 mIU/mL) and a serum anti-Müllerian hormone (AMH) level higher than 2 pmol/L. Negative predictive values for lack of follicles (in order of importance) were: 45X karyotype, serum AMH less than 2 pmol/L, lack of spontaneous pubertal onset, an FSH value greater than 15 IU/L, and the presence of structural chromosomal abnormalities. These recent data confirm the overall impression that the presence of follicles in Turner syndrome patients will manifest itself in the data commonly obtained as part of clinical evaluation and care. These are the patients who should be considered for fertility preservation.

Although a normal FSH concentration is a positive predictive factor, the presence of an elevated FSH level does not preclude spontaneous ovulation, pregnancy, and successful birth. One such case with elevated FSH has been described in a patient

**Table 2**
**Finding among three groups of Turner patients: those having (1) follicles on ovarian biopsy, (2) no follicles on biopsy, and (3) streak ovaries on laparoscopy and not biopsy**

| Group | 1 | 2 | 3 |
|---|---|---|---|
| N | 15 | 32 | 10 |
| Age range | 11.8–18.3 y | 8–18.8 y | 8.4–17.8 y |
| LH | | | |
| Range, IU/L | 0.1–62.8 (13) | 0.1–96.2 (24) | 1.0–49.6 |
| Median | 3.4 | 7.1 | 14.6 |
| FSH | | | |
| Range, IU/L | 1–122 (13) | 3.3–96.2 (24) | 10.4–123 |
| Median | 6.1 | 19 | 110 |
| AMH | | | |
| Range, pM | 0.75–12.27 | 0.55–5.96 | 0.7–3.66 |
| Median | 2.25 | 1.1 | 1.25 |
| Spontaneous puberty | 11/15 | 8/32 | 0/10 |
| Spontaneous menarche | 8/11 | 0/32 | 0/10 |
| Tanner stage-range | 2–5 | 1 | 1 |
| Median | 5 | | |
| Biopsied | 15/15 | 32/32 | 0-streaks |

N in parentheses if less than total group.

*Abbreviations:* AMH, anti-Müllerian hormone; FSH, follicle-stimulating hormone; LH, luteinizing hormone.

*Data from* Birgit B, Julius H, Carsten R, et al. Fertility preservation in girls with Turner syndrome—prognostic signs of the presence of ovarian follicles. J Clin Endocrinol Metab 2009;94:74–80.

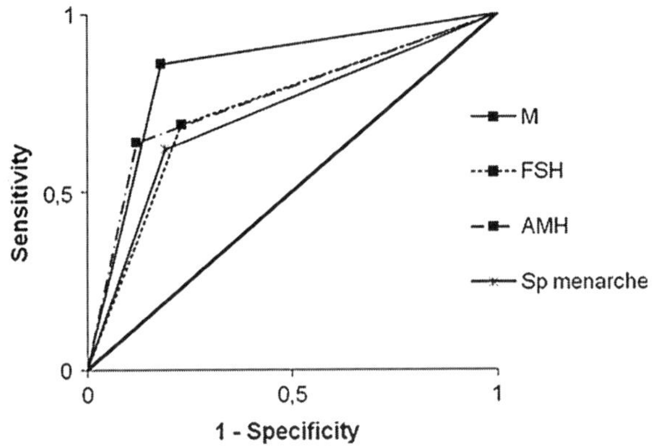


**Fig. 1.** ROC curves showing that there is higher sensitivity than specificity for the following variables: presence of a mosaic karyotype (M), normal FSH for age and stage of development (FSH), normal AMH for age (AMH) and spontaneous menarche (Sp menarche) (*From* Birgit B, Julius H, Carsten R, et al. Fertility preservation in girls with Turner syndrome—Prognostic signs of the presence of ovarian follicles. J Clin Endocrinol Metab 2009;94:74–80; with permission.)

with a mosaic karyotype, spontaneous puberty, and menarche who had a dominant follicle by ultrasonography.[19]

Fertility preservation has been attempted in a 16-year-old adolescent with mosaic Turner syndrome.[20] After laparoscopic wedge resection, visible follicles were aspirated. Eight of the 11 immature oocytes were permitted to mature in vitro and were cryopreserved. However, it is unclear whether this type of a patient is more likely to achieve pregnancy using cryopreservation than she would be without any intervention.

### *Testicular Damage, Including Those with Klinefelter Syndrome*

Boys with the Klinefelter syndrome progressively lose spermatogenic capacity. From early to midpuberty, there is clear histologic change from a testicle showing relatively normal seminiferous tubules, reduced germ cells, and normal Sertoli/Leydig-cell appearance to the adult condition showing extensive fibrosis and hyalinization of the seminiferous tubules.[21,22] As a result of Sertoli cell dysfunction, virtually all men with Klinefelter syndrome are azoospermic or markedly oligospermic by late adolescence or early adulthood. This progressive gonadal failure is correlated with increasing FSH and decreasing inhibin B and AMH levels over time.[21]

In addition to Klinefelter syndrome, if compromised spermatogenesis is found in males with a history of varicocele, cryptorchidism, testicular torsion, or orchitis, procedures of sperm retrieval and cryopreservation may be a worthwhile consideration. Because progression of testicular damage and dysfunction may occur during adolescence, early consideration of fertility preservation is paramount.

## TREATMENTS AND PROCEDURES TO PRESERVE FERTILITY

Efforts to preserve fertility depend on the sex and sexual maturation of the patient. Strategies involve two phases[23]: the first involves removal of gonadal tissue and germ cells, possible in vitro maturation, and cryopreservation, which occurs during childhood; the second phase involves using this previously obtained material in the adult who desires fertility. This may involve auto retransplantation of ovarian or testicular tissue or in vitro fertilization (IVF) using mature oocytes or spermatogonia. Autologous ovarian grafting in an oophorectomized female has resulted in a return of "ovarian" cycling.[24] Successful pregnancies have also been reported using immature spermatozoa and spermatids.[25] These techniques may also be successful in the patient with limited and progressively diminishing fertility, including the pubertal adolescent (**Figs. 2** and **3**). Procedures remain limited for the prepubertal child.

The status of fertility preservation for adult men and women has been reviewed by an expert advisory panel.[26] Techniques may be attempted in patients receiving chemotherapy or radiation therapy for malignancies, autoimmune diseases such as lupus erythematosis, and hematologic conditions such as sickle cell anemia, thalassemia major, and aplastic anemia as well as those who are undergoing gonadectomy. The lack of complete and accurate data concerning the gonadal effects of chemotherapy makes selection of at-risk patients, in which fertility preservation should be strongly considered, difficult.[27] Because of evolving chemotherapeutic regimens, the precise extent of gonadal damage remains difficult to predict. During puberty and thereafter, gonadotropin levels (LH and FSH) as well as AMH and inhibin B levels can be used as indices of gonadal integrity. Because damage may be only transient following chemotherapy or radiation therapy, these hormone measurements should be followed over time to identify trends of recovery or progressive damage.

### *Procedures for Females*

Ovulation induction in anovulatory women has been well documented[28] in those with ovarian pathology. These induction strategies can also be used in those with hypothalamic-pituitary deficiencies (hypogonadotropic or secondary gonadal failure).

Among the technical procedures, embryo cryopreservation remains the most successful and widely available modality for storing germ cells for future pregnancy. This process requires availability of both ova and sperm. For females, this procedure involves ovulation induction, harvesting ova, and storage as ova or fertilized gametes. Obtaining and cryopreserving oocytes involves a complex and time-consuming

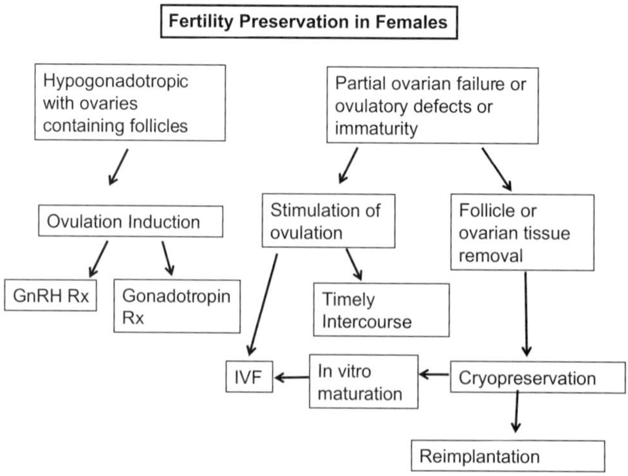


**Fig. 2.** Schematic possibilities for attempted fertility preservation among females, including children and adolescents. GnRH, gonadotropin-releasing hormone (currently unavailable in the United States; IVF, in vitro fertilization).

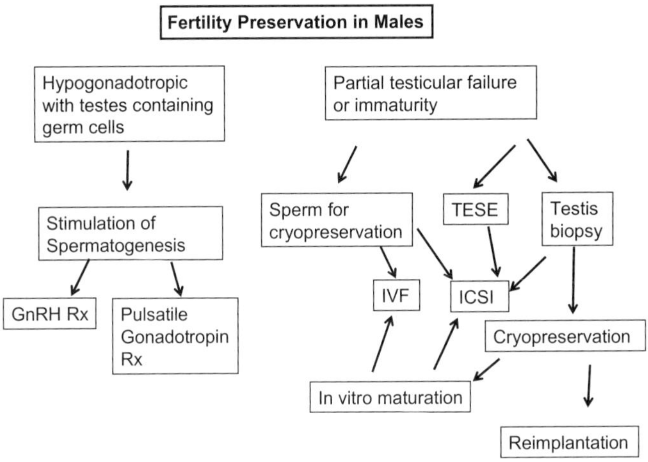


**Fig. 3.** Schematic algorithm for fertility preservation among prepubertal, pubertal and adult males. TESE, testicular sperm extraction; IVF, in vitro fertilization; ICSI, intracytoplasmic sperm injection.

ovarian stimulation called superovulation. Egg fertilization to permit cryopreservation of embryos is appropriate only when the sperm donor has been identified.

In addition to embryo cryopreservation, there have also been recent attempts to cryopreserve ova or sections of ovary. This procedure is done in anticipation of future ovarian tissue autotransplantation[29] and is dependent on type of malignancy, timing of chemotherapy, partner status, and patient's age.

Because both oocyte and embryo freezing require ovarian stimulation, novel stimulation regimens using aromatase inhibitors have been developed for women with estrogen-sensitive cancers that may be exacerbated by estrogen stimulation.[30] In vitro maturation has also been assessed in the unstimulated ovary, which avoids the issues of high cost and potential side effects of ovarian stimulation protocols.[31]

Ovarian tissue cryopreservation, a novel technology, is the only fertility preservation option for prepubertal children and the only treatment strategy allowing restoration of ovarian function. In vitro maturation, if successful, could be used in combination with ovarian tissue cryopreservation to improve fertility rates. Although fertilization of oocytes from unstimulated ovaries has been successful after in vitro maturation,[32] this process may be difficult to use in the prepubertal child, as the factors used to predict success and therefore candidacy for this technique include estradiol and FSH levels and antral follicular count[31]— measurements that would be appropriately low in the prepubertal child.

Although most prepubertal girls receiving therapy for malignancy retain some ovarian function, ovarian tissue harvesting may be appropriate for those patients judged to be at highest risk. Currently, fertilization of the egg and cryopreserving embryos would not be considered appropriate for most adolescent females, because only rarely would a sperm source be identified. The freezing of oocytes remains an option for an adolescent girl; however, the chance of retrieving an oocyte that will result in a live birth is currently very low (3%–5%).[33]

The harvesting and cryopreservation of ovarian cortex tissue for reimplantation is another option; however, limited experience with this technique precludes any meaningful estimation of its success rate. Oocytes retrieved from ovarian tissue excised before chemotherapy or radiotherapy, mature in vitro, and may then be cryopreserved.[34,35] In one report of five women who had ovarian tissue cryopreserved before chemotherapy and who later had this tissue reimplanted showed a restoration of ovarian function, albeit with elevated FSH levels, 4 to 6 months afterward.[36] Unsolved issues include cortical ischemia and follicle loss[37] and the risk of the seeding of malignant cells.[38] However, not only have normal follicles been demonstrated more than a year after autotransplantation of cryopreserved ovarian tissue,[39] but there have also been at least two live births reported following this type of reimplantation.[40,41]

## Procedures for Males

Techniques for males include sperm cryopreservation (the most available technique), sperm retrieval by testicular extraction, testicular tissue freezing, and hormonal suppression. Fertilization is attempted using intracytoplamsic sperm injection (ICSI) obtained from ejaculate, epididymal aspiration, or testicular biopsy using both fresh or cryopreserved germ cells. Fertilization and pregnancy rates using epididymal or testicular spermatozoa are unaffected by the duration of cryopreservation.[42] Germ cell transplantation, germ cell maturation in vitro, stem-cell-to-germ-cell maturation, and spermatogonial stem cells can also be used as a source of sperm.

In the boy in early puberty onward, a semen sample can be collected for sperm cryopreservation. For the boy unable to produce a sample by masturbation, alternative procedures can be used. While these methods are not well developed for prepubertal boys, the goal is to establish procedures to obtain stem cells for storage and potential reimplantation or testicular tissue for storage and culture for in vitro spermatogenesis. Although the retrieval of spermatogonial stem cells, precursors of spermatozoa, have not been attempted in prepubertal boys, studies of animal models[13,43] may form the basis for in vitro maturation of sperm or reimplantation of testicular tissue. Currently, testicular sperm extraction and testicular tissue freezing in the prepubertal child is experimental.

For pubertal or adult men with incomplete primary testicular failure who show rare sperm in the ejaculate, ICSI, a well-established treatment for men with almost any form of infertility[44] can be attempted[45] and a detailed ICSI procedure has been published.[46] The preferred technique in azoospermic men is microdissection testicular sperm extraction (TESE) from which sperm are obtained slightly more than 50% of the time. Using an operating microscope, tubules containing sperm are identified, opened, and biopsied for sperm extraction.[47] Cryopreserved testicular biopsies may also be helpful in men with congenital or acquired reproductive obstruction.

Comparisons between sperm exposed to the maturation process of passing through the reproductive tract and those obtained by TESE show that transit through the male genital tract is unnecessary. In fact, the use of testicular extracted sperm resulted in more conceptions than did ejaculated sperm from severely oligospermic men.[45]

Pretherapy planning is critical for males with malignancy. Depending on patient age and status, procedures include (1) collection and cryopreservation of ejaculated sperm for possible cryopreservation and ICSI,(2) TESE in azoospermic males or early pubertal males to obtain sperm for cryopreservation, and (3) in the future, banking testicular *stem* cells, a technique successful in laboratory animals.[48] TESE and spermatogonial stem cell retrieval[49–51] should be considered for boys with Klinefelter syndrome and other forms of gonadal failure. In a man with nonmosaic Klinefelter syndrome, testicular sperm extraction, cryopreservation, oocyte recovery, and ICSI has been reported.[52]

In men with congenital or acquired hypogonadotropic hypogonadism, pulsatile GnRH administration or intermittent gonadotropin therapy may be used for hypothalamic (GnRH) or pituitary (LH and FSH) deficiency. Both techniques effectively induce spermatogenesis and have resulted in paternity in men with responsive germ cells.[53,54]

## GONADAL PROTECTION DURING AT-RISK THERAPY

Gonad shielding during radiation therapy is a common practice and lead shielding of the testes is used when possible. In females, oophoropexy, a procedure where the ovaries are moved to a different position in the abdomen, out of the radiation field, may be used.

Hormonal suppression techniques, such as gonadotropin-releasing hormone agonist analogs (GnRHa) therapy, can be used to create a hypogonadotropic or prepubertal state and decrease the metabolic activity of the gonad, to attempt to reduce damage to germ cells.[55] Desensitizing the pituitary and indirectly and directly the ovary or testis with GnRHa therapy is a theoretical, but as yet not well demonstrated mechanism to preserve the fertility potential of a pubertal or postpubertal patient. Suggested mechanisms of action for GnRHa in females include decreasing the number of primordial follicles, decreasing vascular supply to the ovary to reduce the exposure to chemotherapeutic agents, and stimulation of antiapoptotic activity within the ovary,[56] and consequent to directly binding to the ovarian follicle, independent of gonadotropin levels.

Amelioration of the gonadotoxic effect of chemotherapy may reduce the incidence of premature ovarian failure.[57] Early data suggest that GnRHa therapy decreases rates of primary ovarian failure and is followed by a higher rate of spontaneous ovulation and menses in women treated for malignant and nonmalignant diseases.[55] A recent randomized, prospective, controlled study in adult women younger than 40 with breast cancer[58] found that 8 months after therapy, in those who received GnRH therapy, 89.6% resumed menses, 69.2% had spontaneous ovulation, and 11.4% developed ovarian failure. In the non-GnRH–treated control group, only 33.3% resumed menses and 25.6% had spontaneous ovulation.

Use of GnRHa involves a delay of 7 to 10 days before therapy for the underlying condition; although the use of a GnRH antagonist used alone, or in combination with GnRHa, would reduce that interval. Because antagonists immediately block GnRH receptors and gonadotropin release, the delay in therapy could be reduced to 3 or 4 days. GnRHa therapy as adjunctive therapy at the time of chemotherapy resulted in a larger number having resumption of cyclic ovarian function and fewer having premature ovarian failure than in the group receiving chemotherapy alone.[59]

It has been suggested that GnRHa be used for fertility preservation in conjunction with other methods, such as embryo cryopreservation after IVF.[56] There are no data that suggest the utility of GnRHa for gonadal protection in the prepubertal individual. Overall, results are encouraging that GnRHa therapy may play a role in fertility preservation in the peripubertal patient. A larger, multicentered, well-defined, age-stratified randomized trial should be considered.

## SUMMARY

Significant advances are being made in optimizing potential for fertility for children and adolescents. Although among adolescents at risk for impaired fertility adult techniques can be used, strong consideration should be given pediatric-aged patients, including prepubertal children, to removal of gonadal tissue for cryopreservation. Success with technique is summarized among adult women.[60] Ovarian cortical slices or primordial follicles obtained in childhood could be reimplanted at a later date, allowing for the possibility of successful pregnancy. In males, isolation of germ cells, either from ejaculate of TESE for future autotransplantation or in vitro maturation and cryopreservation in anticipation of ICSI should be considered. Because the duration of ovarian function following reimplantation may be short lived, transplantation should be done only when fertility is desired. For parents of patients, the parents section in the Web site www.myoncofertility.org may be helpful.

## ACKNOWLEDGMENT

The comments and suggestions of William C. Dodson, MD, Penn State College of Medicine are sincerely appreciated.

## REFERENCES

1. Tulandi T, Huang JY, Tan SL. Preservation of female fertility. An essential progress. Obstet Gynecol 2008;112:1160–72.
2. Wallace WHB, Thomson AB. Preservation of fertility in children treated for cancer. Arch Dis Child 2003;88:493–6.
3. Fallat ME, Hutter J, The Committee on Bioethics, Section on Hematology/Oncology, and Section on Surgery, American Academy of Pediatrics. Preservation of fertility in pediatric and adolescent patients with cancer. Pediatrics 2008;121:e1461–9.
4. Gerris J. Methods of semen collection not based on masturbation or surgical sperm retrieval. Hum Reprod Update 1999;5:211–5.
5. Van Casteren NJ, Dohle GR, Romijn MSC, et al. Semen cryopreservation in puberty; boys before gonadotoxic treatment and the role of endocrinologic evaluation in predicting sperm yield. Fertil Steril 2008;90:1119–25.
6. Müller J, Sønksen J, Sommer P, et al. Cryopreservation of semen from pubertal boys with cancer. Med Pediatr Oncol 2000;34:191–4.
7. Hart R. Preservation of fertility in adults and children diagnosed with cancer. BMJ 2008;337:1045–8.
8. Anderson RA. Fertility preservation techniques: laboratory and clinical progress and current issues. Reproduction 2008;136:667–9.
9. Deepinder F, Agarwal A. Technical and ethical challenges of fertility preservation in young cancer patients. Reprod Biomed Online 2008;16:784–91.
10. Blatt J. Pregnancy outcome in long-term survivors of childhood cancer. Med Pediatr Oncol 1999;33:29–33.
11. Reinmuth S, Lieeskind AK, Wickmann L, et al. Having children after surviving cancer in childhood or adolescence—results of a Berlin survey. Kiln Paediatr 2008;220:159–65.
12. Mackie EJ, Radford M, Shalet SM. Gonadal failure following chemotherapy for childhood Hodgkin's disease. Med Pediatr Oncol 1996;27:74–8.
13. Revel A, Revel-Vilk S. Pediatric fertility preservation: is it time to offer testicular tissue cryopreservation? Mol Cell Endocrinol 2008;66:784–9.
14. Edgar AB, Wallace WHB. Pregnancy in women who had cancer in childhood. Eur J Cancer 2007;43:1890–4.
15. Lahteenmäki PM, Arola M, Suominen J, et al. Male reproductive health after childhood cancer. Acta Paediatr 2008;97:935–42.

16. Van Casteren NJ, ver der Linden GHM, Hakvoort-Cammel FGAJ, et al. Effect of childhood cancer treatment on fertility markers in adult male long-term survivors. Pediatr Blood Cancer 2009;52:108–12.
17. Cools M, Rooman RPA, Wauters J, et al. A nonmosaic 45, X karyotype in a mother with Turner's syndrome and in her daughter. Fertil Steril 2004;82:923–5.
18. Birgit B, Julius H, Carsten R, et al. Fertility preservation in girls with Turner syndrome—prognostic signs of the presence of ovarian follicles. J Clin Endocrinol Metab 2009;94:74–80.
19. Livadas S, Xekouki P, Kafiri G, et al. Spontaneous pregnancy and birth of a normal female from a woman with Turner syndrome and elevated gonadotropins. Fertil Steril 2005;83:769–72.
20. Huang JYJ, Tulandi T, Holzer H, et al. Cryopreservation of ovarian tissue and in vitro matured oocytes in a female with mosaic Turner syndrome: case report. Humanit Rep 2008;23:336–9.
21. Bastida MG, Rey RA, Bergada I, et al. Establishment of testicular endocrine function impairment during childhood and puberty in boys with Klinefelter syndrome. Clin Endocrinol 2007;67:863–70.
22. Alsglaede L, Wikstrom AM, Rajpert-De Meyts, et al. Natural history of seminiferous tubule degeneration in Klinefelter syndrome. Hum Reprod Update 2006; 12:39–48.
23. Nidker J, Baylis K, McLeod C. Choice of fertility preservation in girls and adolescent women with cancer. Cancer 2006;107(Suppl):1686–9.
24. Oktay K, Karlikaya G. Ovarian function after transplantation of frozen, banked, autologous ovarian tissue. N Engl J Med 2000;342:1919.
25. Tesarik J. Fertilization of oocytes by injecting spermatozoa, spermtids, and spermatocytes. Rev Reprod 1996;1:149–52.
26. Lamar CA, DeCherney AH. Fertility preservation: state of the science and future research directions. Fertil Steril 2009;91:316–9.
27. Anderson RA, Wallace WHB, Baird DT. Ovarian cryopreservation for fertility preservation: indications and outcomes. Reproduction 2008;136:681–9.
28. The Practice Committee of the American Society for Reproductive Medicine. Use of exogenous gonadotropins in anovulatory women: a technical bulletin. Fertil Steril 2008;90(Suppl 3):S7–12.
29. Donnez J, Martinez-Madrid B, Jadoul P, et al. Ovarian tissue cryopreservation and transplantation: a review. Hum Reprod Update 2006;12:519–35.
30. Sonmezer M, Oktay K. Assisted reproduction and fertility preservation techniques in cancer patients. Curr Opin Endocrinol Diabetes Obes 2008;15:514–22.
31. Fadini R, Dal Canto MB, Renzini MM, et al. Predictive factors in in-vitro maturation in unstimulated women with normal ovaries. Reprod Biomed Online 2009;18:251–61.
32. Zhao JZ, Zhou W, Zhang W, et al. In vitro maturation and fertilization of oocytes from unstimulated ovaries in infertile women with polcystic ovary syndrome. Fertil Steril 2009;91:2568–71.
33. Gook DA, Edgar DH. Human oocyte cryopreservation. Hum Reprod Update 2007;20:591–605.
34. Huang JYJ, Tulandi T, Holzer H, et al. Combining ovarian tissue cryobanking with retrieval of immature oocytes followed by in vitro maturation and vitrification: an additional strategy of fertility preservation. Fertil Steril 2008;89:567–72.
35. Huang JYJ, Buckett WM, Gilbert L, et al. Retrieval of immature oocytes followed by in vitro maturation and vitrification: a case report on a new strategy of fertility preservation in women with borderline ovarian malignancy. Gynecol Oncol 2007; 105:542–4.

36. Donnez J, Squifflet J, Van Eyck AS, et al. Restoration of ovarian function in orthotopically transplanted cryopreserved ovarian tissue: a pilot experience. Reprod Biomed Online 2008;16:694–704.
37. Newton H, Aubard Y, Rutherford A, et al. Low temperature storage and grafting of human ovarian tissue. Humanit Rep 1996;11:1487–91.
38. Meirow D, Hardan I, Dor J, et al. Searching for evidence of disease and malignant cell contamination in ovarian tissue stored from hematologic cancer patients. Humanit Rep 2008;23:1007–13.
39. Camboni A, Martinez-Madrid B, Dolmans MM, et al. Autotransplantation of frozen-thawed ovarian tissue in a young woman: ultrastructure and viability of grafted tissue. Fertil Steril 2007;90:1215–8.
40. Donnez J, Dolmans MM, Demyalle D, et al. Live birth after orthotopic transplantation of cryopreserved ovarian tissue. Lancet 2004;364:1405–10.
41. Demeestere I, Simon P, Emiliani S, et al. Fertility preservation: successful transplantation of cryopreserved ovarian tissue in a young patient previously treated for Hodgkin's disease. Oncologist 2007;12:1437–42.
42. Wood S, Sephton V, Searle T, et al. Effect on clinical outcome of the interval between collection of epididymal and testicular spermatozoa and intracytoplamsic sperm injection in obstructive azoopsermia. J Androl 2003;24:67–72.
43. Ehmcke J, Schlatt S. Animal models for fertility preservation in the male. Reproduction 2008;136:717–23.
44. Silber SJ, Van Steirtegehem A, Liu J, et al. Normal pregnancies resulting from testicular sperm extraction and intracytoplasmic sperm injection for azoospermia due to maturation arrest. Fertil Steril 1996;66:110–7.
45. Bendikson BA, Neri QV, Takeuchi T, et al. The outcome of intracytoplasmic sperm injection using occasional spermatozoa in the ejaculate of men with spermatogenic failure. J Urol 2008;180:1060–4.
46. Palermo GD, Schlegel PN, Colombero LT, et al. Aggressive sperm immobilization prior to intracytoplasmic sperm injection with immature spermatozoa improves fertilization and pregnancy rates. Humanit Rep 1999;15:1023–9.
47. Schlegel PN. Male infertility: evaluation and sperm retrieval. Clin Obstet Gynecol 2006;49:55–72.
48. Zhang Z, Renfree MB, Short RV. Successful intra- and interspecific male germ cell transplantation in the rat. Biol Reprod 2003;68:961–7.
49. Paduch DA, Fine RG, Bolyakov A, et al. New concepts in Klinefelter syndrome. Curr Opin Urol 2008;18:621–7.
50. Krausz C, Forti G. Sperm cryopreservation in male infertility due to genetic disorders. Cell Tissue Bank 2006;7:105–12.
51. Tournaye H, Goosens E, Verheven G, et al. Preserving the reproductive potential of men and boys with cancer: current concepts and future prospects. Hum Reprod Update 2004;10:525–32.
52. Greco E, Iacobelli M, Rienzi L, et al. Birth of a healthy boy after fertilization if cryopreserved oocytes with cryopreserved testicular spermatozoa from a man with nonmosaic Klinefelter syndrome. Fertil Steril 2008;89:e5–7.
53. Büchter D, Behre HM, Kliesch S, et al. Pulsatile GnRH or human chorionic gonadotropin/human menopausal gonadotropin as effective treatment for men with hypogonadotropic hypogonadism: a review of 42 cases. Eur J Endocrinol 1998;139: 298–303.
54. Zitzmann M, Nieschlag E. Hormone substitution in male hypogonadism. Mol Cell Endocrinol 2000;161:73–88.

55. Lee PA, Houk CP. Recommendation on the use of GnRH in pediatrics. In: Lunenfeld B, editor. GnRH analogs in human reproduction. London: Taylor & Francis; 2005. p. 89–100. Chapter 6.
56. Blumenfeld Z. How to preserve fertility in young women exposed to chemotherapy? The role of GnRH agonist cotreatment in addition to cryopreservation of embryos, oocytes, or ovaries. Oncologist 2007;12:1044–54.
57. Blumenfeld Z. GnRH-agonist in fertility preservation. Curr Opin Endocrinol Diabetes Obes 2008;15:523–8.
58. Badawy A, Elnashar A, El-Ashry M, et al. Gonadotropin-releasing hormone agonists for prevention of chemotherapy-induced ovarian damage: prospective randomized study. Fertil Steril 2008;91:694–7.
59. Blumenfeld Z, Avivi I, Eckman A, et al. Gonadotropin-releasing hormone agonist decreases chemotherapy-induced gonadotoxicity and premature ovarian failure in young female patients with Hodgkin lymphoma. Fertil Steril 2008;89:166–73.
60. Meirow D. Fertility preservation in cancer patients using stored ovarian tissue: clinical aspects. Curr Opin Endocrinol Diabetes Obes 2008;15:536–47.

# Prevention of Type 1 Diabetes

Diane K. Wherrett, MD, FRCPC, Denis Daneman, MBBCh, FRCPC*

**KEYWORDS**

- Type 1 diabetes • Autoimmunity • Prevention • Immunology
- Genetics • Clinical trials

Type 1 diabetes (T1D) is an autoimmune disease in which the β cells of the pancreatic islets are destroyed, rendering the individual increasingly incapable of mounting a normal insulin response to ingested nutrients.[1,2] In the early 1980s, Eisenbarth[2] enunciated the main phases in the pathogenesis of T1D (**Fig. 1**), a framework which continues to be useful in considering approaches to the prevention or cure of this disorder:

1. Susceptibility to T1D is inherited through a series of genes, the most important of which relate to the HLA class II locus on chromosome 6, with lesser contribution from several others, including the insulin gene, CTLA4 and others (see later discussion). Susceptibility genes are essential, but insufficient in explaining the immune pathogenesis of T1D, that is, most individuals with these susceptibility genes never develop the disorder.
2. Exposure to 1 or more environmental triggers alters the immune system in such a way that susceptibility is converted to pathophysiology and destruction of β cells begins. Despite intensive searches for environmental triggers, the number of candidates being assessed in clinical trials remains small, for example, cow's milk proteins, relative lack of vitamin D, and supplementation with omega-3 fatty acids.[3–7]
3. Although attack on the β cells is mediated in large part by T cells, it is the presence of humoral (B-cell) markers that punctuates the next phase: normal glucose homeostasis in the presence of 1 or more T1D-specific autoantibodies; ICA512/IA-2, insulin autoantibody (IAA) and glutamic acid decarboxylase (GAD) are the main ones available for measurement. The progression to clinical T1D is highly predictable based on the number of antibodies present.[8]
4. The earliest metabolic abnormality detected is loss of first phase insulin secretion in response to an intravenous glucose load. Glucose levels remain normal in response to meal challenges at this stage. Later, impaired glucose tolerance develops. This leads inexorably to the next phases of clinical diabetes.

Division of Endocrinology, Department of Pediatrics, The Hospital for Sick Children and University of Toronto, 555 University Avenue, Toronto, Ontario M5G 1X8, Canada
* Corresponding author.
*E-mail address:* denis.daneman@sickkids.ca (D. Daneman).

Endocrinol Metab Clin N Am 38 (2009) 777–790
doi:10.1016/j.ecl.2009.08.006 endo.theclinics.com
0889-8529/09/$ – see front matter 

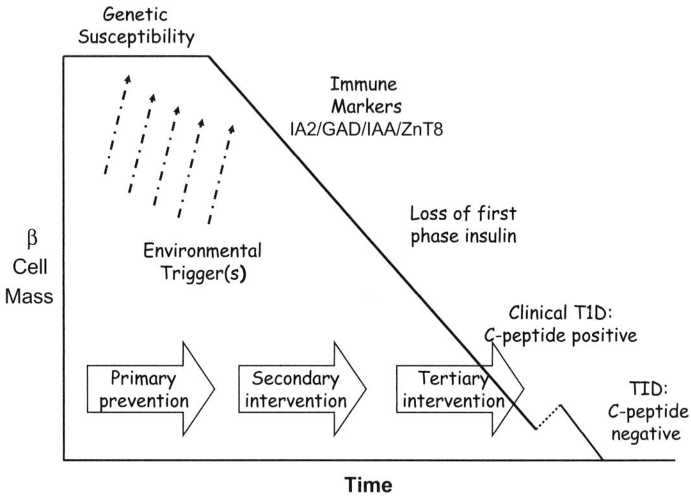


**Fig. 1.** The natural history of T1D.

5. When β-cell mass is significantly decreased, insulin secretory capacity is damaged to such a degree that it is no longer sufficient to maintain normoglycemia and clinical diabetes supervenes. This phase includes the honeymoon or remission period of T1D when some β-cell function is retained, also called the C-peptide–positive phase of clinical diabetes.
6. Finally, in most, but not all, individuals with T1D, β cell function is eventually completely lost and C-peptide levels become undetectable. There is a relationship between the presence of diabetic ketoacidosis at disease onset and the rapidity of loss of β cells, and between the presence of residual β-cell function and the ability to achieve and maintain better metabolic control.

A few additional facts are important in considering targets for prevention or early intervention in the pathogenesis of T1D[9]: Firstly, the incidence of this condition is increasing by 2% to 5% per year worldwide, especially in the youngest age group (<5 years of age).[10] Secondly, there is enormous variability in incidence of T1D around the world, from less than 4 per 100,000 in a population younger than 14 years in much of Africa and Asia to more than 20, in Canada, Australia, and parts of Europe, with the highest incidence being in Finland (>50 per 100,000 in the population reported in 2008).[11] Thirdly, migrating populations take on the increased incidence of their new countries fairly rapidly, for example, Asian immigrants to the United Kingdom, immigrants from the Horn of Africa (Somalia, Eritrea, and Ethiopia) to North America.[12] Fourthly, there is evidence that genetically similar populations may have enormously dissimilar incidence rates, for example, Finland and Russian Karelia.[13] These factors strongly indicate an important role for environmental factors in the cause of T1D, because genetic drift cannot explain the rapidity of these changes. Furthermore, where incidence is increasing most rapidly, the contribution of genetic susceptibility seems to be less.[14]

## GENETICS OF T1D

T1D is 15 times more common in siblings of those with T1D, with the general population prevalence of approximately 0.4% and the sibling prevalence of approximately 6%.[15] Genes located within the HLA class II region on chromosome 6p21 account for approximately 50% of genetic risk of T1D.[16,17] Haplotypes associated with T1D include DQ2 (DQB1*0201–DQA1*0501–DRB1*03) and DQ8 (DQB1*0302–DQA1*0301–DRB1*04).[18] Other HLA alleles, DQA1*0102, DQB1*0602 confer protection from T1D.[19] A region in the regulatory region of the insulin gene (INS) locus has also been shown to provide approximately 10% of the genetic susceptibility to T1D.[18] A polymorphism in the PTPN22 (protein tyrosine phosphatase non-receptor type 22) gene has been found to be associated with several autoimmune diseases, including T1D and autoimmune thyroid disease.[18] The gene product, a lymphoid tyrosine phosphatase, inhibits the T-cell receptor signaling pathway. Polymorphisms in the cytotoxic T-lymphocyte–associated gene (CTLA4) are also associated with T1D and several other autoimmune diseases.[20] Signaling through CTLA4 is critical in the down-regulation of T-cell responses. Over 40 genes/regions have been confirmed to be associated with T1D. Identification of these genes provides investigative targets for new understanding of disease pathogenesis.

Although there have been important discoveries in the genetics of T1D and the autoimmune processes involved, little progress has been made in identifying highly specific environmental factors pivotal in triggering this disorder. Two hypotheses remain prominent in this respect: (1) the hygiene hypothesis suggests that in modern society, the lack of exposure to pathogens early in life prevents the genetically predisposed immune system from protecting itself from autoimmune phenomena, (2) the accelerator hypothesis suggests that increasing worldwide obesity stresses the susceptible β-cell, thereby triggering its early demise.[21–27] The only environmental trigger undergoing active investigation is early exposure to cow's milk proteins, which may be important in T1D pathogenesis; conversely, breast milk may protect against triggering of the autoimmune attack. The effort to better identify environmental factors is currently being led by The Environmental Determinants of Diabetes in the Young study. This study is scheduled to enroll 7800 infants by the end of 2009 with high-risk HLA genotypes for serial assessment of islet autoimmunity and environmental exposures, such as diet, infectious diseases, and immunizations.[28]

## TARGETS FOR PREVENTION OR EARLY INTERVENTION

Prevention of T1D would require interventions aimed at (1) avoiding exposure to environmental triggers early in life—primary prevention; (2) interfering with the autoimmune cascade that occurs during β-cell destruction—secondary prevention or intervention; or (3) halting or reversing β-cell loss after clinical presentation of T1D—tertiary intervention. Once full-blown clinical T1D has developed, the only approach to disease reversal would be physiologic insulin replacement using either an artificial pancreas or β-cell replacement with islet or pancreatic transplantation. T1D is seen as one of the disorders most likely to be amenable to stem cell therapy in the future.

## PRIMARY PREVENTION

An environmental role in the pathophysiology of T1D is supported by a number of factors: low concordance rate of the disorder in identical twins (20%–50%); different incidence rates in populations of similar genetic makeup but significantly different socioeconomic status (eg, Finland and Russian Karelia); and rapid shifts in incidence in different areas of the world and with population migration. The specific environmental factors involved remain largely unproven, although epidemiologic and animal-model data suggest a potential role for dietary factors, more specifically, early exposure to cow's milk and low vitamin D concentrations, with much more data pointing to a role for cow's milk proteins.[3–7,29]

There are good data to indicate that the pathogenetic processes leading to T1D may begin very early in life. This data, with animal-model and epidemiologic data, has provided the impetus to evaluate carefully the role of weaning diets on the evolution of T1D, especially the role of early exposure to cow's milk proteins. A more detailed description of the supporting data is beyond the scope of this article but can be found in references.[3–7,29]

The Trial to Reduce IDDM (insulin-dependent diabetes mellitus) in the Genetically at Risk (TRIGR) is a double-blind, randomized placebo-controlled trial that is intended for definitively testing the hypothesis that weaning to a hydrolyzed diet, thereby avoiding early cow's milk protein exposure, protects high-risk newborns from initiation of the β-cell–specific autoimmune response, and therefore prevents T1D.[30] This international multicenter study is powered to meet these objectives. The recruitment of high-risk neonates allows for concentration of subjects more likely to develop T1D, the criterion being that their mother, father, or sibling has T1D. They are screened for high-risk HLA haplotypes. If results are positive, the neonates are randomly assigned to 1 of 2 groups: feeding up to 6 to 8 months of age with a regular cow's milk-based formula, or an extensively hydrolyzed cow's milk formula. Breast feeding is encouraged and noted as a potential confounder in the study. The study design is shown in **Fig. 2** and inclusion and exclusion criteria are listed below:

Neonates with a first-degree relative (ie, mother/father/sibling) with T1D are eligible.

Inclusion criteria

1. The infant has one of the following genotypes:
   a. HLA-DQB1*0302/DQA1*05-DQB1*02
   b. HLA-DQB1*0302/x (ie, excluding DQB1*02, DQB1*0301, DQB1*0602)
   c. HLA-DQA1*05–DQB1*02/y (ie, excluding DQA1*0201-DQB1*02, DQB1*001, DQB1*0602/3)
   d. HLA-DQA1*03–DQB1*02/y (ie, excluding the same ones as in [c]. above)
2. Family able to provide written informed consent

Exclusion criteria

1. An older sibling in TRIGR intervention
2. Multiple gestation
3. Parents unwilling or unable to give study formula
4. Newborn has recognizable severe illness
5. Inability of family to participate in the study

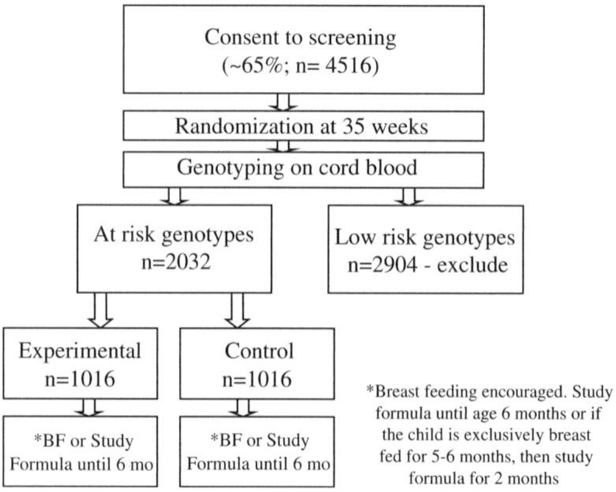


**Fig. 2.** TRIGR design.

6. Infant received any formula other than Nutramigen before randomization
7. Infant older than 7 days at randomization
8. No HLA sample before 8 days of age.

The major outcome for the first phase of TRIGR is the frequency of T1D-associated autoantibodies and/or development of diabetes by age 6 years. The outcome of the second phase is the manifestation of diabetes by age 10 years according to standard criteria, obviously the more definitive outcome, although the intervention may delay rather than prevent the manifestation of T1D. This latter outcome would be masked by the final outcome being measured at age 10 years.[30] Screening for TRIGR began in May 2002, with final enrollment completed by September 2006. The antibody data will be available in 2012 and the T1D outcomes in 2016.

A double-blind placebo-controlled pilot study of omega-3 fatty acid supplementation with docosahexaenoic acid (DHA) to prevent islet autoimmunity is being performed by the Type 1 Diabetes TrialNet study group.[31] Diets higher in omega-3 fatty acids have been associated with lower risk of islet autoimmunity and diabetes.[32] DHA is known to have an anti-inflammatory effect. Entry to the study was during the third trimester for pregnant mothers or during the first 5 months of life for infants with a first-degree relative with T1D. At birth, HLA typing was done on cord blood and those with high risk alleles were eligible. Enrollment of 97 infants is complete with results of compliance, levels of whole blood DHA, and inflammatory markers expected in late 2009.

A feasibility study, BABYDIET, of delay of introduction of gluten to prevent islet autoimmunity in infants with a first-degree relative with T1D and high-risk HLA genotypes is under way in Germany.[33] The timing of introduction of cereals to infants has been associated with diabetes.[34] Infants were randomized to introduction of gluten at age 6 or 12 months with follow-up every 3 months up to 36 months of age.

Vitamin D is increasingly recognized as an immunomodulator. Its effects on the immune system are multifold:

1. In acquired immunity, Vitamin D induces an inhibitory response through reduction of T-cell proliferation, interleukin-2 and interferon-$\gamma$ production, and CD8-mediated cytotoxicity. This results in a reduction of T-helper 1 responses and a promotion of T-helper 2 responses. In this way, it improves T-regulatory forces and provides for a more balanced and tolerogenic milieu[35];
2. In the innate immune system, Vitamin D inhibits dendritic cell function at multiple levels and mediates antibacterial actions through cathelicidin and the toll-like receptor 4 pathway.[35]

Animal models show that treatment with 1,25$(OH)_2$Vitamin $D_3$ or its analogs can prevent T1D and other immune-modulated disorders.[35] Furthermore, there are data on humans that suggest that Vitamin D may also play a role. For example, the incidence of T1D increases with increasing distance from the equator suggesting a role for sun exposure. A published meta-analysis examined the association between vitamin D supplementation and the development of T1D. It found a significantly reduced risk of developing T1D in those supplemented with vitamin D (OR 0.71).[36] A definitive prospective study on the effect of vitamin D supplementation on the development of diabetes remains to be performed.

## SECONDARY PREVENTION

The goal of secondary prevention studies is to prevent the progression of islet destruction that will lead to overt T1D. To carry out these studies, reliable prediction models are required. Current prediction models use combinations of autoantibodies and measures of glucose tolerance to stratify risk. It is known that autoantibodies typically develop years before onset of diabetes. These antibodies include ICA, IAA, and antibodies to GAD, tyrosine phosphatase (IA-2/ICA512), and zinc transporter 8 (ZnT8).[37] The presence of 2 or more antibodies indicates a significantly increased risk of developing diabetes, with some studies reporting increasing risk with increasing number of antibodies. One study showed that relatives with 1 or more antibodies had a 25% risk of disease development over a 5-year period, 2 or more antibodies had a 39% risk of developing T1D within 3 years, and those with 3 or more antibodies had a 75% risk of disease development over a 5-year period.[38] As β-cell destruction progresses, subclinical glucose abnormalities develop. Evidence from the Diabetes Prevention Trial - Type 1 (DPT-1), showed that fasting and 2-hour glucose levels rise gradually, as stimulated C-peptide levels slowly decline in the 30 months before diagnosis.[39] Type 1 Diabetes TrialNet, an international study group performing research in the prevention and early treatment of T1D, is running a large longitudinal observational study of relatives of those with T1D to further improve prediction.[40]

Three large multi-center trials of diabetes prevention in autoantibody-positive subjects have been completed. The European Nicotinamide Diabetes Intervention Trial used nicotinamide as a secondary preventative agent. Despite promising animal data and evidence from a previous study, nicotinamide administration in ICA-positive relatives did not delay the onset of T1D when compared with placebo.[41] In DPT-1, insulin was given orally or parenterally to alter the immune response toward insulin.[42,43] Subjects at high risk (>50% over 5 years with ICA positive and low first-phase insulin response) of developing T1D received parenteral insulin. Those at moderate risk (25%–50% over 5 years with ICA and IAA but normal first-phase insulin secretion) received insulin orally. The primary analysis of both arms of DPT-1 did not show an effect on the development of T1D.[42] Post hoc analysis of DPT-1 oral insulin arm, however, suggested a beneficial effect in the subgroup with high titers of insulin autoantibodies.[43] The results of the T1D Prediction and Prevention Study were recently published.[44] In this study, newborns from the general population and siblings of those with diabetes had HLA genotyping done at birth. Those with 2 or more islet antibodies and high-risk HLA alleles were treated with nasal insulin or placebo. The study was stopped early as the treatment had no effect. The results of these studies, though disappointing, demonstrate that large scale prevention studies are feasible and provide significant insight into planning for future studies.

There are currently 3 diabetes prevention trials underway. The first is the Type 1 Diabetes TrialNet study, "Oral Insulin For Prevention of Diabetes In Relatives at Risk for Type 1 Diabetes Mellitus." This study is further investigating the suggestion of oral insulin benefit as seen in the DPT-1 subjects with high IAA titers. Subjects have insulin autoantibodies and one of ICA, GAD antibodies, or ICA512 antibodies. The study intervention is oral insulin 7.5 mg/d or placebo for the study's duration with the endpoint, the development of diabetes. Recruitment began in 2007. The Pre-POINT trial is an international multicenter study that is examining intervention with nasal and oral insulin in children aged 18 months to 7 years who have a sibling or 2 or more relatives with T1D.[45] These children also have high-risk HLA alleles but no islet autoantibodies. The effects of 4 doses of oral and nasal insulin are being studied to determine whether autoimmunity will be affected. If the study is successful, a larger trial is planned.

The Intranasal Insulin Trial is based in Australia and New Zealand and is assessing the effect of intranasal insulin in first- and second-degree relatives aged 4 to 30 years who are at increased risk of diabetes based on data from an earlier pilot study.[46] Treatment continues for one year with follow-up for the development of diabetes for 4 years.

## TERTIARY PREVENTION

It has long been recognized that most individuals presenting with T1D have little residual insulin secretion (as measured by C-peptide secretion) at the time of diagnosis.[47,48] However, in the weeks to months after diagnosis and initiation of insulin treatment, there can be substantial recovery of β-cell function with falling insulin requirements, increasing C-peptide concentrations, and easily controlled blood glucose levels.[47,48] This "honeymoon" or remission period of diabetes may last from weeks to months and occasionally years.[49] The honeymoon period is believed to be the result of the recovery of residual β cells unable to cope with the metabolic demands of the body. With institution of insulin treatment and reestablishment of glycemic control, these cells recover their capacity for insulin secretion only to be finally destroyed by the underlying autoimmune process. In addition, changes in insulin sensitivity probably also play a role in the expression of the honeymoon period, with decreased sensitivity at the time of diagnosis due to the hyperglycemia, with improvement after establishment of metabolic control.[50]

The ability to measure C-peptide concentrations in those receiving insulin therapy allows an accurate assessment of residual β-cell function, and it can be used as a marker of the efficacy of therapeutic intervention.[51] Prolongation of the honeymoon period has the potential to have significant beneficial effects in those with T1D. Metabolic control is much easier to establish in the presence of some residual insulin secretion. As a result, long-term diabetes-related complications are significantly less prevalent in those with residual insulin secretion. This was well demonstrated in the Diabetes Control and Complications Trial in which those subjects with sustained C-peptide production were found to have rates of nephropathy, retinopathy, and hypoglycemia that were half that of those without any residual insulin.[52] The population of newly diagnosed T1D patients therefore represents an important group for future study of promising new interventions. Therapies that can safely maintain endogenous insulin secretion in the longer term would represent an important clinical advance.

Several agents, including, cyclosporine, azathioprine, and prednisone, were studied in the 1980s for their efficacy in maintaining insulin production after the diagnosis of diabetes.[53–56] Some beneficial effects were observed, but toxicity concerns made further use of these agents unfavorable. Several immunomodulatory monoclonal antibodies have been studied. The monoclonal antibody hOKT3γ1 (Ala-Ala), interferes with T-cell activation by binding the T-cell receptor, CD3.[57] Herold and colleagues[58,59] showed that this modified anti-CD3 monoclonal antibody maintained C-peptide production over 2 years after 1 course administered in newly diagnosed patients within 6 weeks of diagnosis. A reduction in HbA1c and lower insulin doses were found in the treated group when compared with the untreated group. A European multicenter trial showed that a single course of a very similar modified anti-CD3 antibody, ChAglyCD3, in newly diagnosed patients resulted in higher C-peptide production and reduced insulin doses for 18 months following treatment when compared with placebo.[60] These results were most pronounced among patients with C-peptide production at, or higher than, the 50th percentile. Another study of this modified CD3 molecule has recently completed enrollment through the Immune Tolerance Network. In this study, new onset subjects between 3 and 30 years of age within 8 weeks of diagnosis will receive 2 doses of hOKT3γ1 (Ala-Ala), one at the initiation of the study and a second dose one year later. The study will follow C-peptide production over 2 years from the initiation of treatment. In addition, the manufacturers of these modified CD3 molecules are sponsoring trials of these agents, the DEFEND-1 and Protégé studies, in recent-onset patients.

**Table 1**
**Active studies with ongoing enrollment and their eligibility criteria**

| Study | Eligibility criteria |
|---|---|
| Natural History Study of the Development of Type 1 Diabetes<br>Sponsor: TrialNet Study Group | • Does not have diabetes<br>• 1–45 years of age and first-degree relative of a person with T1D<br>• 1–20 years of age and second- or third-degree relative of a person with T1D |
| Oral Insulin For Prevention of Diabetes In Relatives at Risk for Type 1 Diabetes Mellitus<br>Sponsor: TrialNet Study Group | • 3[a]–45 years of age with a relative with T1D<br>• Insulin autoantibodies and one other diabetes autoantibody<br>• Normal glucose tolerance |
| Effects of Recombinant Human Glutamic Acid Decarboxylase Formulated in Alum on the Progression of T1D in New Onset Subjects<br>Sponsor: TrialNet Study Group | • 3–45 years of age<br>• Within 3 months of diagnosis of diabetes<br>• GAD antibodies<br>• Stimulated C-peptide levels $\geq$0.2 pmol/mL[a] |
| Study of Thymoglobulin to Arrest Newly Diagnosed Type 1 Diabetes (START)<br>Sponsor: Immune Tolerance Network | • 12–35 years of age<br>• Diagnosis of diabetes within the 12 weeks before study entry<br>• Positive for 1 or more autoantibodies (anti-GAD, anti-insulin, or IA-2 autoantibodies)<br>• Stimulated C-peptide level >0.4 pmol/mL |
| Trial of Intranasal Insulin in Children and Young Adults at Risk of Type 1 Diabetes (INIT II)<br>Sponsor: Melbourne Health/Diabetes Vaccine Development Center | • Age 4–30 years if first-degree relative of a person with T1D<br>• Age 4–20 years if second-degree relative of a person with T1D<br>• Two or more diabetes autoantibodies<br>• Normal glucose tolerance<br>• First phase insulin relase more than threshold |

| | |
|---|---|
| Primary Intervention with Oral/Nasal Insulin for Prevention of Type 1 Diabetes in Infants at High Genetic Risk to Develop Type 1 Diabetes (Pre-POINT)<br>Sponsor: Juvenile Diabetes Research Foundation | • Ages between 18 months and 7 years<br>• High-risk HLA genotype<br>• Sibling or both parents with diabetes<br>• Does not have diabetes or diabetes autoantibodies |
| Phase 3 Trial of Otelixizumab for Adults With Newly Diagnosed Type 1 Diabetes Mellitus (Autoimmune): DEFEND-1<br>Sponsor: Tolerx/Juvenile Diabetes Research Foundation | • Ages 18–35 years<br>• Diagnosis of diabetes mellitus, no more than 90 days between diagnosis and administration of study drug<br>• Stimulated C-peptide level greater than 0.20 nmol/L and less than or equal to 3.50 nmol/L<br>• Positive for one or both of the following antibodies: ICA (anti-IA2) and/or GAD autoantibodies |
| The Protégé Study - Clinical Trial of Teplizumab in Children and Adults With Recent-Onset Type 1 Diabetes Mellitus<br>Sponsor: MacroGenics | • Ages 8–35 years<br>• Diagnosis of T1D mellitus within 12 weeks<br>• Detectable fasting or stimulated C-peptide level<br>• Positive for ICA512/IA-2, GAD autoantibodies, or IAA (if present during the first 2 weeks, but not beyond 2 weeks, of insulin treatment) |

[a] Currently 16–45, will be changed to 3–45 after regulatory approval.

The TrialNet study group is performing several trials in individuals newly diagnosed with T1D. The first such TrialNet study assessed the role of mycophenolate mofetil (MMF) and dacluzimab (DZB) in maintaining C-peptide production. MMF and DZB have been shown to be effective in transplantation regimens and are well characterized and tolerated. This study was stopped early when analysis of C-peptide production one year after initiation of treatment revealed no difference between the groups receiving both drugs or placebo.

TrialNet is also investigating the use of the anti-B lymphocyte monoclonal antibody, rituximab, in preserving C-peptide production in 8- to 40-year-olds with new onset diabetes. Rituximab depletes mature B cells thereby reducing antigen presentation to T cells. It has been shown to be effective in other autoimmune diseases including lupus and rheumatoid arthritis.[61] Eighty-seven subjects were randomized to this study with results available in mid-2009.

CTLA4, a costimulatory molecule expressed on T cells is an important negative regulator of T-cell activation. CTLA4-Ig is a monoclonal antibody that binds to the costimulatory molecules CD80 and CD86, blocking the costimulation that is required for full T-cell activation. This antibody is approved for use in rheumatoid arthritis. In the ongoing TrialNet study, CTLA4-Ig (abatacept) is being used in a placebo-controlled study in new-onset subjects. Treatment is being given to 112 subjects with two-thirds receiving active therapy and one-third receiving placebo infusions over 2 years, with recruitment completed in 2009 and results expected in 2011.

GAD is an important antigen in T1D. Animal studies have shown that administration of GAD to induce immune tolerance can prevent diabetes.[62] A recent study showed that 2 doses of GAD formulated in alum given within 6 months of diagnosis slowed the decrease of C-peptide production over the first 30 months after initiation of therapy.[63] This study involved 70 subjects aged between 10 and 18 years with fasting C-peptide greater than 0.1 mmol/L. TrialNet has launched a trial of 2 or 3 injections of GAD in alum versus placebo in 126 new-onset subjects that will include children as young as 3 years. The primary endpoint of this study will be C-peptide production at 1 year after initiation of treatment.

A small randomized placebo-controlled pilot study of the antitumor necrosis factor drug, etanercept, was recently reported.[64] The drug was given by subcutaneous injection twice weekly for 24 weeks in 18 children within 4 weeks of diagnosis. C-peptide production was significantly greater in the treatment group with lower HbA1c and smaller insulin doses. Other interventions currently under investigation or planned for study in this patient population, are anakinra, thymoglobulin, antithymocyte globulin, GAD/lansoprazole/sitagliptin, efalizumab, intensive metabolic control, and atorvastatin. **Table 1** lists active studies and their eligibility criteria.

### *"Curing" Established T1D*

Once full-blown T1D has developed, immune interventions are unlikely to be effective because the vast majority of β cells have been destroyed. At this stage, effective interventions would include β-cell implantation as part of pancreatic or islet cell transplantation, or of gene therapy using implanted cells capable of producing insulin in response to glycemia, or of stem-cell–derived β cells. Pancreatic transplantation has been successfully applied, particularly in combination with kidney transplantation necessitated by diabetes-related end-stage renal failure. The paucity of donors and the need for lifelong immune suppression to prevent organ rejection have limited the application of these transplants. Islet cell transplantation enjoyed a period of success when investigators in Edmonton were able to show prolonged graft survival and an insulin-free period. However, limited supply of islets, side effects of the immunosuppression, and eventual return to insulin dependence all challenge the ability of this approach to have a broad impact.

Genetic engineering and stem cell biology hold out the most hope in the long run for a cure for T1D and elimination of the need to inject insulin. With respect to gene therapy, cells have been created in which insulin secretion is possible. However, insulin is produced in small amounts and unregulated by blood sugar concentrations. Stem cells are currently under intensive evaluation; however, successful therapy for diabetes and other immune disorders remains elusive.

## REFERENCES

1. Devendra D, Liu E, Eisenbarth GS, et al. Type 1 diabetes: recent developments. BMJ 2004;328(7442):750–4.
2. Eisenbarth GS. Type I diabetes mellitus. A chronic autoimmune disease. N Engl J Med 1986;314(21):1360–8.
3. Akerblom HK, Vaarala O, Hyoty H, et al. Environmental factors in the etiology of type 1 diabetes. Am J Med Genet 2002;115(1):18–29.
4. Helgason T, Jonasson MR. Evidence for a food additive as a cause of ketosis-prone diabetes. Lancet 1981;2(8249):716–20.
5. Thorsdottir I, Ramel A. Dietary intake of 10- to 16-year-old children and adolescents in central and northern Europe and association with the incidence of type 1 diabetes. Ann Nutr Metab 2003;47(6):267–75.
6. Vaarala O, Knip M, Paronen J, et al. Cow's milk formula feeding induces primary immunization to insulin in infants at genetic risk for type 1 diabetes. Diabetes 1999;48(7):1389–94.
7. Virtanen SM, Laara E, Hypponen E, et al. Cow's milk consumption, HLA-DQB1 genotype, and type 1 diabetes: a nested case-control study of siblings of children with diabetes. Childhood diabetes in Finland study group. [erratum appears in Diabetes 2000;49(9):1617]. Diabetes 2000;49(6):912–7.
8. Barker JM, Yu J, Yu L, et al. Autoantibody "subspecificity" in type 1 diabetes: risk for organ-specific autoimmunity clusters in distinct groups. Diabetes Care 2005; 28(4):850–5.
9. Daneman D. State of the world's children with diabetes. Pediatr Diabetes 2009; 10(2):120–6.
10. International Diabetes Federation. Diabetes atlas. 3rd edition. Brussels. (Belgium): International Diabetes Federation; 2006. Available at: http://www.eatlas.idf.org.
11. Tuomilehto J, Karvonen M, Pitkaniemi J, et al. Record-high incidence of type I (insulin-dependent) diabetes mellitus in Finnish children. The Finnish Childhood Type I Diabetes Registry Group. Diabetologia 1999;42(6):655–60.
12. Raymond NT, Jones JR, Swift PG, et al. Comparative incidence of type I diabetes in children aged under 15 years from South Asian and White or other ethnic backgrounds in Leicestershire, UK, 1989 to 1998. Diabetologia 2001;44(Suppl 3):B32–6.
13. Kondrashova A, Reunanen A, Romanov A, et al. A six-fold gradient in the incidence of type 1 diabetes at the eastern border of Finland. Ann Med 2005; 37(1):67–72.
14. Gillespie KM, Bain SC, Barnett AH, et al. The rising incidence of childhood type 1 diabetes and reduced contribution of high-risk HLA haplotypes. Lancet 2004; 364(9446):1699–700.
15. Redondo MJ, Eisenbarth GS. Genetic control of autoimmunity in type I diabetes and associated disorders. Diabetologia 2002;45(5):605–22.

16. Atkinson MA, Eisenbarth GS. Type 1 diabetes: new perspectives on disease pathogenesis and treatment. Lancet 2001;358(9277):221–9.
17. Achenbach P, Bonifacio E, Koczwara K, et al. Natural history of type 1 diabetes. Diabetes 2005;54(Suppl 2):S25–31.
18. Huber A, Menconi F, Corathers S, et al. Joint genetic susceptibility to type 1 diabetes and autoimmune thyroiditis: from epidemiology to mechanisms. Endocr Rev 2008;29(6):697–725.
19. Barker JM. Clinical review: type 1 diabetes-associated autoimmunity: natural history, genetic associations, and screening. J Clin Endocrinol Metab 2006; 91(4):1210–7.
20. Cooper JD, Smyth DJ, Smiles AM, et al. Meta-analysis of genome-wide association study data identifies additional type 1 diabetes risk loci. Nat Genet 2008; 40(12):1399–401.
21. Ball TM, Castro-Rodriguez JA, Griffith KA, et al. Siblings, day-care attendance, and the risk of asthma and wheezing during childhood. N Engl J Med 2000; 343(8):538–43.
22. Betts P, Mulligan J, Ward P, et al. Increasing body weight predicts the earlier onset of insulin-dependant diabetes in childhood: testing the 'accelerator hypothesis' (2). Diabet Med 2005;22(2):144–51.
23. Daneman D. Is the 'Accelerator Hypothesis' worthy of our attention? Diabet Med 2005;22(2):115–7.
24. Gale EA. A missing link in the hygiene hypothesis? Diabetologia 2002;45(4): 588–94.
25. Kaila B, Taback SP. The effect of day care exposure on the risk of developing type 1 diabetes: a meta-analysis of case-control studies. Diabetes Care 2001;24(8):1353–8.
26. von Mutius E, Martinez FD, Fritzsch C, et al. Skin test reactivity and number of siblings. BMJ 1994;308(6930):692–5.
27. Wilkin TJ. The accelerator hypothesis: weight gain as the missing link between type I and type II diabetes. Diabetologia 2001;44(7):914–22.
28. Group TS. The environmental determinants of diabetes in the young (TEDDY) study. Ann N Y Acad Sci 2008;1150:1–13.
29. Merriman TR, Merriman TR. Type 1 diabetes, the A1 milk hypothesis and vitamin D deficiency. Diabetes Res Clin Pract 2009;83(2):149–56.
30. Group TS. Study design of the trial to reduce IDDM in the genetically at risk (TRIGR). Pediatr Diabetes 2007;8(3):117–37.
31. Chase HP, Lescheck E, Rafkin-Mervis L, et al. Nutritional Intervention to Prevent (NIP) type 1 diabetes a Pilot Trial. ICAN: Infant, Child, Adolescent Nutrition 2009;1(2):98–107.
32. Norris JM, Yin X, Lamb MM, et al. Omega-3 polyunsaturated fatty acid intake and islet autoimmunity in children at increased risk for type 1 diabetes. JAMA 2007; 298(12):1420–8.
33. Schmid S, Buuck D, Knopff A, et al. BABYDIET, a feasibility study to prevent the appearance of islet autoantibodies in relatives of patients with Type 1 diabetes by delaying exposure to gluten. Diabetologia 2004;47(6):1130–1.
34. Norris JM, Barriga K, Klingensmith G, et al. Timing of initial cereal exposure in infancy and risk of islet autoimmunity. JAMA 2003;290(13):1713–20.
35. Moro JR, Iwata M, von Andriano UH, et al. Vitamin effects on the immune system: vitamins A and D take centre stage. Nat Rev Immunol 2008;8(9):685–98.
36. Zipitis CS, Akobeng AK. Vitamin D supplementation in early childhood and risk of type 1 diabetes: a systematic review and meta-analysis. Arch Dis Child 2008; 93(6):512–7.

37. Wenzlau JM, Juhl K, Yu L, et al. The cation efflux transporter ZnT8 (Slc30A8) is a major autoantigen in human type 1 diabetes. Proc Natl Acad Sci U S A 2007; 104(43):17040–5.
38. Verge CF, Gianani R, Kawasaki E, et al. Number of autoantibodies (against insulin, GAD or ICA512/IA2) rather than particular autoantibody specificities determines risk of type I diabetes. J Autoimmun 1996;9(3):379–83.
39. Sosenko JM, Palmer JP, Greenbaum CJ, et al. Patterns of metabolic progression to type 1 diabetes in the Diabetes Prevention trial-type 1. Diabetes Care 2006; 29(3):643–9.
40. Mahon JL, Sosenko JM, Rafkin-Mervis L, et al. The TrialNet Natural History Study of the Development of Type 1 Diabetes: objectives, design, and initial results. Pediatr Diabetes 2009;10(2):97–104.
41. Gale EA, Bingley PJ, Emmett CL, et al. European Nicotinamide Diabetes Intervention Trial (ENDIT): a randomised controlled trial of intervention before the onset of type 1 diabetes. Lancet 2004;363(9413):925–31.
42. Diabetes Prevention Trial–Type 1 Diabetes Study Group. Effects of insulin in relatives of patients with type 1 diabetes mellitus. N Engl J Med 2002;346(22):1685–91.
43. Skyler JS, Krischer JP, Wolfsdorf J, et al. Effects of oral insulin in relatives of patients with type 1 diabetes: the diabetes prevention trial–type 1. Diabetes Care 2005;28(5):1068–76.
44. Nanto-Salonen K, Kupila A, Simell S, et al. Nasal insulin to prevent type 1 diabetes in children with HLA genotypes and autoantibodies conferring increased risk of disease: a double-blind, randomised controlled trial. Lancet 2008; 372(9651):1746–55.
45. Achenbach P, Barker J, Bonifacio E, et al. Modulating the natural history of type 1 diabetes in children at high genetic risk by mucosal insulin immunization. Curr Diab Rep 2008;8(2):87–93.
46. Harrison LC, Honeyman MC, Steele CE, et al. Pancreatic beta-cell function and immune responses to insulin after administration of intranasal insulin to humans at risk for type 1 diabetes. Diabetes Care 2004;27(10):2348–55.
47. Bonfanti R, Bazzigaluppi E, Calori G, et al. Parameters associated with residual insulin secretion during the first year of disease in children and adolescents with Type 1 diabetes mellitus. Diabet Med 1998;15(10):844–50.
48. Sochett EB, Daneman D, Clarson C, et al. Factors affecting and patterns of residual insulin secretion during the first year of type 1 (insulin-dependent) diabetes mellitus in children. Diabetologia 1987;30(7):453–9.
49. Pozzilli P, Manfrini S, Buzzetti R, et al. Glucose evaluation trial for remission (GETREM) in type 1 diabetes: a European multicentre study. Diabetes Res Clin Pract 2005;68(3):258–64.
50. Yki-Jarvinen H, Koivisto VA. Natural course of insulin resistance in type I diabetes. N Engl J Med 1986;315(4):224–30.
51. Palmer JP, Fleming GA, Greenbaum CJ, et al. C-peptide is the appropriate outcome measure for type 1 diabetes clinical trials to preserve beta-cell function: report of an ADA workshop, 21–22 October 2001. [Erratum appears in Diabetes 2004;53(7):1934]. Diabetes 2004;53(1):250–64.
52. Steffes MW, Sibley S, Jackson M, et al. Beta-cell function and the development of diabetes-related complications in the diabetes control and complications trial. Diabetes Care 2003;26(3):832–6.
53. Cyclosporin-induced remission of IDDM after early intervention. Association of 1 yr of cyclosporin treatment with enhanced insulin secretion. The Canadian-European Randomized Control Trial Group. Diabetes 1988;37(11):1574–82.

54. Feutren G, Papoz L, Assan R, et al. Cyclosporin increases the rate and length of remissions in insulin-dependent diabetes of recent onset. Results of a multicentre double-blind trial. Lancet 1986;2(8499):119–24.
55. Harrison LC, Colman PG, Dean B, et al. Increase in remission rate in newly diagnosed type I diabetic subjects treated with azathioprine. Diabetes 1985;34(12): 1306–8.
56. Silverstein J, Maclaren N, Riley W, et al. Immunosuppression with azathioprine and prednisone in recent-onset insulin-dependent diabetes mellitus. N Engl J Med 1988;319(10):599–604.
57. Chatenoud L, Bluestone JA, Chatenoud L, et al. CD3-specific antibodies: a portal to the treatment of autoimmunity. Nat Rev Immunol 2007;7(8):622–32.
58. Herold KC, Gitelman SE, Masharani U, et al. A single course of anti-CD3 monoclonal antibody hOKT3gamma1(Ala-Ala) results in improvement in C-peptide responses and clinical parameters for at least 2 years after onset of type1 diabetes. Diabetes 2005;54(6):1763–9.
59. Herold KC, Hagopian W, Auger JA, et al. Anti-CD3 monoclonal antibody in new-onset type 1 diabetes mellitus. N Engl J Med 2002;346(22):1692–8.
60. Keymeulen B, Vandemeulebroucke E, Ziegler AG, et al. Insulin needs after CD3-antibody therapy in new-onset type 1 diabetes. N Engl J Med 2005;352(25): 2598–608.
61. Levesque MC, St Clair EW, Levesque MC, et al. B cell-directed therapies for autoimmune disease and correlates of disease response and relapse. J Allergy Clin Immunol 2008;121(1):13–21 [quiz 22–3].
62. Tisch R, Wang B, Serreze DV. Induction of glutamic acid decarboxylase 65-specific Th2 cells and suppression of autoimmune diabetes at late stages of disease is epitope dependent. J Immunol 1999;163(3):1178–87.
63. Ludvigsson J, Faresjo M, Hjorth M, et al. GAD treatment and insulin secretion in recent-onset type 1 diabetes. N Engl J Med 2008;359(18):1909–20.
64. Mastrandrea L, Yu J, Behrens T, et al. Etanercept treatment in children with new onset type 1 diabetes: pilot randomized, placebo-controlled, double blind study. Diabetes Care 2009;32(7):1244–9.

# The Role of Complementary and Alternative Therapies in Pediatric Diabetes

Sofia Shapiro, MD*, Robert Rapaport, MD

**KEYWORDS**

• Complementary medicine • Alternative medicine
• Integrative medicine • Diabetes • Pediatrics

Complementary and alternative medicine (CAM), also referred to as holistic, or integrative, medicine, describes a heterogeneous collection of nontraditional therapies, from chemical substances, to biofeedback, to prayer. A recent survey conducted by the Centers of Disease Control and Prevention along with National Department of Health found that Americans spend roughly $34 billion a year out-of-pocket on alternative therapies.[1] The use of CAM in pediatrics has increased in the past decade.[2,3] Randomized prospective trials studying the safety and efficacy of a particular therapy are few in children with diabetes as most such trials are performed in adult patients with type 2 diabetes.

This review focuses on CAM in pediatric patients with type 1 and type 2 diabetes. CAM prevalence in this population and the specific modalities that have been studied in children are described. Randomized, placebo-controlled, prospective studies in young adults are evaluated for their applicability to pediatric patients. CAM's "complementary" role is emphasized, as there is evidence of significant morbidity when CAM replaces standard-of-care therapy.

## PREVALENCE

Complementary medicine is gaining a stronger focus across many agencies that influence pediatric diabetes, including government and private organizations, medical associations and community groups. In 1992, the Office of Alternative Medicine was established by a congressional mandate as part of the National Institutes of Heath (NIH), and became the National Center for Complementary and Alternative Medicine (NCCAM) in 1998. NCCAM defined CAM as "a group of diverse medical and health

Division of Pediatric Endocrinology and Diabetes, Mount Sinai School of Medicine, Box 1616, One Gustave L. Levy Place, New York, NY 10029, USA
* Corresponding author.
*E-mail address:* sofia.shapiro@mssm.edu (S. Shapiro).

Endocrinol Metab Clin N Am 38 (2009) 791–810
doi:10.1016/j.ecl.2009.09.004
0889-8529/09/$ – see front matter. Published by Elsevier Inc.

care systems, practices, and products that are not presently considered to be part of conventional Western medicine."[4] In the winter 2007 issue of its quarterly publication, NCCAM addressed CAM use in young people. In a national survey of approximately 1300 adolescents aged 14–19 years, 80% had used CAM at least once in their life, and as many as 50% had used it within the past month.[2]

Reasons for children using CAM include: one or both parents using it; word-of-mouth; cultural or ethnic tradition; to try to improve qualify of life; dissatisfaction with complexity, discomfort, risks, and/or costs of conventional medical treatment; all options in conventional medicine have been tried; spiritual need; desire for a more "natural," holistic approach; or effects of advertising.[2] NCCAM acknowledged that despite its prevalence, few rigorous studies have been done in children, and emphasized that health care providers discuss CAM use with patients. A survey conducted in 2001 by the American Academy of Pediatrics found that fewer than 5% of providers felt comfortable or knowledgeable discussing CAM therapies.[4]

The American Academy of Pediatrics (AAP) convened the Task Force on Complementary and Alternative Medicine in 2000.[4] The task force provided a comprehensive assessment of CAM use in children, discussing all aspects of CAM, from epidemiology to insurance coverage, from physician awareness to classification of CAM into groups, such as acupuncture, homeopathy, and biofeedback.[3] CAM products such as herbal supplements are not regulated by the Food and Drug Administration (FDA) as are medications. This allows for substantial heterogeneity between products and lots of same-label products, raising uncertainty about the components of the product. The Dietary Supplements Health and Education Act (DSHEA) of 1994 defined a dietary supplement as a vitamin, a mineral, a herb or other botanic, or an amino acid intended to supplement the diet. According to the DSHEA, no data are required from the manufacturers about safety and efficacy of a CAM supplement; instead, the FDA must rely on the Med-Watch voluntary reporting system for adverse events reporting, and must prove that it is unsafe before recalling a product. DSHEA made it mandatory for the supplement label to include the name and quantity of each ingredient, and to have a disclaimer: "This statement has not been evaluated by the FDA. This product is not intended to diagnose, treat, cure, or prevent any disease."[5] The task force provided a "common-sense guide" to CAM: (1) if the therapy is effective and safe, recommend; (2) if the therapy is not effective but safe, tolerate; (3) if the therapy is effective but not safe, monitor closely or discourage; and (4) if the therapy is neither effective nor safe, discourage. Important tips for talking to children and parents about CAM are: ask families about CAM use; respect family's perspectives; monitor response to treatment; and include the family's CAM provider in the care team.[3] The challenge, of course, lies in finding objective evidence whether a specific therapy is effective or safe.

CAM use in children with chronic medical conditions has been studied worldwide and reported to be up to 3 times as frequent as in healthy children.[6] NCCAM proposed a figure as high as 50% of CAM use is children with chronic conditions, a heterogeneous group including diabetes, asthma, cancer, cystic fibrosis, among others.[2] Children with diabetes mellitus were found to have one of the lowest prevalence rates. A Canadian study surveyed 194 children with chronic disease, of whom 49 had diabetes mellitus. Whereas overall prevalence of CAM use was 23%, it was only 6% in children with type 1 diabetes.[7]

Recently, more studies focused on CAM use particularly in children with diabetes. Prevalence will change depending on what is included or excluded in the definition of CAM, such as vitamins or modified diets. A study that surveyed parents of 228 children with type 1 diabetes across 4 pediatric diabetes centers in Germany found that 18.4% used CAM.[8] The most common CAM modalities were homeopathy, vitamins and minerals, modified diet, aloe vera and cinnamon. Reasons behind CAM use were motivation to "try everything" and low side effects. No parents questioned the need for insulin therapy but sought "improved well-being." Two-thirds of parents of CAM users saw an improved overall well-being for their child; more than half of the children noticed no change, positive or negative. There was no improvement in hemoglobin $A_{1c}$ ($HbA_{1c}$) or blood glucose levels during CAM use. The majority (62%) of families informed their medical doctor of CAM use.[8]

Parents of children with diabetes treated at an urban clinic of Children's Memorial Hospital, Chicago, IL, were anonymously asked about specific CAM use for the child's diabetes, perceived effectiveness, communication with provider, and demographics.[9] The survey response rate was 33%, and identified 86 children with type 1 diabetes, aged 7 to 14 years, with duration of diabetes averaging 4.5 years. Seventy-one percent of children were white, 6% black, and 16% Hispanic. Sixteen children, or 19%, had used CAM: faith healing, herbs and nutritional supplements most frequently. None of the responders felt CAM was harmful to their child, and 45% of parents used CAM themselves. CAM use in these children was more frequent if parents used CAM and if parents were foreign-born. There was no association found based on insurance, ethnicity, education level, or diabetes duration. Among CAM users, only 23% of families discussed CAM with the child's pediatrician, and 43% with their diabetes clinician.[9] Neither of the studies reported any severe side effects from CAM.[8,9]

The prevalence of CAM was only 19% among children with type 1 diabetes, lower than for other chronic conditions, and similar to the prevalence found in the German study. Exclusion of multivitamin use from the definition of CAM may have contributed to the low prevalence.[9] However, a more likely reason is that in type 1 diabetes patients, insulin is required for survival, and this dependence on long-standing, standard medical therapy may make CAM much less effective in comparison, thus less appealing to use. Insulin treatment was considered satisfactory in approximately three-quarters of families, and CAM users sought alternative therapies as complementary only, not because of disappointment in insulin efficacy.

A group in Turkey also used a questionnaire to study the prevalence of CAM among children with type 1 diabetes. Among 100 children, 42% used CAM, mostly herbals such as aloe vera, stinging nettle, or leaves; 25% used prayer or spiritual practices. Less frequent therapies were natural water and rabbit brain. As many as 23% of parents in the Turkey cohort reported having used CAM to cure diabetes in their child.[10] Cultural demographic factors inevitably influence the prevalence of CAM and the type of therapies used most frequently.

Association of CAM use and sociodemographic characteristics is controversial. Most studies exploring this were on adults with diabetes. In the United States, there have been inconsistent findings among pediatric patients between CAM use and parental income, education level, family ethnicity, and insurance coverage. A study looking into CAM in a general pediatric clinic found no sociodemographic differences between users and nonusers of CAM.[11] Focusing specifically on children with type 1 diabetes, CAM use also did not vary significantly by insurance type, education level, or ethnicity.[9] In Germany, more CAM use was found among families with higher income and parental tertiary education.[8] In Turkish children with type 1 diabetes, no association was found between CAM use and sociodemographic characteristics.[10]

## NICOTINAMIDE

Nicotinamide is a component of vitamin $B_3$ that is believed to protect $\beta$ cells from free radical damage. It is a potent inhibitor of poly-(ADP-ribose)-polymerase

(PARP), an action that protects against depletion of nicotinamide adenine dinucleotide (NAD); a greater amount of NAD in β cells promotes proinsulin synthesis. It is the dual role of being a free radical scavenger and a protector of NAD that made it a reasonable candidate for improving remission rate, glycemic control, and residual β cell function. Several large prospective trials, and numerous small and pilot studies, have investigated the role of nicotinamide in type 1 diabetes; the large trials are the focus of this section. Nicotinamide was tested in 2 types of patients: patients with new-onset type 1 diabetes and autoantibody-positive, at-risk children without diabetes.

The IMDIAB study group from Italy has published several prospective studies on nicotinamide in children with new-onset type 1 diabetes (**Table 1**). IMDIAB I compared nicotinamide with nicotinamide and cyclosporin in children with recent-onset type 1 diabetes, in achieving disease remission (defined as suspension of insulin therapy for $\geq$2 weeks and normal glycemic parameters). Ninety children with diabetes of less than 4 weeks duration were randomized to either nicotinamide 25 mg/kg/d, or nicotinamide and cyclosporin 5 mg/kg/d, in addition to insulin; both were compared with children solely taking insulin. After 1 year of intervention, 4/27 and 2/25 children in the nicotinamide and nicotinamide-cyclosporin groups, respectively, achieved remission, which lasted several months longer in the nicotinamide group; none in the control group were in remission.[12]

These results prompted further studies. IMDIAB III compared insulin dose, $HbA_{1c}$ and c-peptide levels in 56 children with newly diagnosed type 1 diabetes. The same dose of nicotinamide, 25 mg/kg/d, was given daily for 1 year in addition to intensive insulin therapy. Neither the insulin dose required, $HbA_{1c}$ or c-peptide levels were different between groups at 1 year after diagnosis.[13] IMDIAB VI was a double-blind, multicenter, randomized trial in which 2 different doses of nicotinamide were given to children with new-onset diabetes: 25 mg/kg versus 50 mg/kg. No significant differences in $HbA_{1c}$, c-peptide, and remission rate were noted, and there was actually a tendency toward higher insulin requirements in the 50 mg/d group. The group concluded that the lower dose of 25 mg/d is just as effective; however, there was no control group in this trial as in the IMDIAB I and III trials.[14] Finally, the group extended the observation period to 2 years, comparing nicotinamide plus intensive insulin therapy versus insulin alone in 25 children with recent-onset type 1 diabetes. There was no difference in insulin requirement and c-peptide levels at 2 years after diagnosis; however, $HbA_{1c}$ was noted to be lower in the nicotinamide group.[15] These findings suggest that c-peptide secretion is similarly preserved in children treated solely with insulin, and the reduction in $HbA_{1c}$ warrants further research.

Nicotinamide was combined with vitamin E and calcitriol. The IMDIAB IV study compared vitamin E and nicotinamide, because both are free radical scavengers. In a randomized, prospective, multicenter trial, 84 patients were treated with either vitamin E 15 mg/kg/d or nicotinamide 25 mg/kg/d, in addition to insulin. The ages of patients with newly diagnosed type 1 diabetes ranged from 5 to 35 years. At 1 year, no difference was found between the 2 groups in $HbA_{1c}$, c-peptide, or insulin requirements. The investigators suggested combining the remedies for a possible synergistic effect; however, a control group of patients treated solely with insulin, as seen in earlier studies by the same group, was lacking in this trial.[16] In the IMDIAB IX study by Crino and colleagues,[17] discussed later in the section on vitamin E, children with new-onset type 1 diabetes were treated with either vitamin E or nicotinamide in addition to insulin for 2 years. No significant differences were found between c-peptide and $HbA_{1c}$ levels, and the vitamin E group had a higher insulin requirement than the nicotinamide group. There was no insulin-only control group.

IMDIAB XI focused on comparing vitamin D and nicotinamide in children with new-onset type 1 diabetes (described in detail later in the section on vitamin D). Again, no difference was noted between the 2 groups in insulin dose, $HbA_{1c}$ or c-peptide levels at 1 year of intervention.[18]

Nicotinamide has also been studied in antibody positive, at-risk children without diabetes. In a compelling study by Elliott and colleagues,[19] children without diabetes but with evidence of autoimmunity were treated with nicotinamide. In this prospective, nonrandomized, controlled population trial, 33,568 New Zealand children aged 5 to 7.9 years were screened for Islet cell antibody (ICA) levels of 20 units or greater; those positive were offered treatment with 1.2 g/$m^2$ of nicotinamide daily. ICA was positive in 150 children. After 4.2 years of follow-up, 6 children developed diabetes, compared with 10 new cases in ICA-positive children who refused testing. Another control group was a cohort of 48,335 children not offered ICA testing; at 5.2 years, 55 new cases of diabetes emerged. There was a highly significant difference, expressed as a percent per 100,000 patient years: 8.1% in the treated group versus 21% in the untreated group, and 20.1% in the untested group.[19]

The Deutsche Nicotinamide Intervention Study (DENIS) evaluated the efficacy of high doses of nicotinamide in children at high risk for type 1 diabetes.[20] In this randomized, double-blind, placebo-controlled trial, siblings of type 1 patients aged 3 to 12 years were screened for positive ICA. Nicotinamide doses of 1.2 g/$m^2$ versus placebo were given to 55 ICA-positive children. After 3 years, 6 cases of diabetes were found in the nicotinamide group, compared with 5 cases in the placebo group; no reduction in the incidence of diabetes was shown. The first-phase insulin response to intravenous glucose was lower in the nicotinamide group versus placebo at 2 years. This group, being siblings of type 1 patients and ICA positive, had a more rapid disease progression than in the New Zealand trial.[20]

Eighteen European countries, the United States, and Canada participated in the European Nicotinamide Diabetes Intervention Trial (ENDIT), a randomized, double-blind, placebo-controlled trial on relatives with diabetes antibodies but without diabetes,[21] to investigate whether a nicotinamide group receiving 1.2 g/$m^2$/d would have a lower incidence of diabetes. Subjects ranged in age from 3 to 40 years, and 60% of subjects were less than 20 years. Among 552 ICA-positive patients, 159 developed diabetes within 5 years, 82 in the nicotinamide group and 77 in the placebo group. There was no difference in incidence of diabetes on an intention-to-treat basis. Overall, this large study confirmed prior findings in which no effect of nicotinamide was found. The investigators emphasized the need for large, multicenter, blinded and long-term studies, and cautioned against changing clinical practice based on small pilot studies.[21]

No adverse events were detected in any of the trials mentioned, suggesting that nicotinamide is considered safe up to doses of 3 g/d in adults, or 1.2 g/$m^2$/d in children. Higher doses may cause elevation of liver enzymes and acute jaundice.

The evidence fails to support a role for nicotinamide in preventing or delaying the onset of diabetes in autoantibody-positive relatives of patients with type 1 diabetes. There is also strong and convincing evidence that use of nicotinamide in children with new-onset diabetes less than 4 weeks duration does not alter metabolic parameters such as $HbA_{1c}$, c-peptide, or insulin requirements.

## B VITAMINS: FOLATE AND PYRIDOXAMINE

Within the large complex of vitamin B compounds ($B_1$ [thiamine], $B_2$ [riboflavin], $B_3$ [niacin], $B_6$ [pyridoxine], $B_9$ [folic acid], and $B_{12}$ [cobalamin]), folate and pyridoxamine

**Table 1**
**Clinical trials of vitamins and dietary supplements for glycemic control in pediatric diabetes**

| Supplement | References | Design | Sample | Intervention | Outcomes | Strength[a] | Adverse Events |
|---|---|---|---|---|---|---|---|
| Nicotinamide | Elliott et al (1993) | Nonrandomized; prospective | 33,658 (20,195 tested for ICA) | 1.2 g/m$^2$/d | Fewer new diabetes cases | B | Reported: no effects on liver, no weight or height changes |
| | Lampeter et al (1998) | Randomized; double-blind; placebo-controlled; sequential design | 55 at-risk siblings | 1.2 g/m$^2$/d | No preventative effect; decrease of first-phase insulin release to IVGT | A | Reported: none, no effects on liver or growth |
| | Gale et al (2004) | Randomized; double-blind; placebo-controlled | 552 relatives of type 1, +ICA | 1.2 g/m$^2$/d | No effect on diabetes progression | A | Reported: increased transaminases, no differences between groups |
| | Pozzilli et al (1994) | Randomized; multicenter | 90 recent-onset type 1 | 25 mg/kg/d, cyclosporin 5 mg/kg/d | Longer clinical remission at 1 year | B | Reported: flushing in 1 patient after first dose of nicotinamide |
| | Pozzilli et al (1995) | Randomized; double-blind | 56 recent-onset Type 1 | 25 mg/kg/d | No difference in $HbA_{1c}$, c-peptide, insulin requirement | B | Reported: none |
| | Visalli et al (1999) | Randomized; single-blind | 74 recent-onset Type 1 | 25 mg/kg/d versus 50 mg/kg/d | No difference in $HbA_{1c}$, c-peptide, insulin dose | B | Not reported |
| | Crino et al (2005) | Retrospective | 52 recent-onset Type 1 | 25 mg/kg/d | Lower $HbA_{1c}$, no difference in c-peptide, insulin dose | C | Reported: none |

| | | | | | | | |
|---|---|---|---|---|---|---|---|
| Nicotinamide + vitamin E | Pozzilli et al (1997) | Randomized; multicenter; nonblinded | 84 recent-onset type 1 | 25 mg/kg/d | No difference in $HbA_{1c}$, c-peptide, insulin requirement | B | Reported: leukopenia in 1 patient treated with vitamin E |
| Folate | Pena et al (2004) | Randomized; double-blind; placebo-controlled; crossover | 36 type 1, >1 yr duration | 5 mg daily | Increased flow-mediated dilatation; no change in $HbA_{1c}$ | B | Reported: none |
| Folate and pyridoxamine | MacKenzie et al (2006) | Randomized, double-blind; placebo-controlled | 124 type 1, >1 yr duration | Folate 5 mg/d +/$B_6$ 100 mg/d | Increased flow-mediated dilatation, no additional benefit from combination, irrespective of $HbA_{1c}$, c-peptide, glucose | A | Reported: none |
| Vitamin D | Zipitis et al (2008) | Meta-analysis | 6455 nondiabetic children | N/A | Reduction in risk of developing type 1 diabetes | B | Not reported |
| Vitamin D + nicotinamide | Pitocco et al (2006) | Randomized; open-label | 70 recent-onset type 1 | Calcitriol 0.25 μg every 48 h, nicotinamide 25 mg/kg/d | No difference in $HbA_{1c}$, c-peptide, insulin dose | B | Not reported |
| Cod liver oil | Stene et al (2003) | Case-control | 2213 (545 type 1, 1668 controls) | N/A | Lower risk of type 1 diabetes | B | Not reported |
| | Stene et al (2000) | Case-control | 1876 (85 type 1, 1071 controls) | N/A | Lower risk of type 1 diabetes | B | Not reported |

(*continued on next page*)

**Table 1**
***(continued)***

| Supplement | References | Design | Sample | Intervention | Outcomes | Strength[a] | Adverse Events |
|---|---|---|---|---|---|---|---|
| Omega-3 fatty acid | Norris et al (2007) | 1. Longitudinal 2. Case-subcohort | 1. 1770 and 2. 244 at-risk first-degree relatives of type 1 or +HLA | N/A | Reduced risk of islet autoimmunity | B | Not reported |
| Vitamin E | Jain et al (2000) | Randomized; double-blind; placebo-controlled | 50 (21 type 1, 29 controls) | 100 IU/d | Decrease in $HbA_{1c}$, increase in glutathione | B | Not reported |
| | Giannini et al (2007) | Randomized; placebo-controlled; double-blind; crossover | 10 type 1 + microalbuminuria | 1200 mg/d | No difference in $HbA_{1c}$, microalbuminuria, oxidative stress | C | Reported: none |
| | Chiarelli et al (2004) | Nonrandomized; prospective | 30 (22 type 1, 10 nondiabetes) | 600 mg twice a day | No decrease in angiopathy | C | Reported: none |
| | Uusitalo et al (2008) | Prospective cohort | 4297 newborns | N/A | No decreased risk in autoimmunity | B | N/A |
| Vitamin E + nicotinamide | Crino et al (2004) | Randomized; multicenter; nonblinded | 64 recent-onset type 1 | Vitamin E 15 mg/kg/d | No difference in $HbA_{1c}$, c-peptide; higher insulin requirement in nicotinamide versus vitamin E | B | Reported: none |

| | | | | | | | |
|---|---|---|---|---|---|---|---|
| Cinnamon | Altschuler et al (2007) | Randomized; double-blind; placebo-controlled | 72 type 1 diabetes >18 mo | 1 g/d | No difference in $HbA_{1c}$, insulin dose, hypoglycemia | B | Reported: urticaria in 1 patient with family history of cinnamon allergy |
| | Baker et al (2008) | Meta-analysis | 282 (210 type 2 adults, 72 type 1 adolescents) | 1–6 g/d | No difference in $HbA_{1c}$, fasting glucose, lipids | B | Not reported |
| | de Sena et al (2005) | Nonrandomized; prospective | 37 (20 type 1,17 control) | 7.5–15 mg/d | Increased $HbA_{1c}$ | C | Reported: increased appetite, weight |
| | Uusitalo et al (2008) | Prospective cohort | 4297 newborns | N/A | No decreased risk in autoimmunity | B | N/A |
| α-Lipoic acid | Huang et al (2008) | Randomized; double-blind; placebo-controlled | 40 type 1 | 14–21 mg/kg/d | No difference in $HbA_{1c}$, insulin dose, antioxidant status | B | No adverse events noted |

*Abbreviation:* IVGT, intravenous glucose tolerance test.

[a] A, randomized controlled trials and meta-analyses; B, well-designed controlled and uncontrolled studies; C, retrospective studies or nonrandomized studies with smaller sample size.

have been the main B vitamins studied in pediatric diabetes. B vitamins are believed to ameliorate the development of atherosclerosis; the precise mechanism is unknown. B vitamins may act as antioxidants and reduce homocysteine, which contributes to endothelial dysfunction. Pyridoxine was recently shown to inhibit the formation of advanced glycation end products (AGEs), markers of oxidative stress, and limit progression of vascular disease in animal models.[22]

A randomized, double-blind, placebo-controlled crossover trial in 36 pediatric subjects evaluated the effect of folate supplementation on endothelial function in children and adolescents with type 1 diabetes.[23] Folic acid 5 mg/d versus placebo were given for 8 weeks each, and endothelial function was assessed using brachial artery responses to flow, or flow-mediated dilatation (FMD). An increased FMD in the folic acid group, with no change in the $HbA_{1c}$ or homocystine, was noted, suggesting that short-term high-dose folic acid improves endothelial function in children with type 1 diabetes, independently of homocystine.[23] The same study group compared folate and pyridoxamine supplementation in 124 children with type 1 diabetes.[24] In a similar randomized, double-blind, placebo-controlled study design, the investigators compared 4 groups: (1) folate 5 mg/d versus placebo; (2) pyridoxamine 100 mg/d versus placebo; (3) folate 5 mg/d and pyridoxamine 100 mg/d, and (4) 2 placebo tablets, with 30 subjects in each group. After 8 weeks of interventions, an improvement in FMD was noted in all 3 intervention groups, with no additional benefit from combination treatment. Similar to the initial study, the beneficial effect was independent of $HbA_{1c}$ and homocystine levels, and glucose and c-peptide.[24]

Despite evidence that folate and pyridoxamine seem to improve short-term endothelial function in children with type 1 diabetes, larger studies with longer follow-up are needed. The effect sought is on endothelial function and not on $HbA_{1c}$. Because vascular disease among children with diabetes is an occult process, large, prospective, randomized, placebo-controlled studies are needed to show long-term benefit of B vitamins as an intention-to-treat analysis.

## VITAMIN D, COD LIVER OIL, AND OMEGA-3 FATTY ACIDS

There has been a growing interest in vitamin D and its preventive role in autoimmune diabetes. Vitamin D and its metabolites were shown to have immunomodulatory properties in in vitro studies,[25] and in nonobese diabetic mice, 1,25-dihydroxyvitamin $D_3$ was found to delay the autoimmune progression of diabetes.[26] Hypercalcemia was a side effect that correlated with increased T cell adaptivity and type 1 diabetes protection.[26] Similar to nicotinamide trials, vitamin D studies can be grouped into those addressing children with newly diagnosed type 1 diabetes and preventative studies seeking to delay the onset in high-risk subjects.

In an open-label, randomized, prospective trial, 70 children with recent-onset type 1 diabetes, older than 5 years with at least 1 positive diabetes antibody, used calcitriol (the active form of vitamin D) 0.25 μg on alternate days or nicotinamide 25 mg/kg daily for 1 year.[18] $HbA_{1c}$ and c-peptide did not differ between groups. Insulin dose at 3 and 6 months was lower in the calcitriol-treated group, but this was transient. A higher calcitriol dose may have elicited a different response, at a higher risk of hypercalcemia.[18] One limitation of this study is that 25-hydroxyvitamin $D_3$ was not measured at diagnosis. Hypovitaminosis D is believed to be more prevalent in children with new-onset type 1 diabetes compared with normal children.[27–29]

Most studies relating to vitamin D in pediatric diabetes have focused on the preventive role of vitamin D in decreasing the risk of type 1 diabetes. Zipitis and Akoberg[30] reviewed whether vitamin D supplementation in infancy results in a lesser risk of type 1 diabetes later in life. No prospective, randomized, control studies were found; among retrospective studies, 4 case-control and 1 cohort study were included, totaling 1429 cases (supplemented) and 5026 controls (not supplemented), from many different European countries. The meta-analysis found a 29% risk reduction in infants who received vitamin D supplement. Because the dose of the supplemented vitamin D could not be determined, the investigators of individual studies speculated that, when cod liver oil containing 10 μg of vitamin $D_3$ was used, there was some evidence of a dose-response effect. Similarly, duration of supplementation was not available for all studies. In the EURODIAB study, no effect on type 1 diabetes risk was seen after more than 1 year of vitamin D supplementation compared with only 1 year.[31] These data are prone to recall bias and need to be interpreted with caution, as there are potential confounding factors: breast-feeding and environmental factors; lack of confirmation of antibody-negative status among controls; and combination of cod liver oil and vitamin D (cod liver oil's other components may play a protective role).[30]

The Norwegian Childhood Diabetes Study Group, included in the meta-analysis discussed earlier, investigated cod liver oil in particular; in Norway, this form of vitamin D is the preferred supplement in infancy. Cod liver oil, in addition to vitamin D, has long-chain n-3 fatty acids, docosahexaenoic acid (DHA) and eicosapentaenoic acid (EPA), and these acids are believed to decrease the expression of human leukocyte antigen (HLA) class II molecules on activated human monocytes[32] and reduce expression of interleukins.[33] The group found an association between cod liver oil use in infancy and lower risk of type 1 diabetes, adjusting for potential confounders such as breast-feeding, maternal age and education level, and family history of diabetes. No association was found between maternal use of cod liver oil or other vitamin D supplements during pregnancy and decreased risk of type 1 diabetes in children,[34] even though in an earlier retrospective study by the same group, such an association was described.[35] The investigators were not certain of the cause of such difference, and proposed greater bioavailability of cod liver oil versus other forms of vitamin D during pregnancy.[34]

Omega-3 fatty acids have been studied in adults with diabetes and coronary artery disease, but studies on their use in pediatric subjects with diabetes is limited. A symposium titled "Beyond cholesterol: prevention and treatment of coronary heart disease with n-3 fatty acids" recommended a modest consumption of EPA plus DHA (250–500 mg/d) for adults with diabetes considered to be at risk for cardiovascular disease; and even among adults, dose-response studies are needed.[36]

In a longitudinal observational study, the Diabetes Autoimmunity Study in the Young (DAISY), conducted in Denver, Colorado, 1770 children at increased risk for type 1 diabetes were followed for 6 years.[37] Reported dietary intake of polyunsaturated fatty acids (PUFAs), such as omega-3 fatty acids, starting at 1 year was assessed. Islet autoimmunity was defined as at least 1 positive diabetes antibody at 2 or more visits. The study group found fatty acid intake was inversely associated with risk of islet autoimmunity, and had a stronger association with children positive for 2 or more autoantibodies.[37]

Several prospective studies are underway, evaluating the effect of vitamin D supplementation and the risk of developing type 1 diabetes. The PREVEFIN study in Italy is currently using 2 interventions in newborns: vitamin D 500 units/d, and β-casein-free diet for 12 months.[38] A preliminary report showed a low rate of antibody positivity, some of which is transient, but the large cohort of newborns will be followed for a longer time. In the TrialNet network, the Nutritional Intervention to Prevent (NIP) Type 1 Diabetes study is underway to test whether DHA supplementation during pregnancy for babies at risk of developing type 1 diabetes will delay or prevent the onset of autoimmunity.[39] NIP is a multicenter, 2-arm, randomized, double-masked trial. In 1 arm, pregnant women will take 800 mg/d of DHA versus placebo; in the second arm, HLA-eligible infants and toddlers will take 150 mg/d and 400 mg/d, respectively. Infants and toddlers will be followed up to 3 years, and entered into the Natural History section of TrialNet to be followed for development of diabetes autoimmunity.[40,41]

In summary, use of vitamin D in children newly diagnosed with type 1 diabetes has not been shown to improve glycemic control, but studies with longer follow-up are needed. The preventive role of vitamin D, cod liver oil, and fatty acids (DHA and EPA) are conflicting, and studies with retrospective dietary reporting are prone to recall bias. The ongoing prospective studies of PrevenFin and TrialNet will better answer the question of whether vitamin D and omega-3 fatty acids have a protective role against development of type 1 diabetes.

## VITAMIN E

Vitamin E is a lipid-soluble antioxidant vitamin believed to provide protection against oxidative stress. By inhibiting lipid peroxidation, vitamin E is believed to protect β cells from inflammatory factors such as interleukin 1, tumor necrosis factor, and gamma interferon. Several prospective, randomized, placebo-controlled studies were performed in children with type 1 diabetes using vitamin E. In addition to glycemic control, the focus has been on microvascular complications (retinopathy and nephropathy). Because these complications occur after substantial duration of type 1 diabetes, it is understandable how data in pediatric populations are limited.

In a randomized trial of vitamin E in children with new-onset type 1 diabetes, 32 children aged 4 to 18 years, with type 1 diabetes of less than 4 weeks duration, received either (1) vitamin E, 15 mg/kg, with nicotinamide, 25 mg/kg, or (2) nicotinamide alone, for 2 years.[17] C-peptide levels found at diagnosis were preserved with no difference between the groups, irrespective of age and puberty. Investigators noted that at some time points during the study, patients receiving combination therapy for vitamin E and nicotinamide had a lesser insulin requirement compared with nicotinamide alone.[17] A limitation of this study was that no control group comprised solely of insulin-treated patients was used; however, the investigators did make such a comparison for nicotinamide versus insulin alone [15] (see section on nicotinamide).

One study did find an improvement in $HbA_{1c}$ in children with type 1 diabetes after 3 months of vitamin E supplementation. In a randomized, prospective, placebo-controlled double-blind trial, Jain and colleagues[42] gave 100 IU/d (670 mg/d) of vitamin E to 29 children with type 1 diabetes and 21 age-matched controls. A 16% decrease in $HbA_{1c}$ was found between the vitamin E supplemented group versus the placebo group after 3 months, confirming their earlier study on 13 children with type 1 diabetes.[43] Vitamin E was also shown to increase cellular glutathione and lower malondialdehyde, achieving a more favorable antioxidant profile in 29 children with type 1 diabetes.[42] Limitations of these studies were the small number of subjects and lack of specifics on age parameters, diabetes duration, and insulin regimens.

A randomized, placebo-controlled, double-blind crossover study in 10 young adults with type 1 diabetes and microalbuminuria (albumin excretion rate >20 μg/min) used vitamin E 1200 mg/d for 6 months. Low density lipoprotein peroxidation was improved, but there was no significant difference in $HbA_{1c}$, blood pressure, microalbuminuria, transforming-growth factor-β (TGF-β), or vascular endothelial growth factor (VEGF).[44]

In a study of 12 adolescents with type 1 diabetes of 10 to 18 years duration and microangiopathy who received 1200 mg/d of vitamin E for 3 months, researchers analyzed skin fibroblasts for antioxidant enzyme production (AEP).[45] Vitamin E increased AEP only in control subjects and adolescents without diabetic angiopathy, not in adolescents with diabetic angiopathy. The investigators concluded that in adolescents with type 1 diabetes and early angiopathy, the antioxidant defense mechanism may be impaired and unresponsive to vitamin E.[45]

A double-masked, randomized, placebo-controlled, crossover adult trial of vitamin E 1800 IU/d (1200 mg/d) versus placebo for 4 months in 36 patients aged 18 to 45 years with diabetes for less than 10 years and no or minimal diabetic retinopathy or microalbuminuria, showed no difference in $HbA_{1c}$ before and after vitamin E supplementation. There was a significant increase in retinal blood flow; subjects with worse retinopathy had the greatest increase.[46]

The role of vitamin E during pregnancy to decrease the risk of autoimmunity has been studied in Finland, as part of the Type 1 Diabetes Prediction and Prevention Project.[47] Using a comprehensive questionnaire, mothers of 4297 children at risk for type 1 diabetes based on major histocompatibility complex HLA-DQB1 were asked to retrospectively recall diet and dietary supplements used during pregnancy. The main sources of vitamin E, in addition to supplements, were vegetable oils and cereal products. Among multiple supplements with proposed antioxidant properties used during pregnancy, including vitamin E, selenium, zinc, vitamin C, retinol, β-carotene, and manganese, none was associated with a decreased β-cell autoimmunity in the offspring.[47]

In summary, vitamin E supplementation in 2 small studies of children and adolescents with type 1 diabetes was shown to decrease $HbA_{1c}$. Several small trials assessing oxidative stress and microangiopathy did not find an improvement after vitamin E intake. Larger trials with longer follow-up are needed to validate these results. Vitamin E supplementation in pregnancy did not decrease the risk of diabetes autoimmunity in the offspring, but prospective studies are lacking.

## CINNAMON

The theory that cinnamon improves glycemic control was prompted by in vitro studies showing that cinnamon plays a role in insulin signaling. The bioactive compounds are water-soluble, double-linked A-type polyphenol polymers that have been shown to potentiate insulin receptor action in rat models.[48,49] A recent study proposed activation of glucose transport and increasing GLUT4 by a P13-K-independent pathway.[50]

In adult patients with type 2 diabetes, no improvement in glycemic control indices or increased insulin sensitivity were observed.[51,52] Very few studies have evaluated the role of cinnamon in pediatric patients with diabetes. In a prospective, double-blind, placebo-controlled trial, 72 adolescents with type 1 diabetes took 1g/d of cinnamon for 90 days. Adolescents were 13 to 18 years of age, with diabetes of at least 18 months duration, and average $HbA_{1c}$ of 8.5 ± 1.3%. One patient in the cinnamon group developed hives; there was a family history of cinnamon allergy. Similarly, no statistical differences in $HbA_{1c}$, daily insulin requirements, weighted Z-scores, or hypoglycemic episodes were found in 72 pediatric patients.[53] These findings dampened the initial optimism regarding the benefits of cinnamon as a complementary therapy in diabetes.

A recent meta-analysis in Diabetes Care by Baker and colleagues[54] included 5 clinical trials using cinnamon as complementary therapy in diabetes mellitus. Only 1 of the 5 studies was performed in a pediatric population, the study by Altschuler and colleagues[54] described earlier; the other studies were on adults with type 2 diabetes. Cinnamon doses varied from 1 to 6 g/d, and follow-up ranged from 5.7 to 16 weeks. Data from 282 subjects were analyzed, and the results confirmed that cinnamon had no effect on $HbA_{1c}$, fasting blood glucose, or lipid parameters.

The length of the cinnamon treatment may not have been long enough to alter the $HbA_{1c}$. The duration of the study in adolescents was 90 days, and the median duration in the meta-analysis was 12 weeks; however, the lifespan of a red blood cell is approximately 120 days. The investigators acknowledged this and proposed that, if a lowering effect of cinnamon on $HbA_{1c}$ truly exists, it would likely at least have shown a trend toward a lower $HbA_{1c}$ value compared with placebo. Thus, current evidence does not support use of cinnamon in children with type 1 or type 2 diabetes to improve glycemic control.

## CHROMIUM

Chromium is believed to alter glucose metabolism by lowering insulin resistance. Apochromomodulin is an oligopeptide chromium-binding substance, which is an intracellular apolipoprotein that influences the insulin receptor.[55] There is ongoing controversy whether chromium supplementation improves glycemic control in adult patients with type 2 diabetes. However, no prospective, randomized clinical trials in children with type 1 or type 2 diabetes are known to date. A study is currently underway to evaluate chromium's effects on $HbA_{1c}$ and lipid profiles in type 1 and type 2 adolescents.[56]

Different forms of chromium have been studied in adults: chromium picolinate, chromium yeast, among others. A meta-analysis of herbs and dietary supplements by Yeh and colleagues[57] in type 2 diabetes found no difference between chromium and placebo groups with respect to $HbA_{1c}$. Subsequent studies showed conflicting results, some showing no effect,[58] others detecting a decrease in the $HbA_{1c}$ [59,60]; some research groups used chromium and biotin combinations.[59–61] Baseline insulin resistance, assessed by the hyperinsulinemic-euglycemia clamp, correlated with improved insulin sensitivity in the chromium group.[62]

The controversial role of chromium in improving diabetes control in adults with type 2 diabetes does not support its use in that population. Studies to prospectively assess chromium's effect on glycemic control in children with type 1 and type 2 diabetes are lacking.

## ZINC

Zinc has been shown to attenuate hyperglycemia in animal models by a mechanism that is not clearly established. One proposed mechanism is that zinc increases sensitivity to glucose uptake in muscle tissues.[63] Increased urinary loss of zinc, or hyperzincuria, has been found in children with diabetes,[64] and was shown to normalize as better control was achieved.[64–67] In the review of herbs and dietary supplements in adults with diabetes,[57] one study compared zinc versus chromium versus both versus placebo, and found no change in fasting blood glucose, $HbA_{1c}$, insulin, weight, or body mass index.[66]

In a prospective, nonrandomized study, 20 Brazilian children aged 4 to 16 years with type 1 diabetes received daily zinc supplementation 1.5 to 1.8 times the recommended dietary allowances for 4 months.[68] The study found an increase in $HbA_{1c}$ after zinc supplementation, attributing this to poor metabolic control. Increased appetite and weight were side effects reported by participants, and agreed with findings of increased $HbA_{1c}$ in 7 young adults with type 1 diabetes after a month of zinc supplementation.[69]

Uusitalo and colleagues,[47,70] as part of the Type 1 Diabetes Prediction and Prevention Project, assessed maternal zinc intake, along with other antioxidants, This large, prospective, population-based, cohort study elicited dietary data of mothers whose children had the major histocompatibility complex HLA-DQB1, signifying advanced risk of β cell autoimmunity. The self-administered food-frequency questionnaire was prone to recall bias. High maternal intake of zinc did not protect the child from developing diabetes autoantibodies (islet cell Ab plus at least 1 other diabetes antibody). None of the other antioxidant vitamins and trace elements studied, namely, retinol, β-carotene, vitamin C, vitamin E, selenium, or manganese, protected the child from this advanced β cell autoimmunity.[47]

Thus, zinc supplementation was not shown to have a role in improving metabolic control or preventing β cell autoimmunity after disease onset or in the prenatal period.

## α-LIPOIC ACID

α-Lipoic acid is a potent antioxidant that functions as a cofactor in mitochondrial dehydrogenase complexes. In adults, intravenous α-lipoic acid was found to be an effective treatment of diabetic neuropathy.[71] In a double-blind, randomized, placebo-controlled pilot study, oral controlled-release α-lipoic acid (CRLA) of 17 mg/kg/d versus placebo was given to 30 versus 10 adolescents with type 1 diabetes.[72] After 90 days, there was no significant change in any measurement of oxidative damage, total antioxidant status, or $HbA_{1c}$. Further investigations with more subjects and longer duration of treatment are warranted.

## "COMPLEMENTARY" MEDICINE: ITS STRICTLY ADJUVANT ROLE

This article reviews objective evidence regarding alternative therapies used in pediatric diabetes. In all of the studies mentioned, children continued their standard-of-care diabetes treatments; specifically, all subjects with type 1 diabetes remained on insulin regimens. The importance of providing insulin replacement in children and adolescents with type 1 diabetes cannot be overemphasized. If an alternative treatment is sought and tried, even if it does not yield benefit, it will unlikely cause harm, especially if doses given have already been reported as safe in research studies. Interruption of insulin therapy in a child with type 1 diabetes, however, is certain to lead to diabetic ketoacidosis, a dangerous complication that can be fatal if untreated. There are case reports in the literature where alternative therapies have been tried as a replacement for insulin, based not on scientific evidence but on cultural beliefs. A 6-year-old boy with type 1 diabetes had his insulin reduced by more than 70% and was given an ayurvedic herbal preparation; he came into the hospital with severe ketoacidosis and coma.[73] An 11-year-old girl was given a herbal product "goldenseal" (*Hydrastis canadensis*) as treatment of evolving diabetic ketoacidosis that caused severe hypernatremia and hyperosmolality.[74] Recent news reported the death of a child deprived of insulin treatment, as the family sought other means of cure and did not bring her to a doctor.[75] Although there are fewer studies on alternative therapies in children than adults with diabetes mellitus, more studies are emerging. Today, when technology makes it possible to find the latest evidence-based medicine on the Internet, it is more important than ever for a physician to serve as an educator and to guide families and children with diabetes toward reputable sources of information. We must protect patients and families from numerous catchy advertisements and anecdotal success stories that have not been adequately tested. Finally, it is the health care team's responsibility to learn about various alternative therapies; to be confident in searching the literature and communicating the known benefits and risks to our patients; and to accept a family's decision to use complementary therapies when no harm has been shown.

## SUMMARY

The use of CAM is increasing among children and adolescents with diabetes. Most studies focus on type 1 rather than type 2 diabetes. The strongest evidence comes from nicotinamide trials; among children newly diagnosed with type 1 diabetes and relatives at risk for type 1 diabetes, nicotinamide neither altered diabetes control nor delayed the onset of type 1 diabetes. Folate and pyridoxamine similarly had no effect on $HbA_{1c}$ and c-peptide levels, and possible improvement seen in endothelial function needs further research. Vitamin D supplementation was not shown to improve $HbA_{1c}$ or residual $\beta$ cell function in children newly diagnosed with type 1 diabetes. Transient reductions in $HbA_{1c}$ found in small studies after supplementation with vitamin E need to be confirmed in larger trials. Cinnamon use in children with type 1 diabetes did not show evidence of improved markers of glycemic control. Chromium's role in pediatric diabetes has not yet been widely studied. Zinc supplementation was not shown to improve glycemic control in children with type 1 diabetes. Pilot studies of $\alpha$-lipoic acid also showed no effect in children with type 1 diabetes. As preventative therapy, among supplements taken during pregnancy (including vitamin D, vitamin E, selenium, zinc, vitamin C, retinol, $\beta$-carotene, and manganese) none was shown to reduce type 1 diabetes risk in the offspring. What was reassuringly consistent across all studies was that the complementary therapies were safe when used at the doses previously reported, even at high doses in some trials; this held true for the risk of hypercalcemia with vitamin D. Finally, the strictly adjuvant role of these alternative therapies is discussed. The unquestionable need for insulin therapy in youth with type 1 diabetes cannot be overemphasized.

## REFERENCES

1. Pleis JR, Lucas JW. Summary health statistics for US adults: National Health Interview Survey, 2007. Vital Health Stat 1 2009;240:1–159.
2. Thinking about CAM therapies for young people. CAM at the NIH 2007;14(1): 1, 4–7.
3. Kemper KJ, Vohra S, Walls R, et al. The use of complementary and alternative medicine in pediatrics. Pediatrics 2008;122(6):1374–86.
4. National Institutes of Health. National Center for Complementary and Alternative Medicine. Available at: http://ncam.nih.gov. Accessed August 19, 2009.
5. Food and Drug Administration. Dietary Supplement Health and Education Act of 1994. 1994; Public Law Number:103–417.
6. McCann LJ, Newell SJ. Survey of paediatric complementary and alternative medicine use in health and chronic illness. Arch Dis Child 2006;91(2):173–4.
7. Samdup DZ, Smith RG, Il Song S. The use of complementary and alternative medicine in children with chronic medical conditions. Am J Phys Med Rehabil 2006;85(10):842–6.
8. Dannemann K, Hecker W, Haberland H, et al. Use of complementary and alternative medicine in children with type 1 diabetes mellitus–prevalence, patterns of use, and costs. Pediatr Diabetes 2008;9(3 Pt 1):228–35.
9. Miller JL, Binns HJ, Brickman WJ. Complementary and alternative medicine use in children with type 1 diabetes: a pilot survey of parents. Explore (NY) 2008;4(5):311–4.

10. Arykan D, Sivrikaya SK, Olgun N. Complementary alternative medicine use in children with type 1 diabetes mellitus in Erzurum, Turkey. J Clin Nurs 2009; 18(15):2136–44.
11. Jean D, Cyr C. Use of complementary and alternative medicine in a general pediatric clinic. Pediatrics 2007;120(1):e138–41.
12. Pozzilli P, Visalli N, Boccuni ML, et al. Randomized trial comparing nicotinamide and nicotinamide plus cyclosporin in recent onset insulin-dependent diabetes (IMDIAB 1). The IMDIAB Study Group. Diabet Med 1994;11(1):98–104.
13. Pozzilli P, Visalli N, Signore A, et al. Double blind trial of nicotinamide in recent-onset IDDM (the IMDIAB III study). Diabetologia 1995;38(7):848–52.
14. Visalli N, Cavallo MG, Signore A, et al. A multi-centre randomized trial of two different doses of nicotinamide in patients with recent-onset type 1 diabetes (the IMDIAB VI). Diabetes Metab Res Rev 1999;15(3):181–5.
15. Crino A, Schiaffini R, Ciampalini P, et al. A two year observational study of nicotinamide and intensive insulin therapy in patients with recent onset type 1 diabetes mellitus. J Pediatr Endocrinol Metab 2005;18(8):749–54.
16. Pozzilli P, Visalli N, Cavallo MG, et al. Vitamin E and nicotinamide have similar effects in maintaining residual beta cell function in recent onset insulin-dependent diabetes (the IMDIAB IV study). Eur J Endocrinol 1997;137(3):234–9.
17. Crino A, Schiaffini R, Manfrini S, et al. A randomized trial of nicotinamide and vitamin E in children with recent onset type 1 diabetes (IMDIAB IX). Eur J Endocrinol 2004;150(5):719–24.
18. Pitocco D, Crino A, Di Stasio E, et al. The effects of calcitriol and nicotinamide on residual pancreatic beta-cell function in patients with recent-onset Type 1 diabetes (IMDIAB XI). Diabet Med 2006;23(8):920–3.
19. Elliott RB, Pilcher CC, Stewart A, et al. The use of nicotinamide in the prevention of type 1 diabetes. Ann N Y Acad Sci 1993;696:333–41.
20. Lampeter EF, Klinghammer A, Scherbaum WA, et al. The Deutsche Nicotinamide Intervention Study: an attempt to prevent type 1 diabetes. DENIS Group. Diabetes 1998;47(6):980–4.
21. Gale EA, Bingley PJ, Emmett CL, et al. European Nicotinamide Diabetes Intervention Trial (ENDIT): a randomised controlled trial of intervention before the onset of type 1 diabetes. Lancet 2004;363(9413):925–31.
22. Jain SK. Vitamin B6 (pyridoxamine) supplementation and complications of diabetes. Meta 2007;56(2):168–71.
23. Pena AS, Wiltshire E, Gent R, et al. Folic acid improves endothelial function in children and adolescents with type 1 diabetes. J Pediatr 2004;144(4): 500–4.
24. MacKenzie KE, Wiltshire EJ, Gent R, et al. Folate and vitamin B6 rapidly normalize endothelial dysfunction in children with type 1 diabetes mellitus. Pediatrics 2006; 118(1):242–53.
25. Mathieu C, Gysemans C, Giulietti A, et al. Vitamin D and diabetes. Diabetologia 2005;48(7):1247–57.
26. Driver JP, Foreman O, Mathieu C, et al. Comparative therapeutic effects of orally administered 1,25-dihydroxyvitamin D(3) and 1alpha-hydroxyvitamin D(3) on type-1 diabetes in non-obese diabetic mice fed a normal-calcaemic diet. Clin Exp Immunol 2008;151(1):76–85.
27. Littorin B, Blom P, Scholin A, et al. Lower levels of plasma 25-hydroxyvitamin D among young adults at diagnosis of autoimmune type 1 diabetes compared with control subjects: results from the nationwide Diabetes Incidence Study in Sweden (DISS). Diabetologia 2006;49(12):2847–52.

28. Pozzilli P, Manfrini S, Crino A, et al. Low levels of 25-hydroxyvitamin D3 and 1,25-dihydroxyvitamin D3 in patients with newly diagnosed type 1 diabetes. Horm Metab Res 2005;37(11):680–3.
29. Greer RM, Rogers MA, Bowling FG, et al. Australian children and adolescents with type 1 diabetes have low vitamin D levels. Med J Aust 2007;187(1):59–60.
30. Zipitis CS, Akobeng AK. Vitamin D supplementation in early childhood and risk of type 1 diabetes: a systematic review and meta-analysis. Arch Dis Child 2008; 93(6):512–7.
31. Vitamin D supplement in early childhood and risk for Type I (insulin-dependent) diabetes mellitus. The EURODIAB Substudy 2 Study Group. Diabetologia 1999; 42(1):51–4.
32. Hughes DA, Pinder AC. n-3 Polyunsaturated fatty acids inhibit the antigen-presenting function of human monocytes. Am J Clin Nutr 2000;71(Suppl 1): 357S–60S.
33. Endres S, Meydani SN, Ghorbani R, et al. Dietary supplementation with n-3 fatty acids suppresses interleukin-2 production and mononuclear cell proliferation. J Leukoc Biol 1993;54(6):599–603.
34. Stene LC, Joner G, Norwegian Childhood Diabetes Study Group. Use of cod liver oil during the first year of life is associated with lower risk of childhood-onset type 1 diabetes: a large, population-based, case-control study. Am J Clin Nutr 2003; 78(6):1128–34.
35. Stene LC, Ulriksen J, Magnus P, et al. Use of cod liver oil during pregnancy associated with lower risk of Type I diabetes in the offspring. Diabetologia 2000;43(9): 1093–8.
36. Deckelbaum RJ, Leaf A, Mozaffarian D, et al. Conclusions and recommendations from the symposium, beyond cholesterol: prevention and treatment of coronary heart disease with n-3 Fatty acids. Am J Clin Nutr 2008;87(6): 2010S–2S.
37. Norris JM, Yin X, Lamb MM, et al. Omega-3 polyunsaturated fatty acid intake and islet autoimmunity in children at increased risk for type 1 diabetes. JAMA 2007; 298(12):1420–8.
38. Lorini R, Minicucci L, Napoli F, et al. Screening for type 1 diabetes genetic risk in newborns of continental Italy. Primary prevention (Prevefin Italy)–preliminary data. Acta Biomed 2005;76(Suppl 3):31–5.
39. Chase HP, Butler-Simon N, Garg S, et al. A trial of nicotinamide in newly diagnosed patients with type 1 (insulin-dependent) diabetes mellitus. Diabetologia 1990;33(7):444–6.
40. Chase PH, Lescheck E, Rafkin-Mervis L, et al. Nutritional Intervention to Prevent (NIP) Type 1 Diabetes: a pilot trial. ICAN 2009;1(98):99–107.
41. Type 1 Diabetes trial net. Available at: http://www.diabetestrialnet.org/patientinfo/studies/nutritional/htm. Accessed July 27, 2009.
42. Jain SK, McVie R, Smith T. Vitamin E supplementation restores glutathione and malondialdehyde to normal concentrations in erythrocytes of type 1 diabetic children. Diabetes Care 2000;23(9):1389–94.
43. Jain SK, McVie R, Jaramillo JJ, et al. Effect of modest vitamin E supplementation on blood glycated hemoglobin and triglyceride levels and red cell indices in type I diabetic patients. J Am Coll Nutr 1996;15(5):458–61.
44. Giannini C, Lombardo F, Curro F, et al. Effects of high-dose vitamin E supplementation on oxidative stress and microalbuminuria in young adult patients with childhood onset type 1 diabetes mellitus. Diabetes Metab Res Rev 2007;23(7): 539–46.

45. Chiarelli F, Santilli F, Sabatino G, et al. Effects of vitamin E supplementation on intracellular antioxidant enzyme production in adolescents with type 1 diabetes and early microangiopathy. Pediatr Res 2004;56(5):720–5.
46. Bursell SE, Clermont AC, Aiello LP, et al. High-dose vitamin E supplementation normalizes retinal blood flow and creatinine clearance in patients with type 1 diabetes. Diabetes Care 1999;22(8):1245–51.
47. Uusitalo L, Kenward MG, Virtanen SM, et al. Intake of antioxidant vitamins and trace elements during pregnancy and risk of advanced beta cell autoimmunity in the child. Am J Clin Nutr 2008;88(2):458–64.
48. Qin B, Nagasaki M, Ren M, et al. Cinnamon extract (traditional herb) potentiates in vivo insulin-regulated glucose utilization via enhancing insulin signaling in rats. Diabetes Res Clin Pract 2003;62(3):139–48.
49. Kim SH, Hyun SH, Choung SY. Anti-diabetic effect of cinnamon extract on blood glucose in db/db mice. J Ethnopharmacol 2006;104(1–2):119–23.
50. Lakshmi BS, Sujatha S, Anand S, et al. Cinnamic acid, from the bark of *Cinnamomum cassia*, regulates glucose transport via activation of GLUT4 on L6 myotubes in a phosphatidylinositol 3-kinase-independent manner. J Diabetes 2009;1(2): 99, 100–106.
51. Mang B, Wolters M, Schmitt B, et al. Effects of a cinnamon extract on plasma glucose, HbA, and serum lipids in diabetes mellitus type 2. Eur J Clin Invest 2006;36(5):340–4.
52. Vanschoonbeek K, Thomassen BJ, Senden JM, et al. Cinnamon supplementation does not improve glycemic control in postmenopausal type 2 diabetes patients. J Nutr 2006;136(4):977–80.
53. Altschuler JA, Casella SJ, MacKenzie TA, et al. The effect of cinnamon on A1C among adolescents with type 1 diabetes. Diabetes Care 2007;30(4):813–6.
54. Baker WL, Gutierrez-Williams G, White CM, et al. Effect of cinnamon on glucose control and lipid parameters. Diabetes Care 2008;31(1):41–3.
55. Davis CM, Vincent JB. Chromium oligopeptide activates insulin receptor tyrosine kinase activity. Biochemistry 1997;36(15):4382–5.
56. Kordella T. Research profile. Chromium. Can it help kids with type 2? Sushil K. Jain, PhD. Diabetes Forecast 2004;57(7):83–5.
57. Yeh GY, Eisenberg DM, Kaptchuk TJ, et al. Systematic review of herbs and dietary supplements for glycemic control in diabetes. Diabetes Care 2003;26(4):1277–94.
58. Kleefstra N, Houweling ST, Bakker SJ, et al. Chromium treatment has no effect in patients with type 2 diabetes in a Western population: a randomized, double-blind, placebo-controlled trial. Diabetes Care 2007;30(5):1092–6.
59. Singer GM, Geohas J. The effect of chromium picolinate and biotin supplementation on glycemic control in poorly controlled patients with type 2 diabetes mellitus: a placebo-controlled, double-blinded, randomized trial. Diabetes Technol Ther 2006;8(6):636–43.
60. Albarracin CA, Fuqua BC, Evans JL, et al. Chromium picolinate and biotin combination improves glucose Meta in treated, uncontrolled overweight to obese patients with type 2 diabetes. Diabetes Metab Res Rev 2008;24(1):41–51.
61. Geohas J, Daly A, Juturu V, et al. Chromium picolinate and biotin combination reduces atherogenic index of plasma in patients with type 2 diabetes mellitus: a placebo-controlled, double-blinded, randomized clinical trial. Am J Med Sci 2007;333(3):145–53.
62. Wang ZQ, Qin J, Martin J, et al. Phenotype of subjects with type 2 diabetes mellitus may determine clinical response to chromium supplementation. Meta 2007;56(12):1652–5.

63. Song MK, Hwang IK, Rosenthal MJ, et al. Anti-hyperglycemic activity of zinc plus cyclo (his-pro) in genetically diabetic Goto-Kakizaki and aged rats. Exp Biol Med (Maywood) 2003;228(11):1338–45.
64. Hagglof B, Hallmans G, Holmgren G, et al. Prospective and retrospective studies of zinc concentrations in serum, blood clots, hair and urine in young patients with insulin-dependent diabetes mellitus. Acta Endocrinol (Copenh) 1983;102(1): 88–95.
65. Pedrosa LF, Ferreira SR, Cesarini PR, et al. Influence of glycemic control on zinc urinary excretion in patients with type 1 diabetes. Diabetes Care 1999;22(2): 362–3.
66. Anderson RA, Roussel AM, Zouari N, et al. Potential antioxidant effects of zinc and chromium supplementation in people with type 2 diabetes mellitus. J Am Coll Nutr 2001;20(3):212–8.
67. Chausmer AB. Zinc, insulin and diabetes. J Am Coll Nutr 1998;17(2):109–15.
68. de Sena KC, Arrais RF, das Gracas Almeida M, et al. Effects of zinc supplementation in patients with type 1 diabetes. Biol Trace Elem Res 2005;105(1-3):1–9.
69. Cunningham JJ, Fu A, Mearkle PL, et al. Hyperzincuria in individuals with insulin-dependent diabetes mellitus: concurrent zinc status and the effect of high-dose zinc supplementation. Meta 1994;43(12):1558–62.
70. Uusitalo L, Nevalainen J, Niinisto S, et al. Serum alpha- and gamma-tocopherol concentrations and risk of advanced beta cell autoimmunity in children with HLA-conferred susceptibility to type 1 diabetes mellitus. Diabetologia 2008; 51(5):773–80.
71. Ziegler D, Nowak H, Kempler P, et al. Treatment of symptomatic diabetic polyneuropathy with the antioxidant alpha-lipoic acid: a meta-analysis. Diabet Med 2004;21(2):114–21.
72. Huang EA, Gitelman SE. The effect of oral alpha-lipoic acid on oxidative stress in adolescents with type 1 diabetes mellitus. Pediatr Diabetes 2008;9(3 Pt 2):69–73.
73. Vanelli M, Chiari G, Gugliotta M, et al. [Diabetes and alternative medicine: diabetic patients experiences with Ayur-Ved, "clinical ecology" and "cellular nutrition" methods]. Minerva Pediatr 2002;54(2):165–9 [in Italian].
74. Bhowmick SK, Hundley OT, Rettig KR. Severe hypernatremia and hyperosmolality exacerbated by an herbal preparation in a patient with diabetic ketoacidosis. Clin Pediatr (Phila) 2007;46(9):831–4.
75. Glauber B. Faith, medicine collide, and a young girl dies: parents chose to pray rather than get medical help for sick child. Journal Sentinel Online, Milwaukee Wisconsin March 27, 2008. Available at: http://www.jsonline.com/news/wisconsin/29545619.html. Accessed August 19, 2009.

# Recent Consensus Statements in Pediatric Endocrinology: A Selective Review

Michelle Klein, MD*, Anpalakan Sathasivam, MD,
Yeray Novoa, MD, Robert Rapaport, MD**

**KEYWORDS**

- Consensus statements • Diabetic ketoacidosis
- Small for gestational age • Idiopathic short stature
- Intersex disorders

Jo Rycroft-Malone,[1] PhD, a leading expert in the field of evidence-based medicine, said, "to achieve clinically effective care we must access three strands of evidence: knowledge from research findings, knowledge from clinical experience, and patient-specific information (including preferences and acceptability of an intervention to individuals."

Clinical guidelines and consensus statements serve to summarize and organize current knowledge on diverse subjects, and provide practical guidelines for proper clinical management. Recommendations should be based on research and evidence derived from appropriate sources. Randomized controlled trials and systematic reviews of randomized controlled trials are usually the preferred sources.[2] When a certain aspect of treatment or care has not been covered adequately in the literature, expert opinion is considered in developing guidelines.

In 2008, more than 20 consensus statements were published in the pediatric literature alone. To acquaint the reader in pediatric endocrinology with some of the major findings, the authors summarize the salient points of the latest consensus statements jointly developed by multiple endocrine societies including the Lawson Wilkins Society for Pediatric Endocrinology (LWPES) and the European Society for Pediatric Endocrinology (ESPS). Common to all of the reviewed consensus statements is the bringing together of experts in the field to review the literature, evaluate the evidence, and formulate statements representing the views of many. As much as possible, the

Division of Pediatric Endocrinology and Diabetes, Mount Sinai Hospital, One Gustave Levly Place, Box 1616, New York, NY 10029, USA
* Corresponding author.
** Corresponding author.
*E-mail address:* michelle.klein@mssm.edu (M. Klein); robert.rapaport@mssm.edu (R. Rapaport).

Endocrinol Metab Clin N Am 38 (2009) 811–825
doi:10.1016/j.ecl.2009.09.003 endo.theclinics.com
0889-8529/09/$ – see front matter 

original intent and language of the statements was respected and paraphrased. For more information and for review of sources used for the consensus statements, the reader is referred to the original published articles.

## CONSENSUS STATEMENT ON THE MANAGEMENT OF DIABETIC KETOACIDOSIS IN CHILDREN AND ADOLESCENTS

The purpose was to explore management and complications of diabetic ketoacidosis (DKA) in children and adolescents to formulate a consensus on prevention and reduction of DKA.[3]

The statement was endorsed by LWPES, ESPS, International Society for Pediatric and Adolescent Diabetics (ISPAD), Juvenile Diabetes Research Foundation International (JDRF), World Federation of Pediatric Intensive and Critical Care Societies (WFPICCS), European Society for Pediatric Critical Care (ESPCC), European Society for Pediatric and Neonatal Intensive Care (ESPNIC), and Australian Pediatric Endocrine Group (APEG).

Later guidelines published by the American Diabetes Association (ADA)[4] and by the ISPAD[5] included recommendations of this consensus statement.

### *Definition of DKA*

DKA occurs when there is a disruption in the homeostatic balance between insulin and counter-regulatory hormones secondary to a deficiency in circulating insulin and an increase in levels of catecholamines, glucagon, growth hormone, and cortisol. The result is a state of hyperglycemia, hyperosmolarity, increased lipolysis, ketonemia, and metabolic acidosis secondary to increased ketone body production. Osmotic diuresis, dehydration, and loss of electrolytes are further consequences of the hyperglycemia and acidosis.

The major biochemical diagnostic criteria for DKA include hyperglycemia (blood glucose: greater than 11 mmol/L [approximately 200 mg/dL]) with a venous pH less than 7.3 or bicarbonate less than 15 mmol/L.[6] There are associated minor criteria including glycosuria, ketonuria, and ketonemia. DKA is classified further by the degree of the acidosis:

Mild (venous pH: less than 7.30; HCO3: less than 15 mmol/L)
Moderate (pH: less than 7.2; HCO3: less than 10 mmol/L)
Severe (pH: less than 7.1; HCO3: less 5 mmol/L)

Clinical features of DKA include dehydration, Kussmaul breathing, severe abdominal pain, nausea, and vomiting; additionally, patients may have fever if infection is also present.[4]

### *Frequency of DKA*

The more prevalent type I diabetes mellitus (TIDM) is in a given region, the less likely it is for DKA to be present at diagnosis. It is more common to see DKA at the onset of diabetes in children less than 4 years of age, children who do not have a first-degree relative with TIDM, and children from families of lower socioeconomic status or without ready access to medical care. Certain medications including glucocorticoids, atypical antipsychotics, and Diazoxide have been indicted as causative agents of DKA in patients not previously diagnosed with TIDM.

Factors such as poor metabolic control, a history of DKA, poor family structure, a psychiatric history, or being a peripubertal or adolescent female increase the risk of DKA in patients with TIDM. The most common reason for the occurrence of DKA

(75% of cases) in these patients is either incorrect insulin dosing or absence of insulin. Other causes include insufficient amounts of insulin during stress or illness to balance counter-regulatory hormones and inappropriate cessation of insulin pump therapy.

### *Cerebral Edema*

The first signs of cerebral edema (CE) can be subtle and nonspecific and include headache, mental status changes, bradycardia, and hypertension. Studies have shown that CE usually occurs 4 to 12 hours after management of DKA has begun, but it can occur any time before or during treatment. The incidence of CE is up to 1% in all cases of DKA.

Increased risk for CE is seen in patients who present with DKA at diagnosis, are younger, and have symptoms of DKA for a longer amount of time. Other risk factors include degree of acidosis at presentation, greater hypocapnia at presentation after adjusting for the severity of acidosis, bicarbonate treatment during DKA, elevated serum urea nitrogen at presentation, and a slower rise in measured serum sodium concentrations during treatment of DKA. Neither the severity of hyperglycemia at presentation of DKA nor the concentration of sodium in intravenous fluids has been shown to increase the risk of cerebral edema.

### *Management of DKA*

Mild cases of DKA, in which patients have hyperglycemia and ketosis, but can tolerate oral (PO) and are not dehydrated, do not require inpatient or emergency room management. Patients who are vomiting, cannot tolerate fluids by mouth, or are dehydrated should be evaluated in an emergency room or inpatient setting. Admission to an ICU should be advised in children with severe DKA (prolonged duration of symptoms, mental status changes, or vascular compromise) or patients who are at increased risk of cerebral edema.

The initial assessment of DKA requires a detailed history and physical examination. Degree of dehydration should be assessed using weight, pulse, blood pressure and respiratory effort, capillary refill, and skin turgor. Samples for measurement of glucose, electrolytes, osmolality, venous or arterial pH and pCO2, hemoglobin and hematocrit, and HbA1c should be obtained, as well as a urinalysis for ketones.

Management of DKA in the ICU should include hourly measurement of the vital signs including strict fluid input and output, capillary blood glucose, and neurologic examinations (looking for Cushing's triad and other signs of cerebral edema). Every 2 to 4 hours, blood gases and chemistries should be done to evaluate electrolytes, serum urea nitrogen (BUN), hematocrit, and blood glucose. More frequent testing is warranted if the patient is critically ill. An electrocardiogram should be considered if potassium measurement is delayed.

### *Hydration Status and Fluid Replacement*

Hemodynamic instability and shock are rare in pediatric DKA. Chemical measurements, as a means of assessing fluid deficit, can be unreliable at diagnosis. The extracellular fluid has higher osmolality and fluid shifts from the intracellular to extracellular compartments. Therefore, sodium measured on a blood chemistry is usually lower than the total body sodium. The effective osmolality at the time of presentation is usually in the range of 300 to 350 mOsm/L. Hemoconcentration leads to an increased BUN and hematocrit and may help to differentiate severe extracellular fluid (ECF) contraction from true hyponatremia.

Goals of therapy in DKA include replacement of diminished circulatory volume, repletion of electrolytes, recovery of the glomerular filtration rate (GFR) to further eliminate glucose and ketones from the circulation, and avoidance of complications including cerebral edema. Slower correction of overall fluid deficit with isotonic or near-isotonic fluids can lead to quicker resolution of acidosis. The risk of using large amounts of normal saline is hyperchloremic metabolic acidosis. There is no evidence supporting the use of colloids over crystalloids for DKA therapy.

Fluids given to the child before assessment should be factored into calculation of deficit. Initial intravenous fluid administration should begin immediately with an isotonic solution, which can be given if needed in a 10 to 20 cc/kg bolus over 1 to 2 hours. The remainder replacement intravenous fluid should be given evenly over at least 48 hours. Subsequent fluid management should be with a solution with a tonicity greater than or equal to 0.45% saline. In addition to clinical assessment of dehydration, calculation of effective osmolality may be valuable to guide fluid and electrolyte therapy. Because the severity of dehydration may be difficult to determine and can be overestimated, fluid infusion should not exceed a rate of 1.5 to 2 times the usual daily requirement based on age, weight, or body surface area. Urinary losses should not be added to the calculation of replacement fluids.

### *Insulin*

After the fluid deficit and electrolyte losses are calculated, low-dose intravenous insulin administration is standard of care. The goal of insulin therapy is to inhibit lipolysis and ketogenesis and decrease the blood glucose levels. A bolus of insulin is not necessary, and its use is controversial. The dose of insulin should be maintained at 0.1 U/kg/h until resolution of ketoacidosis (pH: greater than 7.30; HCO3: greater than 15 mmol/L) or until the anion gap is closed. If the patient has hypoglycemia on maximum amounts of intravenous dextrose, then the insulin drip should be lowered, but not less than 0.05 U/kg/h.

To prevent hypoglycemia, glucose should be added to the intravenous fluid when the plasma glucose falls to approximately 14 to 17 mmol/L (250 to 300 mg/dL), because the resolution of acidemia usually takes longer than the normalization of blood glucose. Five percent glucose can be used initially and then slowly increased to maintain euglycemia on the insulin drip. Reassessment of the patient, review of insulin therapy, and consideration of other possible causes of impaired response to insulin should be considered (eg, infection, errors in insulin preparation, or adhesion of insulin to tubing with very dilute solutions) if biochemical parameters of ketoacidosis do not improve. In the rare event that intravenous insulin cannot be given, insulin may be administered subcutaneously or intramuscularly every hour at the same dose.

### *Electrolyte Replacement*

In DKA, potassium is lost from the intracellular compartment as a result of insulin deficiency, hypertonicity, and the exchange of hydrogen ions within the cell. Potassium also is lost secondary to vomiting and osmotic diuresis. Therefore, serum levels of potassium are not reliable in the initial work-up of DKA. Once insulin is given, potassium will move from the extracellular to intracellular space, and serum levels will decrease. Repletion of potassium is necessary and should be started once the serum levels are no longer elevated and the patient has urinated.

In DKA, phosphate deficit also occurs as a result of osmotic diuresis and movement across the cell. Treatment with insulin results in movement of phosphate back into the intracellular space and a subsequent drop in serum phosphate. Although studies have not shown significant clinical benefit from phosphate repletion in DKA and its use remains controversial, potassium phosphate may be used safely together with potassium chloride to avoid hyperchloremia. Calcium levels should be monitored closely.

### *Acidosis*

Fluid replacement and insulin are the first-line agents for treating acidosis. Insulin prevents ketoacid production and breaks it down into bicarbonate. Fluid replacement improves tissue perfusion and increases GFR to aid in acid excretion.

The use of bicarbonate in treating DKA remains controversial. Some studies have shown that bicarbonate may worsen electrolyte abnormalities in DKA by contributing to hypokalemia and hypernatremia via increased sodium load. Bicarbonate also can increase the synthesis of ketones in the liver and thereby slow down the time to recovery from ketoacidosis. Still, a subset of patients with severe DKA (arterial pH: less than 6.9) who have impaired cardiac contractility, peripheral vasodilatation, poor tissue perfusion, and life-threatening hyperkalemia may benefit from judicious use of bicarbonate.

### *Treatment of Cerebral Edema*

The clinician should have high suspicion for CE in patients with DKA, and therapy should commence immediately once diagnosed. The head of the bed should be elevated. Intravenous fluids should be reduced, and intravenous mannitol should be given. If Mannitol is not available, 3% hypertonic saline may be used instead. Mechanical ventilation may be required if the patient's respiratory status is compromised. Studies have shown poor outcomes in patients with CE associated with DKA who were aggressively ventilated (pCO2 less than 22 mm Hg). The role of glucocorticoids in treatment of CE in DKA has not been supported.

### *Prevention of DKA*

Education and early detection remain the ultimate tools in prevention. Genetic and immunologic diagnostic testing in patients at higher risk for T1DM has been shown to decrease the occurrence of DKA at onset of diabetes. In patients with TIDM, studies have shown that comprehensive health care and education including plans for sick day management and continuous subcutaneous insulin pump malfunction can help to decrease the incidence of DKA.

## CONSENSUS STATEMENT ON IDIOPATHIC SHORT STATURE

The purpose was to summarize the advances in the management of children with idiopathic short stature (ISS).[7]

The statement was endorsed by: Growth Hormone Research Society (GHRS), LWPES, European Society for Pediatric Endocrinology (ESPE), Latin American Society of Pediatric Endocrinology (SLEP), Japanese Society of Pediatric Endocrinology (JSPE), Canadian Pediatric Endocrine Group (CPEG), Asia Pacific Pediatric Endocrine Society (APPES), and APEG.

### *Definition*

ISS was defined as

> *"a height more than two standard deviation scores (SDS) below the corresponding mean for a given age, sex, and population group without evidence of systemic, endocrine, nutritional, or chromosomal abnormalities"*

This includes constitutional delay of growth and puberty (CDGP) and familial short stature. Children born small for gestational age, children with syndromes involving short stature, and children with chronic medical conditions that interfere with growth should be excluded from this definition.

ISS can be subdivided into two groups based on the midparental height (calculated by average of parents' heights + 6.5 cm for boys/- 6.5 cm for girls.)[8] One group is children whose adult height is about the same as the midparental height, and the other is children whose adult height is below the midparental height.

### *Assessment of the Short Child*

Each evaluation of a short child should begin with a comprehensive history:

Birth history (including in utero events, anthropomorphic data at birth, amniocentesis, gestational age, and complications)
Medical history including hospitalizations, surgeries, medications, chronic diseases, dietary history, developmental history including dentition, which can parallel bone maturation
Family history focusing on stature, onset of puberty, and chronic diseases of first- and second-degree family members; consanguinity should be documented
Pubertal history of the patient
Prior growth point or curves

The physical examination should include the general appearance, any dysmorphic features, and body disproportions. A length should be obtained in all children under 3 years of age with a recumbent stadiometer. A standing stadiometer can be used in cooperative children over 3 years of age. Arm span, sitting height or upper-to-lower segment ratios, body mass index (BMI), and for children younger than 4 years measurement of the head circumference should be included. Pubertal status using Tanner staging should be documented.

## DIAGNOSTIC STUDIES

If the history and physical examination do not reveal a specific diagnosis, the following screening tests are indicated:

A complete blood count
Sedimentation rate
A complete metabolic panel
Screening for celiac disease
Thyroid function tests
Insulin-like growth factor (IGF)-1 level
A radiograph for bone age (BA)

In a female with unexplained short stature or in any male with genital abnormalities, a karyotype should be done. Skeletal survey should be reserved for patients with suspicion of a skeletal dysplasia.

It is strongly recommended that IGF-1 levels be obtained as part of the evaluation. Insulin-like growth factor binding protein (IGFBP-3) measurements add little to the evaluation of short stature except in children younger than 3 years. Measures of spontaneous growth hormone (GH) secretion are not indicated. GH stimulation testing should be performed in any patient with a history and physical examination suggestive of GH deficiency, a low growth velocity or low IGF-1 levels. A peak stimulated GH value less than 10 ng/dL is considered GH deficiency (and thus excludes ISS). If a diagnosis of ISS is made, a head magnetic resonance imaging (MRI) scan is not indicated. Genetic testing including short stature homeobox (SHOX) gene analysis should be considered in appropriate clinical settings.

## TREATMENT

The primary goal of treatment is to reach a normal adult height. A secondary goal is to reach a more socially acceptable height during childhood. In the United States, GH treatment has been approved for children shorter than -2.25 SDS (1.2 percentile). Children whose heights are -2 SDS and who are more than 2 SDS below their midparental target height (TH) or their predicted adult height (PAH) also should be considered for treatment. There are no laboratory criteria for starting GH therapy. Optimal age for initiating treatment is 5 years to early puberty (most studies examined children older than 3 to 4 years). The role of PAH in the decision to treat with GH is unclear. The PAH may be inaccurate, but it can be a helpful tool together with other factors (BA, family height and pubertal history, and midparental target height) in deciding to treat.

### *Dosing and Duration of GH Treatment*

Current US Food and Drug Administration (FDA)-approved dosing for GH in children with ISS is up to 0.3 to 0.37 mg/kg/wk (42 to 52 μg/k/d).[9] There are no data on long-term safety of doses higher than 0.35 mg/k/wk (50 μg/k/d) in children with ISS. The dose of GH is adjusted based on weight gain and interval growth velocity. IGF-1 measurements are also useful in assessing efficacy, safety, and compliance. Increased short-term growth is achieved with higher IGF-1 values, but there are no long-term studies to asses the safety or ultimate effect of these elevated levels. The current recommendation is if IGF-1 levels are consistently above 2.5 SDS, the dose of GH should be reduced.

There are two groups with differing ideas about when to stop treatment with GH. One group recommends stopping GH when near-adult height is reached (height velocity less than 2 cm/y or BA greater than 16 years in boys or greater than 14 years in girls). The other group recommends stopping GH when the height is in the normal adult range (above -2 SDS) or has reached another cut-off for the reference adult population. The individual patient's desire to terminate treatment should be considered at each visit.

### *Response to GH*

Change in height SDS of more than 0.3 to 0.5, height velocity increase of more than 3 cm/y, and height velocity SDS increase of more than 1 suggest a successful first-year response to GH. The dose of GH can be increased if the growth velocity is decreased, and compliance is assured. If the rate of growth is still suboptimal after 1 to 2 years of higher doses of GH, then GH treatment should be stopped and other treatment options considered.

Children with ISS on GH therapy (average duration 4 to 7 years) have a mean increase in adult height of 3.5 to 7.5 cm. Responses are highly variable and are dose-dependent. Children who are younger, heavier, who receive higher doses per kilogram, and who are shortest relative to target height have the best growth response. Adult height outcome is influenced negatively by older age at the start of treatment and is influenced positively by a taller midparental height, a taller height at the start of treatment, a greater BA delay, and a greater first-year response to GH therapy.

### *Monitoring*

Adverse effects noted in children receiving GH for ISS are generally the same as those previously reported in children receiving GH for other indications, although they occur less frequently.[10] Height, weight, pubertal development, and adverse effects to GH should be monitored every 3 to 6 months in children treated with GH. Regular evaluations for scoliosis, tonsillar hypertrophy, papilledema, and slipped capital femoral epiphysis should be performed. After 1 year of treatment, the response to GH should be assessed by calculating height velocity SDS and the change in height SDS. A BA may be obtained periodically. No instances of elevated blood glucose in GH-treated patients with ISS have been reported.

### *Alternative to GH Treatment*

Anabolic steroids, such as oxandrolone (given orally) and testosterone (patch or gel) are alternative treatment options. Both have been shown useful in boys with CDGP and short stature greater than -2.5 SDS. If the adult height prediction is close to the target height, then testosterone has been shown to be the most appropriate treatment. Oxandrolone has not been shown to significantly increase predicted or measured adult height.

IGF-1 is FDA-approved for short stature associated with severe IGF deficiency and normal GH secretion. Children first should be given a trial of GH, and if they do not respond, IGF-1 should be considered. Data are lacking regarding efficacy and safety.

GnRH analogs (GnRHa) are not recommended to be used alone in children with ISS, but in combination with GH it has potential value if it is used for at least 3 years. Its use might be considered if the PAH is below 2 SDS at the time of onset of puberty. When using GnRHa, one must consider the psychological effects of delaying puberty.

Studies using aromatase inhibitors (AIs) for at least 2 years have shown that males with ISS on GH have an increase in PAH.[11,12] The long-term efficacy and safety of AI in males have not been demonstrated. No data support the use of AI in females.

## CONSENSUS STATEMENT ON THE MANAGEMENT OF THE CHILD BORN SMALL FOR GESTATIONAL AGE THROUGH TO ADULTHOOD

The purpose was to identify key health issues facing children born small for gestational age (SGA) and to propose management strategies.[13]

The statement was endorsed by: ESPE, LWPES, GHRS, SLEP, APPES, APEG, JSPE.

### *Definition*

To diagnose a child as SGA the following information must be obtained:

- Gestational age (preferably calculated from the first trimester ultrasound examination)
- Birth weight, length, and head circumference
- Reference cut-off defined by a comparable population of patients, below which the definition lies

The definition of SGA is birth weight or birth length less than -2 SD below the mean specific for the population. Children born SGA must be monitored for many health issues including heart disease, perinatal morbidity, associated neurodevelopmental disorders, poor growth/short stature, and metabolic irregularities.

### *Early Growth and Development*

Longitudinal studies of growth in children born SGA have shown weight catch-up usually occurs in the first 6 months, while height catch-up can take up to 2 years. Ninety percent of children born SGA do catch-up. Factors that decrease the chance of catch-up growth include severe prematurity, growth retardation, and very low birth weight, while having tall parents increases the likelihood of catch-up.

Children born SGA should be monitored with measurements of length, weight, and head circumference every 3 months for the first year of life and every 6 months thereafter. Pediatricians should be aware of children who do not catch-up in the first 6 months of life or remain short by 2 years of age. These children should be referred to a pediatric endocrinologist.

Children born SGA have increased central adiposity and decreased lean mass. Studies have shown rapid weight gain in infancy is associated with obesity as an adult; therefore earlier dense feedings for SGA infants may not be appropriate.

### *Endocrinopathies and Metabolic Disorders*

Overall, there are no true endocrinopathies associated with SGA. Classic growth GH deficiency usually is not seen. IGF1 and IGFBP3 levels are decreased 1 SDS in SGA children; however, they are not predictive of growth velocity or adult height. Routine evaluation of the hypothalamic-pituitary-adrenal and the thyroid axes are not recommended.

Being born SGA is not associated with late or early puberty. The small population of children who do have early puberty also have rapid puberty, leading to faster bone maturation and ultimately decreased adult height. Bone age is unreliable in children born SGA, and height prediction based on it is not routinely recommended. Hypospadias and cryptorchidism are observed in children born SGA.

Type 2 diabetes mellitus, adolescent hypertension, impaired glucose tolerance, and dyslipidemia have not been shown to occur more frequently in children born SGA. Insulin resistance, however, has been shown to occur as early as 1 year of age. Although the overall prevalence of risk factors is low, young adults born SGA have a higher incidence of metabolic risk factors (2.3%), especially if they are obese, of a certain ethnicity, and have strong family history.

### *Management of Growth and Puberty*

Early evaluation of short children born SGA is recommended. There are over 40 years of research on the use of GH in children with SGA, and its use has been approved by the FDA and the European Agency for the Evaluation of Medicinal Products. The general consensus is that children between the ages of 2 to 4 years born SGA who have not caught up with a height less than 2.5 SD should be treated with GH. If the child is over the age of 4 years and does not show catch-up growth, then a height of 2 SD should be used as the cut-off. The starting dose of GH is 0.24 to 0.49 mg/kg/wk (35 to 70 μg/kg/d), with the higher doses used in those with the most marked growth retardation.[14]

Age and height SDS at the start of treatment, midparental height, and dose of GH all influence the response during the first 2 to 3 years. Children with recognized syndromes respond less well to GH than those with nonsyndromic SGA. A growth velocity of more than + 0.5 SDS in the first year of treatment is considered a positive response to GH treatment. If there is a poor response, re-evaluation is indicated, including consideration of compliance, dose of GH, diagnosis, and the decision to discontinue treatment. In those with a positive response, withdrawal of GH therapy after 2 to 3 years leads to catch-down growth and is not recommended. GH should be stopped in adolescence when the growth velocity falls to less than 2 cm/y.

There is no evidence that the addition of a GnRH analog is associated with additional height gain in children born SGA. Pre-treatment IGF-1 levels may have a role in predicting responsiveness to GH, and in those receiving treatment, IGF-1 monitoring may be a useful tool for dose optimization. Some syndromes, such as Bloom's syndrome or Fanconi syndrome may carry risks that may contraindicate the use of GH therapy. Adverse effects from GH treatment are not seen more commonly in children born SGA compared with other conditions.

### *Consequences in Adulthood*

Studies have shown that children born SGA are at increased risk for metabolic consequences later on in life. Most of the evidence, however, comes from observational studies not limited to children born SGA. A rapid weight gain in infancy has been associated with an increased risk of obesity. Both small and large sizes at birth have been reported to be associated with increased risk of type 2 diabetes and glucose intolerance. Women born SGA are at an increased risk of having an SGA infant, preeclampsia, and gestational diabetes.

## CONSENSUS STATEMENT ON MANAGEMENT OF INTERSEX DISORDERS

The purpose was to review the management of intersex disorders and devise a consensus statement on definitions, diagnosis, and management, and formulated proposals for future studies.[15]

The consensus statement was endorsed by LWPES, ESPE.

### *Introduction and Definitions*

The definitions and nomenclature for intersex disorders are being reviewed and reworked continually as a result of dissatisfaction amongs health care professionals, families, and patients with the current terminology. The term disorders of sex development (DSD), as defined by congenital conditions in which development of chromosomal, gonadal, or anatomic sex is atypical was proposed by the consensus committee. This phrase would replace terminology such as intersex, pseudohermaphroditism, hermaphroditism, and sex reversal, as these terms are potentially imprecise and derogatory (**Table 1**).

Psychosexual development is shaped by both biologic and environmental influences including exposure to androgens, genetics, neuro-anatomy, and family and social history. To understand psychosexual development, one must define its three components:

1. Gender identity—a person's self-representation as male or female (some individuals may not identify exclusively with either)

**Table 1**
**Proposed revised nomenclature**

| Previous | Proposed |
|---|---|
| Intersex | Disorders of sex development (DSD) |
| Male pseudohermaphrodite, undervirilization of an XY male | 46, XY DSD |
| Female pseudohermaphrodite, overvirilization of an XX female, and masculinization of an XX female | 46, XX DSD |
| True hermaphrodite | Ovotesticular DSD |
| XX male or XX sex reversal | 46, XX testicular DSD |
| XY sex reversal | 46, XY complete gonadal dysgenesis |

2. Gender role—the psychological characteristics that are sexually dimorphic within the general population, such as toy preferences and physical aggression
3. Sexual orientation—the direction(s) of erotic interest (heterosexual, bisexual, homosexual)

Gender dissatisfaction occurs more often in people with DSD than in the general population and signifies discontent with sex assignment. Psychosocial care, like medical and surgical care, is an integral part of DSD management.

### *Clinical Management of DSD*

DSD usually is diagnosed in newborns with atypical genitalia, with congenital adrenal hyperplasia (CAH) remaining the most common cause.[16] DSD, however, may be diagnosed in the older child or adult who presents with) gynecomastia or hematuria in a male, inguinal hernia, virilization, or primary amenorrhea in a female, or delayed/partial puberty or previously unrecognized genital ambiguity.

Specifically, criteria suggestive of DSD include:

- Obvious genital ambiguity
- Female genitalia with an enlarged clitoris, posterior labial fusion, or an inguinal/labial mass
- Male genitalia with bilateral undescended testes, micropenis, isolated perineal hypospadias, or mild hypospadias with undescended testis
- Family history of DSD
- Discordance between genital appearance and a prenatal karyotype

In newborns with DSD, gender assignment should not occur until an evaluation is performed by an experienced multidisciplinary team including a pediatric endocrinologist, surgeon/urologist, psychologist/psychiatrist, geneticist, gynecologist, and neonatologist. All individuals should receive a gender assignment. The families should be involved in the decision-making process, and in the case of older children, the patient should be involved also.

A comprehensive history including prenatal and family history should be obtained followed by a complete physical examination. The examination of the genitalia must be thorough and documented well. Anatomy should be compared with published norms.

Initial testing should be tailored to clinical findings depends on availability of testing at the individual center. First-line testing should include:

- Fluorescence in situ hybridization (FISH) with X- and Y-specific probe detection (even when prenatal karyotype is available)
- A full karyotype
- Imaging of the abdomen and pelvis via sonography
- Measurement of 17-hydroxyprogesterone
- Testosterone
- Gonadotropins
- Anti-Müllerian Hormone
- Serum electrolytes
- Urinalysis

The results obtained from these tests should be sufficient for making a diagnosis within the category of DSD. Should the diagnosis remain elusive, additional testing can include

- Human chorionic gonadotropin- and adrenocorticotropin-stimulation tests (to assess testicular and adrenal steroid biosynthesis)
- Urinary steroid analysis by gas chromatography mass spectroscopy
- Imaging studies
- Gonadal biopsies
- DNA analysis of the main genes in the pathway of testis differentiation and functionality

Despite all of the available testing, only 20% of cases of DSD have an identified molecular diagnosis. Only 50% of 46,XY children with DSD will receive a definitive diagnosis.

### *Assigning Gender in Newborns*

After a comprehensive evaluation, deciding on gender assignment is a daunting and stressful task for both the health care team and family. The following evidence from patients with DSD should be used along with individual factors including opinions of the family and their cultural practices, genital appearance and surgical options, a need for lifelong replacement therapy, and potential for fertility . Evidence to assist in sex assignment includes

- Markedly virilized 46, XX infants with CAH should be raised as female, because more than 90% of patients with 46XX CAH identify as female.
- 60% of patients with 5-alpha-reductase-deficiency assigned female as a newborn and who then virilized at puberty lived as males. This along with the potential for fertility as a male should be discussed when deciding on gender assignment. Although fertility is less well documented in 17-beta-hydroxysteroid dehydrogenase deficiency, the same considers should be made.
- 25% of patients with partial androgen insensitivity syndrome (PAIS), androgen biosynthetic defects, and incomplete gonadal dysgenesis were dissatisfied with their assigned sex whether male of female.
- Available data support male rearing in all patients with micropenis, again taking into consideration fertility.
- Potential for fertility on the basis of gonadal differentiation and genital development should be considered in patients with ovotesticular DSD
- Prenatal androgen exposure, testicular function at and after puberty, phallic development, and gonadal location should be considered in patients with mixed gonadal dysgenesis (MGD).
- 65% of individuals with cloacal exostrophy lived as female, but there was still variability in gender identity outcome.

### *Surgical Management*

Surgeons should have both pediatric training and expertise in DSD surgery. Early genitoplasty is acceptable if the cause of DSD has been identified, and severe virilization (Prader 3 to 4) exists. Genitoplasty should be performed in concordance with repair of the common urogenital sinus. The surgical procedure should focus on preservation of erectile function and the innervation of the clitoris. Vaginal dilatation should not be used in childhood. It is expected that revision of surgeries done in infancy will be necessary at the time of puberty or shortly after.

If there is less severe clitoromegaly and no involvement of the urogenital sinus, then surgery should be postponed until adolescence. Once a patient with an absent or inadequate vagina is psychologically motivated and a full partner is involved, then vaginoplasty should be performed. Unfortunately, self-dilatation, skin substitution, and bowel vaginoplasty all have pros and cons, and none has been universally successful.

If hypospadias is associated with a DSD, then surgical repair and testosterone supplementation are recommended. There is no evidence that removal of asymptomatic discordant structures prophylactically is necessary. Symptoms in the future may suggest the need for surgical removal.

The testes in patients with DSD raised female should be removed to prevent malignancy in adulthood. Because the earliest reported malignancy was at 14 years of age, a parents' right to refuse removal of the testes until adolescence is supported. The availability of estrogen-replacement therapy allows for the option of early removal at the time of diagnosis. The streak gonad in a patient with MGD raised male should be removed in early childhood. Females with gonadal dysgenesis (bilateral streak gonads) and Y-chromosome material should have bilateral gonadectomy performed in early childhood. Gonadectomy should be performed before puberty in patients with androgen biosynthetic defects raised female.

Testicular biopsy should be performed at puberty in patients with gonadal dysgenesis to monitor for premalignant lesion termed carcinoma in situ or undifferentiated intratubular germ cell neoplasia. If the biopsy is positive, the patient should be given the option of sperm banking. Treatment with local low-dose radiation is curative.

### *Replacement of Sex Steroids*

The goal of replacement of sex steroids in patients with DSD is to mimic normal pubertal maturation so that the patient experiences a normal pubertal growth spurt, secondary sexual characteristics, and appropriate bone mineral accumulation. Testosterone is available as an intramuscular depot injection, an oral preparation, and transdermal preparations. The depot injection is the most commonly used. Patients with PAIS may require supraphysiologic doses of testosterone for optimal effect.

Females with hypogonadism require estrogen supplementation to induce a pubertal growth spurt, secondary sexual characteristics such as breasts, and menarche. A progestin usually is added after breakthrough bleeding develops or within 1 to 2 years of continuous estrogen. In women without a uterus, there is no evidence that the addition of cyclic progesterone is beneficial.

### *Psychosocial Management and Long-term Outcomes*

Psychosocial care provided by mental health staff with expertise in DSD is an integral part of management of DSD. The earliest age at which gender identity can be assessed accurately remains unclear, but it is thought to begin before the age of 3 years. Atypical gender role behavior is more common in children with DSD. In affected children and adolescents who report significant gender dysphoria, a specialist in psychosexual development is crucial to help the patient identify feelings about gender. If the patient expresses a desire to change gender, the patient's wish should be supported. Patients with DSD often complain of sexual aversion and lack of arousability, which often are misinterpreted as decreased libido. A support network including medical and psychological professionals is crucial to identifying and treating these important issues.

There is much needed follow-up for long-term outcomes for patients with DSD including medical, surgical, and psychological. What is known is related mainly to surgical outcomes and sexual function. Early surgery, while successful in many cases, does run the risk of decreased sexual sensitivity, loss of clitoral tissue, and cosmetic

**Box 1**
**Abbreviations of organizations**

APEG-Australian Pediatric Endocrine Group
APPES-Asia Pacific Pediatric Endocrine Society
CPEG-Canadian Pediatric Endocrine Group
ESPCC-European Society for Pediatric Critical Care
ESPNIC-European Society of Pediatric and Neonatal Intensive Care
ESPE-European Society for Pediatric Endocrinology
GHRS-Growth Hormone Research Society
ISPAD-International Society
JDRF-Juvenile Diabetes Research Foundation International
JSPE-Japanese Society of Pediatric Endocrinology
LWPES-Lawson Wilkins Pediatric Endocrine Society
SLEP-Latin American Society of Pediatric Endocrinology
WFPICCS-World Federation of Pediatric Intensive and Critical Care Societies

concerns. The success of the surgery depends on the experience, skill, and technique of the surgeon. Scarring may need revision to insure proper sexual function. Surgery to construct a neovagina carries a risk of neoplasia. The degree of hypospadias and the amount of erectile tissue play a large role in the surgical result of undermasculinized males with a phallus. Feminizing genitoplasty requires less surgery to achieve an acceptable outcome compared to masculinizing genitoplasty and results in fewer urologic difficulties.

The highest tumor risk is found in TSPY (testis-specific protein Y-encoded) positive gonadal dysgenesis and PAIS with intra-abdominal gonads, whereas the lowest risk (less than 5%) is found in ovotestis and complete androgen insensitivity syndrome (CAIS). For a complete list please refer to the consensus statement (**Box 1**).

### *Addendum to Consensus Statement*

Since publication of the consensus statement on management of intersex disorders, some have recommended the term atypical genitalia replace the previous term ambiguous genitalia.[17,18]

## REFERENCES

1. Rycroft-Malone J. Formal consensus: the development of a national clinical guideline. Qual Health Care 2001;10:238–44.
2. Grimshaw JM, Russel IT. Achieving health gains through clinical guidelines: I. Developing scientifically valid guidelines. Qual Assur Health Care 1993;2:243–8.
3. Dunger DB, Sperling MA, Acerini CL, et al. European Society for Pediatric Endocrinology/Lawson Wilkins Pediatric Endocrine Society consensus statement on diabetic ketoacidosis in children and adolescents. Pediatrics 2004;113:e133–40.
4. Wolfsdorf J, Glaser N, Sperling MA. Diabetic ketoacidosis in infants, children, and adolescents. A consensus statement from the American Diabetes Association. Diabetes Care 2006;29(5):1150–9.

5. Wolfsdorf J, Craig ME, Daneman D, et al. ISPAD Clinical practice consensus guidelines 2006–2007. Diabetic ketoacidosis. Pediatr Diabetes 2007;8:28–43.
6. Dunger DB, Sperling MA, Acerni CL, et al. ESPE/LWPES consensus statement on diabetic ketoacidosis in children and adolescents. Arch Dis Child 2004;89: 188–94.
7. Cohen P, Rogol AD, Deal CL, et al. Consensus statement on the diagnosis and treatment of children with idiopathic short stature: a summary of the Growth Hormone Research Society, the Lawson Wilkins Pediatric Endocrine Society, and the European Society for Paediatric Endocrinology Workshop. J Clin Endocrinol Metab 2008;93(11):4210–7.
8. Lee M. Idiopathic short stature. N Engl J Med 2006;354:2576–82.
9. Wit J, Rekers-Mombarg L, Cutler G, et al. Growth hormone treatment to final height in children with idiopathic short stature: evidence for a dose effect. J Pediatr 2004;146:45–53.
10. Quigley C, Gill A, Crowe B, et al. Safety of growth hormone treatment in pediatric patients with idiopathic short stature. J Clin Endocrinol Metab 2005;90:5188–96.
11. Hero M, Norjavaara E, Dunkel L. Inhibition of estrogen biosíntesis with a potent aromatase inhibitor increases predicted adult height in boys with idiopathic short stature: a randomized controlled trial. J Clin Endocrinol Metab 2005;90: 6396–402.
12. Hero M, Wickman S, Dunkel L. Treatment with the aromastase inhibitor letrozole during adolescence increases near-final height in boys with constitutional delay of puberty. Clin Endocrinol 2006;64:510–3.
13. Clayton PE, Cianfarani S, Czernichow P, et al. Consensus statement: management of the child born small for gestational age through to adulthood: a consensus statement of the International Societies of Pediatric Endocrinology and the Growth Hormone Research Society. J Clin Endocrinol Metab 2007; 92(3):804–10.
14. Rapaport R, Saenger P, Wajnrajch MP, et al. Predictors of first-year growth response to a fixed-dose of growth hormone treatment in children born small for gestational age: results of an open-label, multicenter trial in the United States. J Pediatr Endocrinol Metab 2008;21:411–22.
15. Lee PA, Houk CP, Ahmed SF, et al. Consensus statement on Management of Intersex Disorders. International Consensus Conference on Intersex. Pediatrics 2006;118:e488–500.
16. Hughes I. Disorders of sex development: a new definition and classification. Best Pract Res Clin Endocrinol Metab 2008;22(1):119–34.
17. Rapaport R. Disorders of the gonads. In: Behrman RE, Kliegman RM, Jenson HB, editors. Nelson textbook of pediatrics. 17th edition. Philadelphia: Saunders; 2004. p. 1921–46.
18. Klein G, Rapaport R. Early diagnosis and management of atypical-appearing genitalia. In: Altchek A, Deligdisch L, editors. Pediatric, adolescent and young adult gynecology. West Sussex, UK: Wiley-Blackwell; 2009. p. 14–24.

# Update: Newborn Screening for Endocrinopathies

Kenneth A. Pass, PhD[a,*], Eurico Carmago Neto, PhD[b]

**KEYWORDS**

• Newborn screening • Congenital adrenal hyperplasia
• Congenital hypothyroidism • Dried blood specimen

Congenital hypothyroidism (CH) and congenital adrenal hyperplasia (CAH) are included in many newborn screening (NBS) panels worldwide and in all state-sponsored programs in the United States. They both meet the fundamental prerequisites for NBS: high incidence in the population; biomarkers in the dried blood specimen that are easily detected; and, effective therapies to lessen, if not prevent, the sequelae of absent or late treatment.[1] CH screening uses thyroxin (T4) and/or thyrotrophin (TSH) as indicators, whereas CAH screening uses an increase in 17-hydroxyprogesterone (17OHP). Additional markers for both conditions have been proposed[2,3] with mixed adoption by NBS programs. In this review, the history of NBS is discussed for these 2 conditions. The technologies and protocols used in their detection, and related subjects such as genetics, treatment and outcomes, are also discussed.

## CH

More than a decade after NBS started with testing for phenylketonuria (PKU) and with the new availability of sensitive radioimmunoassays (RIA) for TSH and T4, programs began to add testing for CH in the early 1970s.[4] Most programs in the United States chose to use T4 as the primary screen, with TSH as a second-tier screen to confirm a low T4 value, whereas programs outside the United States predominately chose TSH for the primary screening biomarker. This diversity continues today, with 131 NBS programs worldwide using TSH only for screening and 75 using the T4/TSH protocol, all using a form of immunoassay. In the United States, 4 programs use TSH only and 35 use the T4/TSH strategy (Hannon, Harry, personal communication, 2008). Each method will miss certain CH syndromes. The TSH only protocol will

[a] Biggs Laboratory, Wadsworth Center, NYS Department of Health, PO Box 0509, Albany, NY 12201-2002, USA
[b] Laboratorio Nobel and Centro de Triagem Neonatal, Porto Alegre, RS, Brazil
* Corresponding author.
*E-mail address:* kpass@wadsworth.org (K.A. Pass).

Endocrinol Metab Clin N Am 38 (2009) 827–837
doi:10.1016/j.ecl.2009.08.005 **endo.theclinics.com**
0889-8529/09/$ – see front matter 

miss those infants with central hypothyroidism, that is, of pituitary or hypothalamic origin (estimated at 1 in 50,000 births) (Hannon, Harry, personal communication, 2008). The T4/TSH protocol will miss those infants with minimally functioning or ectopic thyroid glands that seem normal at birth, then decline in function.[5] The preferred protocol would include testing for both biomarkers simultaneously as is done in 5 state programs, a procedure that was prohibitively expensive and time-consuming for large programs until recently. Multi-analyte assays have now been developed that can probe for several biomarkers simultaneously in the same assay well.[6]

### *Screening Protocols and Technology*

There is no consensus regarding the best screening protocol for CH. As noted above, either protocol, by its design, will miss certain occurrences of CH. In an effort to be more comprehensive with this screening tool, some programs screen for both T4 and TSH in the primary test; there are 5 programs in the United States using this protocol. **Table 1** shows data extracted from the National Newborn Screening and Genetics Resource Center (NNSGRC; http://www2.uthscsa.edu/nnsis/, accessed 3 December 2008) for 3 screening protocols: (1) T4 followed by TSH; (2) TSH followed by T4; (3) both T4 and TSH as first screen; and (4) for comparison, the 4 largest programs. The positive predictive value (PPV) is closely correlated with prevalence regardless of the choice of T4 or TSH as the primary screen, so that no protocol shows superior benefit, with 2 exceptions, for reasons that are not apparent. Even those programs using both T4 and TSH in the primary screening show no clear advantage.

Multiplex systems, providing the ability to measure numerous biomarkers simultaneously, offer the possibility of combining 4 markers for CH (T4, TSH, FT4, and thyroid binding globulin [TBG]). In 2000 we reported on the ability to measure T4 and TSH simultaneously from the same 3 mm punch.[7] This platform provides the opportunity for inclusion of additional markers for CH in the assay, for example, TBG and FT4, both of which have been shown to increase the detection of CH when combined with T4 and TSH.[7,8]

### *False-positive Results*

As pointed out recently by Howell,[9] false-positive results, that is, analytically positive but biologically negative results, are "an absolutely critical situation" in NBS and if present in large numbers can generate a sense of distrust by the primary physician. Howell goes on to suggest these problems can be addressed by: adjusting cutoffs, but not so far as to generate false-negatives; using second-tier assays; and improving communication. NBS CH data from the NNSGRC (http://www2.uthscsa.edu/nnsis/) for the most recent year for which full data are available indicate that, with certain caveats, the true-positive rate for CH that year was 3.9% of screen positive results. Stated another way, only 1 in 26 newborns who are screen positive for CH is biologically positive for the condition. Kwon and Farrell[10] reported similar numbers, greater than 1:50 for a collection of 5 conditions, with CH and CAH contributing the greatest number, and an estimated cost of $2 million annually for CH alone. A 2008 report on false-positive CH results indicated followup costs that 43% of children with a finding of CH positive followed by a second specimen some days later with normal TSH have demonstrated subclinical (compensated) hypothyroidism at 5 years of age.[11] These investigators and others[12] recommend therapy with levothyroxine in these children although others strongly argue against its use. The single conclusion from these various studies is that NBS is a screening program, and infants symptomatic of CH or other conditions in the panel should be examined for that condition without regard to the NBS report.[13]

**Table 1**
**CH screening strategies (2006)**

| Protocol | Screened | Screen Positive | % Total | Confirmed Positive | Prevalence (1:) | False-positive | PPV (%) |
|---|---|---|---|---|---|---|---|
| T4 followed by TSH | | | | | | | |
| Arizona | 98,605 | 1141 | 1.2 | 0 | N/A | 1141 | N/A |
| Colorado | 69,974 | 296 | 0.4 | 19 | 3683 | 277 | 6.4 |
| Massachusetts | 73,156 | 981 | 1.3 | 36 | 2032 | 945 | 3.7 |
| Indiana | 89,888 | 1849 | 2.0 | 28 | 3210 | 1821 | 1.6 |
| New Jersey | 111,290 | 2648 | 2.3 | 79 | 1408 | 2569 | 2.9 |
| TSH followed by T4 | | | | | | | |
| Missouri | 44,621 | 123 | 0.3 | 16 | 2788 | 107 | 13.0 |
| Oklahoma | 51,126 | 39 | 0.07 | 15 | 3408 | 24 | 38.5 |
| Oregon | 46,881 | 990 | 2.1 | 23 | 2086 | 967 | 2.3 |
| Virginia | 104,475 | 2513 | 2.4 | 38 | 2749 | 2475 | 1.5 |
| T4 and TSH | | | | | | | |
| West Virginia | 21,356 | 883 | 1.3 | 24 | 889 | 465 | 2.7 |
| Georgia | 145,074 | 3326 | 2.3 | 26 | 5580 | 3300 | 0.8 |
| Kansas | 41,293 | 849 | 2.1 | 40 | 1032 | 309 | 4.7 |
| Louisiana | 61,456 | 524 | 0.8 | 16 | 3849 | 508 | 3.0 |
| South Carolina | 55,530 | 1529 | 2.8 | 27 | 2057 | 1502 | 1.8 |
| TSH only | | | | | | | |
| Arizona | 38,845 | 1546 | 3.9 | 13 | 2984 | 1533 | 0.8 |
| Iowa | 39,529 | 629 | 1.5 | 30 | 1318 | 588 | 4.8 |
| New Mexico | 28,538 | 196 | 0.6 | 15 | 1902 | 181 | 7.6 |
| Minnesota | 72,278 | 191 | 0.3 | 35 | 2605 | 159 | 18.3 |
| T4 largest | | | | | | | |
| California[a] | 656,090 | 789 | 0.1 | 301 | 1847 | 488 | 38.2 |
| Texas[b] | 394,629 | 7688 | 1.9 | 239 | 1819 | 7451 | 2.8 |
| New York[c] | 247,901 | 4539 | 1.8 | 217 | 1037 | 4300 | 5.3 |

[a] TSH only.
[b] T4 followed by TSH.
[c] 2005: T4/TSH.

### *Incidence*

Until recently, the incidence of CH as measured by NBS was around 1:3600 births[14] and this was generally accepted by the world NBS community. However, several reports recently suggest an increase in incidence. Harris and Pass[15] recently reported a doubling of CH incidence in New York compared with that in the initial screening program in 1978 (1:1700 vs 1:3400). An increase in CH was observed in all programs in the United States, but none approached the increase noted in New York. Despite analysis of 5 possible causes, Harris and Pass[15] could not identify the primary factor(s) responsible for the increase. In 2008, a conference was organized by the Centers for Disease Control and Prevention (CDC) to investigate this issue. As recently reported[16] this 2-day conference with international attendees could not agree on the cause(s) of this increase. Factors such as primary care follow-up for CH, prevalence of CH and effects of laboratory technology, observed/expected national rates of CH based on NY prevalence data, race/ethnicity and gender in relation to prevalence of CH, medical management and follow-up of CH and transient hypothyroidism were considered. Attendees formulated plans for further investigation to include examination of changes in the environment with special attention to iodine and possible use of existing data sources (National Birth Defects Prevention Study, NHANES, and matched maternal serum/infant Guthrie specimens in California).

### *Genetics*

It is generally accepted that 80%–85% of CH is the result of thyroid dysgenesis, with 15%–20% of a familial nature. Causes of dysgenesis are largely unknown, but are usually expressed as aplasia, hypoplasia or ectopia, with the classic screening result of low T4 and increased TSH. Genes proposed as operatives in dysgenesis of thyroid follicular cells have been identified (TITF1, TITF2, PAX8 and TSHR).[17] Defects of T4 synthesis as a result of defects in iodide trapping or organification, iodotyrosine coupling or synthesis of TBG display the typical pattern of autosomal recessive inheritance[18] and have been attributed to defects in several genes: the thyroglobulin gene, leading to production of insufficient TBG; thyroperoxidase (TPO) linked to iodide organification defects; sodium/iodide symporter (NIS) mutations leading to insufficiency in iodine uptake, the rate-limiting step in the synthesis of T4 and T3; and, mutations in the ThOX gene, resulting in a deficiency of the $H_2O_2$ necessary for organification in its role as modulation of TPO activity.[19] At this time, we know of no NBS programs using molecular analysis as part of the protocol for CH screening, although a strong case has been made for its use.[20]

### *Treatment and Outcomes*

In its most recent review of NBS for CH, the American Academy of Pediatrics recommends that therapy for all infants with CH should normalize T4 within 2 weeks and TSH within 1 month of life,[21] with a recommended initial dose of 10–15μg/kg of levothyroxine.[21] However, these recommendations are altered in various screening results, such as low T4 and increased TSH (ie, classic CH)[22,23]; normal T4 with increased TSH[24]; low T4 with normal TSH[25]; low T4 and delayed TSH increase[26]; and transient increase in TSH.[27–30] When screening results present normal T4 with increased TSH (hyperthyrotropinemia) the condition is most often a transient event resolving spontaneously,[31] especially if the FT4 is in the upper half of normal.[32,33] However, these newborns cannot be considered false-positive, with many later being diagnosed with thyroid abnormalities and subclinical hypothyroidism.[31] Maruo and colleagues,[34] attributed much of this transient CH to mutations in the DUOX2 gene, finding biallelic mutations in 6 of 8 newborns classified as transient. Even though early initiation of T4 therapy at the dose mentioned earlier is required for the child with CH to attain normal outcomes,[34] even with normalized T4 measurements, children may still exhibit deficits as noted earlier. A logical and easy to follow diagnostic protocol has recently been presented by Jain and colleagues[35] and merits careful consideration.

Salerno and colleagues[36] have raised the question of long-term therapy with levothyroxine in young adults. Looking at the cardiovascular system in adults aged 16–20 years, diagnosed by NBS and maintained with normal TSH levels, and FT4 in the high-normal range, Salerno and colleagues demonstrated dysfunction of left ventricular diastolic action, impaired exercise capacity, and increased intima media thickness. The investigators recommended a thorough cardiovascular workup, especially in those individuals who might have had a brief period of subclinical hyper- and hypothyroidism during therapy.

It is generally agreed that mental retardation caused by CH has been eradicated. However, careful study of children detected by NBS programs indicates mild effects relating to the period of CH during which there was no therapy (pre- and postnatal). These effects are most notable as deficits in visuospatial, motor, language, memory, and attention abilities.[37,38] Children with CH who were identified and treated early as a result of NBS exhibit normal growth rate and height attainment.[39,40] However, it is critical that therapy be instituted within the first 2 weeks of life to avoid deficits in IQ.[41–44] In a recent study of more than 500 births that were near term and had normal T4 measurements in NBS, the investigators reported no association of cognitive outcomes or maternal thyroid function with the T4 level,[44] contrary to earlier reports.[45,46] A recent study noted deficits in perceived quality of life, developmental tasks, and self-esteem by the young adults, and recommended attention to these issues and provision of additional emotional and educational guidance.[47]

## CAH

CAH is a group of disorders in steroid biosynthesis, caused by an enzyme deficiency in the conversion of cholesterol to cortisol.[48] CAH caused by a deficiency of steroid 21-hydroxylase (21OHD) can occur in 2 forms: a severe or classic form, and a mild or nonclassic form. Classic CAH is also divided into salt-wasting and simple-virilizing forms. In 21OHP and 11β-hydroxylase deficiency only adrenal steroidogenesis is affected, whereas a defect in 3β-hydroxysteroid dehydrogenase or 17α-hydroxylase also involves gonadal steroid biosynthesis.[49] This discussion is limited to the most common form of CAH (21OHD). Incidence varies according to ethnicity and geographic area. The highest rates of classic CAH occur in 2 geographically isolated populations: the Yupic Eskimos of Alaska (1:280 births) and the French island of La Réunion (1:2100). High rates have also been reported in Brazil (1:7500) and the Philippines (1:7000).[50] In the United States, the incidence of CAH is lower in African Americans than in the white population (1:42,000 vs 1:15,500).[51] CAH is a monogenic, autosomal recessive disorder[50] and more than 90% of cases of CAH arise from 21OHD. In most cases, females with the classic form of 21OHD are born with ambiguous genitalia caused by overproduction of androgens from the fetal adrenal in which the precursors to the 21-hydroxylase enzyme defect are shunted into the androgen pathway causing virilization of external genitalia. Affected males do not have sexual ambiguity. The nonclassic form of 21OHD does not result in ambiguous genitalia in the 46XX female, as the prenatal level of androgens is not high enough to virilize the external genitalia.[48]

Steroid 21-hydroxylase (CYP21, also termed CYP21A2 and P450c21) is a cytochrome P450 enzyme that catalyzes the conversion of 17OHP to 11-deoxycortisol, a precursor of cortisol, and the conversion of progesterone to deoxycorticosterone, a precursor of aldosterone.[49] Patients with 21OHD cannot synthesize cortisol efficiently and the adrenal cortex stimulated by corticotrophin overproduces cortisol precursors. Some of these precursors are diverted to the biosynthesis of sex androgens, which may cause signs of androgen excess, including ambiguous genitalia in newborn girls and rapid postnatal growth in both sexes. Concomitant aldosterone deficiency may lead to salt-wasting with consequent failure to thrive, hypovolemia, and shock.

Much has been learned about the genetics of the various clinical forms of 21OHD, and correlations between the genotype and the phenotype have been studied extensively in various ethnic and racial groups.[50] The 21-hydroxylase gene (CYP21A2) is located in the human leucocyte antigen (HLA) gene cluster region of chromosome

6p21.3. The first genetic analyses were performed by linkage analysis of HLA haplotypes, with patients in the same family being HLA identical. Direct genetic analysis of CYP21A2 is complicated because the functional gene and a nonfunctional pseudogene (CYP21A1P) are closely adjacent in tandem arrangement with the C4A and C4B genes encoding for the fourth component of the serum complement.[52]

### *Screening Protocols and Technology*

CAH screening uses 17OHP as a marker and is performed in all programs in the United States (http://www.marchofdimes.com/peristats/level1.aspx?reg=99&top=12&stop=233&lev=1&slev=1&obj=20, accessed 26 December 2008). An increase in the levels of 17OHP in a filter paper test requires a rapid confirmatory test because undetected salt-wasting forms can be fatal. NBS for CAH was introduced in 1977 when a specific RIA test became available.[53] Most programs now use enzyme-linked immunosorbant assays (ELISA) to determine levels of 17OHP[54] and, more recently, liquid chromatography-tandem mass spectrometry (MS/MS).[55,56] Compared with other neonatal screening tests, the specificity of screening for CAH by immunoassay is low. Cross--reactivity of the specific antibody with other steroids, particularly pregnenolone, increases the number of false-positive results,[50] which have been reported to be as high as 8% for different steroids and for several medications, greatly reducing discrimination between normal neonates and those with CAH, perhaps because of inhibition of 3β-hydroxysteroid dehydrogenase by maternal estrogens.[57]

### *False-positive Results*

NBS based on 17OHP in a dried blood spot on filter paper is an effective tool for early diagnosis of CAH caused by 21OHD. However, the 17OHP test shows a high false-positive rate and it is difficult to interpret blood spot 17OHP levels because these values change with gestational age.[54] Cutoff values for 17OHP, based on gestational age to reduce the number of false-positive results in preterm babies have been established by different investigators.[51,58–60] Preterm or severely ill babies often show high levels of 17OHP because of stress, poor kidney function, or physiologically delayed expression of the 11β-hydroxylase that causes transiently increased concentrations of 17OHP, among other causes.[55,61] The time after birth at which the blood is collected also has to be taken into account, because this parameter can alter the screening performance.[62]

The introduction of more specific antibodies and of preanalytical processing, such as solvent extraction, has not markedly enhanced the screening efficiency of existing immunoassays.[63] Similarly, cutoff values for 17OHP adjusted for birth weight, gestational age, and stress factors have not significantly improved the PPV of this test, which remains the lowest of all screening conditions.[59,64] To minimize false-positive results attributable to cross-reactivity with other steroids, Wudy and colleagues developed a method to analyze 17OHP and other steroids in blood and urine by gas chromatography[63] and liquid chromatography-mass spectrometry.[65] In CAH screening programs, a clear distinction of true-negative and true-positive results is not evident with the use of a single marker (17OHP). Dhondt[62] has introduced the concept of a priori false-negatives, that is, the acknowledgment before starting the screening program that a missed case is inevitable.

### *Improving CAH Screening*

According to Minutti and colleagues, in a retrospective study of 1220 blood spots collected between the second and fifth day of life in 4 countries, the application of steroid profiling by MS/MS to the NBS for CAH yielded an 89% reduction of false-positive results. The cutoff value for 17OHP determined by MS/MS was lower than by immunoassay.[57] Measuring only the concentration of 17OHP will yield increased results not related to CAH that do not require follow-up investigations. Consideration of additional steroids allows better discrimination between increased 17OHP levels caused by CAH and those caused by stress reactions.[57] This is especially significant in light of a recent review of the magnitude of false-positive results in NBS programs in the United States.[15] This review concluded that among 5 disorders studied (biotinidase deficiency, CAH, congenital hypothyroidism, classic galactosemia, and phenylketonuria), CAH screening had the lowest PPV (111 true-positive cases among 20,647 abnormal screening results in a 2-year period, or 0.53%, compared with 6.36% for biotinidase deficiency, 1.84% for congenital hypothyroidism, 0.56% for classic galactosemia, and 2.9% for phenylketonuria). According to this estimate, 200 unaffected newborns required clinical and laboratory follow-up for every true case of CAH. MS/MS could be used as a second-tier test to follow up abnormal results by immunoassay rather than using it in primary screening.[57] Molecular studies would increase the specificity but not the sensitivity of CAH screening because not all mutations can be reliably detected in a screening setting.[64]

Infants with low or very low 17OHP levels may be screen negative for CAH, but not for congenital adrenal hypoplasia (AHC). As reported by Peter and colleagues,[66] this condition, in which there may be complete functional absence of the adrenal glands, has an estimated incidence of 1:16,000, close to that of CAH. Infants with AHC produce no 17OHP and thus do not appear affected in the immunoassay protocol, unless MS/MS is used as second-tier testing. The NY NBS program has observed 3 occurrences of this condition (unpublished data), which again emphasizes the importance of clinical observations that may not be supported by NBS results.[13]

### *Treatment*

CAH is a chronic disease that requires long-term therapy. In the classic form of the disease, glucocorticoids are required not only to overcome the cortisol deficiency mostly in stress situations but also to suppress the adrenocorticotropic hormone (ACTH)-driven stimulation of adrenal androgens. In 75% of cases, mineralocorticoid substitution is required and salt supplementation is advisable in infancy. Surgical correction of the ambiguous genitalia in girls is also part of the management of these patients. Treatment of infants and children affected by the nonclassic form of the disease is not recommended until, and unless, symptoms and signs of androgen excess become evident.[67] Other studies are under way that show improvement in growth rate and final height prediction with gonadotropin-releasing hormone agonists used alone and in combination with growth hormone.[68] Metformin, an antidiabetic agent, decreases ovarian and adrenal hyperandrogenism, improving menstrual disorders in patients with primary polycystic ovary syndrome and insulin resistance.[69,70] None of these experimental therapies is recommended as the standard of care, but represent potential novel therapeutic approaches not yet ready for human use.[71,72]

Adverse outcomes can occur in babies with false-positive results for CAH who receive treatment. Reviewing the literature Brosco and colleagues[73] identified a case report of iatrogenic injury to a child improperly treated for CAH. After 5 years of treatment with corticosteroids, the patient developed Cushing syndrome, including hirsutism, truncal fat, growth retardation, and glaucoma in his right eye. The child also demonstrated rapid catch-up growth and dramatic change in his physical appearance, and apparently had some damage to his pituitary ACTH feedback system.[73]

Gene therapy may be feasible for 21-hydroxylase deficiency, because the disorder is caused by a single gene defect. Some options, still at the early stage, include transplantation of adrenal cells or tissue, or stem-cell approaches.[52]

## REFERENCES

1. Watson M, Mann M, Lloyd-Puryear M, et al. Newborn screening: toward a uniform screening panel and system—executive summary. Pediatrics 2006;117(5): S296–307.
2. Osotimehin M, Black E, Hoffenbert R. Thyroglobulin concentration in neonatal blood: a possible test for neonatal hypothyroidism. Br Med J 1978;2:1467–8.
3. Gruneiro-Papendieck L, Prieto L, Chiese A, et al. Usefulness of thyroxine and free thyroxine filter paper measurements in neonatal screening for paper measurements in neonatal screening for congenital hypothyroidism of preterm babies. J Med Screen 2000;7:78–81.
4. Fisher D, Dussault J, Foley T, et al. Screening for congenital hypothyroidism: results of screening 1 million North American infants. J Pediatr 1979;94(5):700–5.
5. Djemli A, Van Vliet G, Delvin E. Congenital hypothyroidism: from Paracelsus to molecular diagnosis. Clin Biochem 2006;39:511–8.
6. Bellisario R, Colinas R, Pass K. Simultaneous measurement of thyroxine and thyrotropin from newborn dried blood-spot specimens using a multiplexed fluorescent microsphere immunoassay. Clin Chem 2000;46(9):1422–4.
7. Mitchell M, Hermos R. Measurement of thyroglobulin in newborn screening specimens from normal and hypothyroid infants. Clin Endocrinol 1995;42:523–7.
8. Jones J, Mackenzie J, Croft G, et al. Improvement in screening performance and diagnosis of congenital hypothyroidism in Scotland 1979–2003. Arch Dis Child 2006;91:680–5.
9. Howell R. The high price of false positives. Mol Genet Metab 2006;87:180–3.
10. Kwon C, Farrell P. The magnitude and challenge of false-positive newborn screening test results. Arch Pediatr Adolesc Med 2000;154:714–8.
11. Polizzotti N, Carta A, Gelsomina R, et al. Longitudinal study of thyroid function in children with mild hyperthyrotropinemia at neonatal screening for congenital hypothyroidism. J Clin Endocrinol Metab 2008;93:2679–85.
12. Kohler B, Schnabel D, Biebermann H, et al. Transient congenital hypothyroidism and hyperthyrotropinemina: normal thyroid function and physical development at the ages of 6–14 years. J Clin Endocrinol Metab 1996;81(4):1563–7.
13. Pass K. How reliable is newborn screening for congenital adrenal hyperplasia? Nat Clin Pract Endocrinol Metab 2006;2:74–5.
14. LaFranchi S, Hanna C, Krainz P, et al. Screening for congenital hypothyroidism with specimen collection at two time periods: results of the Northwest Regional Screening Program. Pediatrics 1985;76:734–40.
15. Harris K, Pass K. Increase in congenital hypothyroidism in New York State and in the United States. Mol Genet Metab 2007;91:268–77.
16. Harris K, Pass K, Vogt R, et al. Is congenital hypothyroidism increasing in the newborn population? 2008 Newborn Screening and Genetic Testing Symposium; November 4, 2008; San Antonio, TX.
17. Macchia P. Recent advances in understanding the molecular basis of primary congenital hypothyroidism. Mol Med Today 2000;6:36–42.
18. Niu D, Lin C, Hwang B, et al. Contribution of genetic factors to neonatal transient hypothyroidism. Arch Dis Child Fetal Neonatal Ed 2005;90:F69–72.

19. De Deken X, Wang D, Dumont JE, et al. Characterization of ThOX proteins as components of the thyroid H(2)O(2)-generating system. Exp Cell Res 2002; 273(2):187–96.
20. Green NS, Pass KA. Neonatal screening by DNA microarray: spots and chips. Nat Rev Genet 2005;6:147–51.
21. Rose S, Brown R, Kaplowitz P, et al. Update of newborn screening and therapy for congenital hypothyroidism. Pediatrics 2006;117:2290–303.
22. Kaiserman I, Siebner R, Kletter G, et al. A ten-year temporal analysis of primary congenital hypothyroidism in Israel. Early Hum Dev 1991;26(3):193–201.
23. Bakker B, Kempers M, DeVijlder J, et al. Dynamics of the plasma concentrations of TSH, FT4 and T3 following thyroxine supplementation in congenital hypothyroidism. Clin Endocrinol (Oxf) 2002;57:529–37.
24. Fisher D. Disorders of the thyroid in the newborn and infant. In: Sperling MA, editor. Clinical pediatric and adolescent endocrinology. Philadelphia: Saunders; 2002. p. 164.
25. Rapaport R, Rose S, Freemark M. Hypothyroxinemia in the preterm infant: the benefits and risks of thyroxine treatment. J Pediatr 2001;139:182–8.
26. Larson C, Hermos R, Delaney A, et al. Risk factors associated with delayed thyrotropin elevations in congenital hypothyroidism. J Pediatr 2003;143:587–91.
27. Weber G, Vigone M, Rapa A, et al. Neonatal transient hypothyroidism: aetiological study. Arch Dis Child Fetal Neonatal Ed 1998;79:F70–2.
28. Yang R, Zhu Z, Zhou X, et al. Treatment and follow-up of children with transient congenital hypothyroidism. J Zhejiang Univ Sci B 2005;6(12):1206–9.
29. Evans C, Jordan N, Owens G, et al. Potent thyrotrophin receptor-blocking antibodies: a cause of transient congenital hypothyroidism and delayed thyroid development. Eur J Endocrinol 2004;150:265–8.
30. Ordookhani A, Mirmiran P, Walfish P, et al. Transient neonatal hypothyroidism is associated with elevated serum anti-thyroglobulin antibody levels in newborns and their mothers. J Pediatr 2007;3:315–7.
31. Calaciura F, Motta R, Miscio G, et al. Subclinical hypothyroidism in early childhood: a frequent outcome of transient neonatal hyperthyrotropinemia. J Clin Endocrinol Metab 2002;87(7):3209–14.
32. Bongers-Schokking J, Koot H, Wiersma D, et al. Influence of timing and dose of thyroid hormone replacement on development in infants with congenital hypothyroidism. J Pediatr 2000;136:292–7.
33. Zamproni I, Grasberger H, Cortinovis F, et al. Biallelic inactivation of the dual oxidase maturation factor 2 (DUOXA2) gene as a novel cause of congenital hypothyroidism. J Clin Endocrinol Metab 2008;93:605–10.
34. Maruo Y, Takahashi H, Soeda I, et al. Transient congenital hypothyroidism caused by biallelic mutations of the dual oxidase 2 gene in Japanese patients detected by a neonatal screening program. J Clin Endocrinol Metab 2008;93: 4261–7.
35. Jain V, Agarwal R, Deorari A, et al. Congenital hypothyroidism. Indian J Pediatr 2008;75:363–7.
36. Salerno M, Oliviero U, Lettiero T, et al. Long-term cardiovascular effects of levothyroxine therapy in young adults with congenital hypothyroidism. J Clin Endocrinol Metab 2008;93(7):2486–91.
37. Rovet J. Congenital hypothyroidism: an analysis of persisting deficits and associated factors. Child Neuropsychol 2002;8(3):150–62.
38. Heyerdahl S, Oerbeck B. Congenital hypothyroidism: developmental outcome in relation to levothyroxine treatment variables. Thyroid 2003;13:1029–38.

39. Morin A, Guimarey L, Apezteguia M. Linear growth in children with congenital hypothyroidism detected by neonatal screen and treated early: a longitudinal study. J Pediatr Endocrinol Metab 2002;15:973–7.
40. Oerbeck B, Sundet K, Kase B, et al. Congenital hypothyroidism: influence of disease severity and L-thyroxine treatment on intellectual, motor, and school-associated outcomes in young adults. Pediatrics 2003;112:923–30.
41. Gruters A, Jenner A, Krude H. Long-term consequences of congenital hypothyroidism in the era of screening programmes. Best Pract Res Clin Endocrinol Metab 2002;16:369–82.
42. Oken E, Braverman L, Platek D, et al. Neonatal thyroxine, maternal thyroid function, and child cognition. J Clin Endocrinol Metab 2008;93:2648–53.
43. Bongers-Schokking J. Pre- and postnatal brain development in neonates with congenital hypothyroidism. J Pediatr Endocrinol Metab 2001;14(Suppl 6):1463–8.
44. Kreisner E, Schermann L, Camargo-Neto E, et al. Predictors of intellectual outcome in a cohort of Brazilian children with congenital hypothyroidism. Clin Endocrinol (Oxf) 2004;60:250–5.
45. Cassio A, Cacciari E, Cicognani A, et al. Treatment for congenital hypothyroidism: thyroxine alone or thyroxine plus triiodothyronine? Pediatrics 2003;111:1055–60.
46. Kurinczuk J, Bower C, Lewis B, et al. Congenital hypothyroidism in Western Australia 1981–1998. J Paediatr Child Health 2002;38:187–91.
47. Veer L, Kempers M, Last B, et al. Quality of life, developmental milestones, and self-esteem of young adults with congenital hypothyroidism diagnosed by neonatal screening. J Clin Endocrinol Metab 2008;93:2654–61.
48. Merke DP, Bornstein SR. Congenital adrenal hyperplasia. Lancet 2005;365:125–36.
49. Krone N, Dhir V, Ivison H, et al. Congenital adrenal hyperplasia and P450 oxidoreductase deficiency. Clin Endocrinol 2000;66:162–72.
50. Speiser P, White P. Congenital adrenal hyperplasia. N Engl J Med 2003;349:776–88.
51. Torresani T, Grüters A, Scherz R, et al. Improving the efficacy of newborn screening for congenital adrenal hyperplasia by adjusting the cut-off level of 17β-hydroxyprogesterone to gestational age. Screening 1994;3:77–84.
52. Riepe F, Sippell W. Recent advances in diagnosis, treatment, and outcome of congenital adrenal hyperplasia due to 21-hydroxylase deficiency. Rev Endocr Metab Disord 2007;8:349–63.
53. Pang S, Hotchkiss J, Drash AL, et al. Microfilter paper method for 17β-hydroxyprogesterone radioimmunoassay: its application for rapid screening for congenital adrenal hyperplasia. J Clin Endocrinol Metab 1977;45:1003–8.
54. Dressendorfer R, Strasburger C, Bidlingmaier F, et al. Development of a highly sensitive nonisotopic immunoassay for the determination of salivary 17-hydroxyprogesterone: reference ranges throughout childhood and adolescence. Pediatr Res 1998;44:650–5.
55. Janzen N, Peter M, Sander S, et al. Newborn screening for congenital adrenal hyperplasia: additional steroid profile using liquid chromatography-tandem mass spectrometry. J Clin Endocrinol Metab 2007;92:2581–9.
56. Matern D, Tortorelli S, Oglesbee D, et al. Reduction of the false-positive rate in newborn screening by implementation of MS/MS-based second-tier tests: the Mayo Clinic experience (2004–2007). J Inherit Metab Dis 2007;30:585–92.
57. Minutti C, Lacey J, Magera M, et al. Steroid profiling by tandem mass spectrometry improves the positive predictive value of newborn screening for congenital adrenal hyperplasia. J Clin Endocrinol Metab 2004;89:3687–93.

58. Lee J, Moon Y, Lee M, et al. Corrected 17-alpha-hydroxyprogesterone values adjusted by a scoring system for screening congenital adrenal hyperplasia in premature infants. Ann Clin Lab Sci 2008;38:235–40.
59. Allen D, Hoffman G, Fitzpatrick P, et al. Improved precision of newborn screening for congenital adrenal hyperplasia using weight-adjusted criteria for 17-hydroxyprogesterone levels. J Pediatr 1994;130:128–33.
60. Olgemöller B, Roscher A, Liebl B, et al. Screening for congenital adrenal hyperplasia: adjustment of 17-hydroxyprogesterone cut-off values to both age and birth weight markedly improves the predictive value. J Clin Endocrinol Metab 2003;88:5790–4.
61. Gruneiro-Papendieck L, Prieto L, Chiesa A, et al. Neonatal screening program for congenital adrenal hyperplasia: adjustments to the recall protocol. Horm Res 2001;55:271–7.
62. Dhondt JL. Neonatal screening: from the ‘Guthrie age’ to the ‘genetic age’. J Inherit Metab Dis 2007;30:418–22.
63. Wudy SA, Hartmann M, Svoboda M. Determination of 17-hydroxyprogesterone in plasma by stable isotope dilution/benchtop liquid chromatography-tandem mass spectrometry. Horm Res 2000;53:68–71.
64. Nordenstrom A, Wedell A, Hagenfeldt L, et al. Neonatal screening for congenital adrenal hyperplasia: 17-hydroxyprogesterone levels and CYP21 genotypes in preterm infants. Pediatrics 2001;108:68–74.
65. Wudy S, Wachter U, Homoki J, et al. 17β-Hydroxyprogesterone, 4-androstenedione, and testosterone profiled by routine stable isotope dilution/gas chromatography-mass spectrometry in plasma of children. Pediatr Res 1995;38:76–80.
66. Peter M, Viemann M, Partsch C, et al. Congenital adrenal hypoplasia: clinical spectrum: experience with hormonal diagnosis, and report on new point mutations of the DAX-1 gene. J Clin Endocrinol Metab 1998;83:2666–74.
67. Torresani T, Biason-Lauber A. Congenital adrenal hyperplasia: diagnostic advances. J Inherit Metab Dis 2007;30:563–75.
68. Quintos JB, Vogiatzi MG, Harbison MD, et al. Growth hormone therapy alone or in combination with gonadotropin releasing hormone analog therapy to improve the height deficit in children with congenital adrenal hyperplasia. J Clin Endocrinol Metab 2001;86:1511–7.
69. Arslanian SA, Lewy V, Danadian K, et al. Metformin therapy in obese adolescents with polycystic ovary syndrome and impaired glucose tolerance: amelioration of exaggerated adrenal response to adrenocorticotropin with reduction of insulinemia/insulin resistance. J Clin Endocrinol Metab 2002;87:1555–9.
70. Marca A, Morgante G, Paglia T, et al. Effects of metformin on adrenal steroidogenesis in women with polycystic ovary syndrome. Fertil Steril 1999;72:985–9.
71. Bornstein S, Webster E, Torpy D, et al. Chronic effects of a nonpeptide corticotropin-releasing hormone type I receptor antagonist on pituitary-adrenal function, body weight, and metabolic regulation. Endocrinology 1998;139:1546–55.
72. Webster E, Lewis D, Torpy D, et al. In vivo and in vitro characterization of antalarmin, a nonpeptide corticotropin-releasing hormone (CRH) receptor antagonist: suppression of pituitary ACTH release and peripheral inflammation. Endocrinology 1996;137:5747–50.
73. Brosco J, Seider M, Dunn A. Universal newborn screening and adverse medical outcomes: a historical note. Ment Retard Dev Disabil Res Rev 2006;12:262–9.

# Index

*Note:* Page numbers of article titles are in **boldface** type.

## A

Accelerator hypothesis, of Type 1 diabetes, 779
Acidosis, in diabetic ketoacidosis, 812
management of, 815
Adamantinomatous craniopharyngiomas (ACPs), imaging of, 689–690
Adenohypophysis, pituitary, imaging of, 673
Adenomas, pituitary, imaging of, 685–687
Adjuvant role, of complementary and alternative therapies, for diabetes mellitus, 805–806
Adolescent disorders, hypogonadism as, **719–738**
evaluation of, 729
hypergonadotropic hypogonadism, 724–729
acquired origins of, 728–729
causes of, 724–725
clinical manifestations of, 724–725
congenital origins of, 724–728
hypogonadotropic hypogonadism, 719–724
acquired origins of, 723–724
causes of, 719–721
clinical manifestations of, 719–721
congenital origins of, 720, 722–723
constitutional delay of growth and puberty in, 720
summary overview of, 719, 732
treatment of, 730–732
estrogen replacement for, 730–731
testosterone replacement for, 731–732
primary amenorrhea as, **739–760**
definitions for, 739
duplex/color Doppler sonography for, abnormal findings with, 746–757
advantages of, 739, 746 747, 757
normal anatomy findings vs., 742–746
technique for, 741–742
etiologies of, 740
medical evaluation of, 739–740
normal anatomy review for, 742–746
of ovary, 743–746
of uterus, 742–743
of vagina, 743–744
physical examination for, 740–741
puberty and, 740
summary overview of, 739, 757

Endocrinol Metab Clin N Am 38 (2009) 839–862
doi:10.1016/S0889-8529(09)00102-9 

Adrenal hyperplasia, steroid 21 hydroxylase deficiency in, **699–718**. See also *Congenital adrenal hyperplasia (CAH).*
Adrenal hypoplasia, steroid 17 hydroxylase deficiency in, 833
Adrenal rest tumor, testicular, congenital adrenal hyperplasia associated with, 703–704, 708
Adrenal steroidogenic pathways, 700–701
Adrenocorticotrophic hormone (ACTH), adrenal steroid production regulation by, 700–701
in adrenal hyperplasia. See *Congenital adrenal hyperplasia (CAH).*
Adulthood, transitioning pediatric patient to, with congenital adrenal hyperplasia, 711–712
with small for gestational age, 818–820
consensus statement on, 818
consequences of, 820
definition of, 818
early growth and development in, 818–819
endocrinopathies and, 819
growth management in, 819–820
metabolic disorders and, 819
puberty management in, 819–820
Agenesis, callosal, of pituitary, imaging of, 693–695
$\alpha$-Lipoic acid, for diabetes mellitus, 805
clinical trials of, 799
Ambiguous genitalia, congenital adrenal hyperplasia presenting as, 701, 833
corrective surgery for, 708–709
Amenorrhea, hypothalamic, hypogonadotropic hypogonadism related to, 724
primary, **739–760**. See also *Primary amenorrhea.*
Anabolic steroids, for idiopathic short stature, 818
Androgen suppression, for congenital adrenal hyperplasia, 706, 708, 833
bone mineral density and, 709–710
Anterior lobe, of pituitary, imaging of, 674
Anterior pituitary arterial supply, imaging of, 674
Antibodies, monoclonal, in Type 1 diabetes prevention, 783, 786
Anti-Müllerian hormone (AMH), in Turner syndrome, fertility preservation and, 766–767
Antitumor necrosis factor, in Type 1 diabetes prevention, 786
Arachnoid cysts, imaging of, 691
Arginine vasopressin (AVP), in water balance disorders, 663–665, 669
normal water regulation vs., 663–664
Arterial supply, to ovaries, 746
to pituitary, imaging of, 674
Atresia, vaginal, primary amenorrhea related to, duplex/color Doppler sonography of, 753, 755
Autoantibodies, in Type 1 diabetes, 777–778
secondary prevention and, 782
tertiary prevention and, 783, 786
Autoimmune diseases, fertility preservation with, 768
Type 1 diabetes as, 777–779, 783, 786
zinc impact on, 805
Autoimmune gonadal failure, fertility preservation with, 763–764
hypergonadotropic hypogonadism related to, 729
Autosomal nephrogenic diabetes insipidus (XNDI), as pediatric disorder, 664–666

## B

BABYDIET, Type 1 diabetes prevention and, 781
β-Cells, in Type 1 diabetes, 777–778, 786
secondary prevention and, 781–782
tertiary prevention and, 783
Bicarbonate, for diabetic ketoacidosis, 815
Bicarbonate level, in diabetic ketoacidosis, 812–813
Bicornuate uterus, primary amenorrhea related to, duplex/color Doppler sonography of, 752–753
Biochemical diagnosis, of congenital adrenal hyperplasia, 705–706
Biomarkers, in congenital adrenal hyperplasia screening, 832
in congenital hypothyroidism screening, 828
Biopsy, testicular, for intersex disorders, 823
Bone mineral density (BMD), congenital adrenal hyperplasia treatment effect on, 709–710
Brain, MRI of, for pediatric water balance disorders, 667
traumatic injury to, hypogonadotropic hypogonadism related to, 723

## C

Callosal agenesis, of pituitary, imaging of, 693–695
Callosal hypogenesis, of pituitary, imaging of, 694
Callosal hypoplasia, of pituitary, imaging of, 694–695
Cancers, childhood, long-term survival with, fertility preservation for, 771
outcome studies of, 764–765
trends of, 761–764
Carbohydrate-deficient glycoprotein syndrome, hypergonadotropic hypogonadism related to, 726
Cavernous sinuses, in pituitary imaging, 679
Central diabetes insipidus, as pediatric disorder, 666–667, 669
Central nervous system (CNS), tumors of, hypogonadotropic hypogonadism related to, 723–724
Cerebral edema (CE), in diabetic ketoacidosis, 813
treatment of, 815
Cerebral salt wasting (CSW), syndrome of inappropriate antidiuretic hormone secretion vs., 669
Cerebral spinal fluid (CSF), in pituitary imaging, 677–679, 690–691
Chemotherapy, gonadotoxicity of, 764
fertility preservation for, 768. See also *Cancers.*
hypergonadotropic hypogonadism related to, 728
Chiari hindbrain malformations, pituitary involvement of, imaging of, 694–695
Chromium, for diabetes mellitus, 804
Cinnamon, for diabetes mellitus, 803–804
clinical trials of, 799
Cleft cysts, Rathke, imaging of, 687–688
Clitoromegaly, in intersex disorders, 822
Cod liver oil, for diabetes mellitus, 801
clinical trials of, 797
Complementary and alternative medicine (CAM), for pediatric diabetes, **791–810**
adjuvant role of, 805–806
α-lipoic acid as, 805

Complementary (*continued*)
chromium as, 804
cinnamon as, 803–804
clinical trials of, 796–799
cod liver oil as, 801
folate as, 795, 800
pyridoxamine plus, 797
nicotinamide as, 793–795
vitamin D plus, 795, 797
vitamin E plus, 794, 797
omega-3 fatty acids as, 801
prevalence of, 791–793
pyridoxamine as, 795, 800
folate plus, 797
summary overview of, 791, 806
vitamin B as, 795, 800
vitamin D as, 800–802
nicotinamide plus, 795, 797
vitamin E as, 802–803
nicotinamide plus, 794, 797
zinc as, 804–805
Complete androgen insensitivity syndrome (CAIS), hypergonadotropic hypogonadism related to, 725, 727
intersex disorders and, 824
Computed tomography (CT), of pituitary, pediatric, 676, 693
pelvic, for primary amenorrhea, 742, 746
Congenital adrenal hyperplasia (CAH), disorders of sex development associated with, 702–703, 821
hypergonadotropic hypogonadism related to, 725, 727
newborn screening for, 831–834
false-positive results of, 832
improvement strategies for, 832–833
protocols for, 832
treatment of, 833–834
trends in, 831–832
steroid 21 hydroxylase deficiency in, **699–718**
clinical presentations of, 701–705
classical vs. nonclassical, 699–700
external genitalia and, 701
fertility and, 703
gender role behavior and, 702–703
internal genitalia and, 701–702
nonclassical symptoms in, 704–705
postnatal effects and growth in, 702
puberty and, 702
salt wasting and, 703–704
secondary sexual characteristics in, 702
diagnosis of, 705–707
hormonal, 705–706
molecular genetics in, 705, 707, 833
late-onset, 704–705

newborn screening for, 831–834
pathophysiology of, 700–701
steroid 21 hydroxylase deficiency in, 699–700
summary overview of, 699, 712
treatment of, 706, 708–712
bone mineral density in, 709–710
during pregnancy, 710–711
fertility and, 710–712
gene therapy in, 834
goal of, 706
hormone replacement for, 706, 708, 833
metabolic aspects of, 710
prenatal, 711
stress dosing for, 708
surgery for, 708–709
transitioning to adulthood, 711–712
Congenital anomalies, of uterus and vagina, primary amenorrhea related to, 752–757
Congenital hypothyroidism (CH), newborn screening for, 827–831
false-positive results of, 828
genetics of, 830
incidence of, 829–830
mental retardation and, 831
protocols for, 828–829
technology for, 828
treatment and outcomes of, 830–831
trends in, 827–828
Congenital nephrogenic diabetes insipidus (XNDI), 664–666
Constitutional delay of growth and puberty (CDGP), consensus statement on, 815–818
hypogonadotropic hypogonadism vs., 720
Contraceptives, oral, for congenital adrenal hyperplasia, 708
Corticosteroid replacement therapy, for congenital adrenal hyperplasia, 706, 708, 833
stress dosing of, 708
Cosmetic issues, with intersex disorder surgery, 823–824
Cow's milk proteins, Type 1 diabetes prevention and, 779–780
C-peptide level, in Type 1 diabetes, 778
secondary prevention and, 782
tertiary prevention and, 783, 786
Cranial nerves, in pituitary imaging, 679
Craniopharyngiomas (CPs), imaging of, 689–690
Cryopreservation, for fertility preservation, 767
of embryo, 768–769
of ovarian tissue, 763, 768–770
of testicular tissue, 763, 768, 770
CTLA4 gene, in Type 1 diabetes, 779
tertiary prevention and, 786
Cystic lesions, ovarian. See *Polycystic ovarian syndrome (PCOS).*
pituitary, imaging of, 687–691
Cytotoxic T-lymphocyte–associated gene (CTLA4), in Type 1 diabetes, 779
tertiary prevention and, 786

## D

Dacluzimab (DZB), in Type 1 diabetes prevention, 786
*DAX-1* gene, hypogonadotropic hypogonadism related to, 720–721
de Morsier Syndrome, pituitary involvement of, imaging of, 695
Delayed sexual development, with primary amenorrhea, pelvic duplex/color Doppler sonography of, 747
Desmopressin, for diabetes insipidus, 667, 669
Dexamethasone (DEX), for congenital adrenal hyperplasia, 706, 708
    during prenatal period, 711
Diabetes insipidus (DI), as pediatric disorder, 664–667, 669
    acquired forms of, 667
    central vs. nephrogenic, 664, 666
    diagnosis of, 667
    genetics of, 664–666
    management of, 665, 667, 669
    presenting signs of, 665, 667
Diabetes mellitus, pediatric, complementary and alternative therapies for, **791–810**
        adjuvant role of, 805–806
        α-lipoic acid as, 805
        chromium as, 804
        cinnamon as, 803–804
        clinical trials of, 796–799
        cod liver oil as, 801
        folate as, 795, 800
            pyridoxamine plus, 797
        nicotinamide as, 793–795
            vitamin D plus, 795, 797
            vitamin E plus, 794, 797
        omega-3 fatty acids as, 801
        prevalence of, 791–793
        pyridoxamine as, 795, 800
            folate plus, 797
        summary overview of, 791, 806
        vitamin B as, 795, 800
        vitamin D as, 800–802
            nicotinamide plus, 795, 797
        vitamin E as, 802–803
            nicotinamide plus, 794, 797
        zinc as, 804–805
    Type 1, prevention of, **777–790**. See also *Type 1 diabetes (T1D).*
    Type 2. See *Type 2 diabetes (T2D).*
Diabetic ketoacidosis (DKA), 812–815
  acidosis in, 812
    management of, 815
  cerebral edema in, 813
    treatment of, 815
  consensus statement on, 812
  definition of, 812
  electrolyte replacement for, 814
  fluid replacement for, 813–814

frequency of, 812–813
herbal products for, 805
hydration status and, 813–814
insulin therapy for, 814
management of, 813
prevention of, 815
Dietary factors, of Type 1 diabetes prevention, 779–781
Disorders of sex development (DSDs), 820–824. See also *Intersex disorders.*
assigning gender in newborns, 821–822
clinical management of, 821–822
consensus statement on, 820, 824
criteria suggestive of, 821
definitions for, 820–821
diagnosis of, 821–822
fertility preservation and, 763
hypergonadotropic hypogonadism related to, 725–727
introduction to, 820
long-term outcomes of, 823–824
psychosocial management of, 821, 823–824
sex steroid replacement for, 823
surgical management of, 822–823
Diuretics, thiazide, for nephrogenic diabetes insipidus, 665
Docosahexaenoic acid (DHA), Type 1 diabetes prevention and, 781
Duplex/color Doppler sonography, pelvic, for primary amenorrhea, abnormal findings with, 746–757
advantages of, 739, 746–747, 757
normal anatomy findings vs., 742–746
technique for, 741–742
with delayed sexual development, 747
with gonadal dysgenesis, 748–749
with hypergonadotropic hypogonadism, 748–749
with hypogonadotropic hypogonadism, 747
with pseudointersex, 749–752
with uterine/vaginal obstruction, 752–757
normal anatomy review for, of ovary, 743–746
of uterus, 742–743
of vagina, 743–744
Duplications, of uterus and vagina, primary amenorrhea related to, duplex/color Doppler sonography of, 756–757
Dysgenesis, gonadal, testicular biopsy for, 823
testis-specific protein Y-encoded positive, 824
with primary amenorrhea, pelvic duplex/color Doppler sonography of, 748–749
XY pure, hypergonadotropic hypogonadism related to, 725, 727
primary amenorrhea related to, 749
of pituitary callosa, imaging of, 693–695
of thyroid, genetics of, 830
Dysplasia, fibrous, of pituitary, imaging of, 693–694
gonadal, fertility preservation for, 765–767
septo-optic, pituitary involvement of, imaging of, 695

E


Electrolyte imbalance, in diabetic ketoacidosis, 813–815
Electrolyte replacement, for diabetic ketoacidosis, 814
Embryo cryopreservation, for fertility preservation, 768–769
Embryology, of pituitary gland, imaging of, 675
signaling system in, 675–676
"Empty sella," of pituitary, imaging of, 690
Endocrinopathies, in small for gestational age patient, 819
newborn screening for, **827–837**
congenital adrenal hyperplasia, 831–834
false-positive results of, 832
improvement strategies for, 832–833
protocols for, 832
treatment of, 833–834
trends in, 831–832
congenital hypothyroidism, 827–831
false-positive results of, 828
genetics of, 830
incidence of, 829–830
protocols for, 828–829
technology for, 828
treatment and outcomes of, 830–831
trends in, 827–828
summary overview of, 827
Environmental triggers, of Type 1 diabetes, 777–779
primary prevention and, 779–781
Epithelioid granulomas, pituitary involvement of, imaging of, 691–692
Estrogen replacement, for hypogonadism, in adolescent girls, 730–731
for intersex disorders, 823
Etanercept, in Type 1 diabetes prevention, 786
Ethical issues, of fertility preservation, 762
Euvolemia, in syndrome of inappropriate antidiuretic hormone secretion, 669
Evidence-based medicine, in pediatric endocrinology, 811
External genitalia, congenital adrenal hyperplasia features of, 701, 833
corrective surgery for, 708–709


F


Familial short stature, consensus statement on, 815–818
Family history, in intersex disorders, 821
in primary amenorrhea, 739–740
Feminization, testicular, pelvic duplex/color Doppler sonography of, 749–751
Fertility, congenital adrenal hyperplasia effect on, 703
treatment of, 710–712
prepubertal markers of, 764–765
Fertility preservation, pediatric considerations for, **761–775**
attainment of human potential, 762
diagnoses relevant to, 762–764
ethical issues of, 762
gonadal dysfunction, hypoplasia, or dysplasia and, 765–767
hypothalamic-pituitary dysfunction and, 765, 771

Klinefelter syndrome and, 767
legal issues of, 762
malignancy and, gonadal shielding during therapy, 771
outcome studies of, 764–765
trends of, 761–764
summary overview of, 761, 771–772
testicular damage and, 767
treatment and procedures in, for females, 768–770
for males, 770–771
potential, 762–763, 767–768
protective, during at-risk therapy, 771
Fibrous dysplasia, of pituitary, imaging of, 693–694
Fludrocortisone, for congenital adrenal hyperplasia, 708
Fluid deficit, in diabetic ketoacidosis, 813–814
Fluid replacement, for diabetic ketoacidosis, 813–815
Folate, for diabetes mellitus, 795, 800
clinical trials of, 797
Folate plus pyridoxamine, for diabetes mellitus, 797
Follicle stimulating hormone (FSH), as prepubertal fertility marker, 764–765
in gonadarche physiology, 719
in hypergonadotropic hypogonadism, 725–726
in Turner syndrome, fertility preservation and, 766–767
Follicular development, in fertility preservation, 765–767
attainment of potential, 762
Follicular maturation, in vitro, for fertility preservation, 763, 767–768


## G


Gadolinium, in pituitary imaging, 676–677, 681, 687
Galactosemia, hypergonadotropic hypogonadism related to, 725, 727–728
Gender assignment, for newborns, with intersex disorders, 821–822
Gender identity, psychosocial development and, 820
Gender role/gender role behavior, congenital adrenal hyperplasia effect on, 702–703
psychosocial development and, 821
Gene therapy, for steroid 21-hydroxylase deficiency, in congenital adrenal hyperplasia, 834
Genetic engineering, for Type 1 diabetes, 787
Genetic screening, for congenital adrenal hyperplasia, 832–833
for congenital hypothyroidism, 830
Genetics, of pediatric disorders, diabetes insipidus and, 664–666
midline pituitary lesions and, 695
molecular, congenital adrenal hyperplasia and, 705, 707, 831–833
hypergonadotropic hypogonadism and, 724–728
hypogonadotropic hypogonadism and, 720–723
Type 1 diabetes and, 777–779
Genitalia, congenital adrenal hyperplasia features of, corrective surgery for
ambiguous, 708–709
external, 701, 833
internal, 701–702
Genitoplasty, for intersex disorders, 822, 824
Germ cell maturation, stimulation of, for fertility preservation, 763–764, 767
Germ cell preservation, for fertility preservation, 763–764, 767–768, 770

Germ cell tumors, pituitary, imaging of, 691
Germinomas, pituitary, imaging of, 691
Gliomas, pituitary, imaging of, 691
Glucocorticoid replacement therapy, for congenital adrenal hyperplasia, 708, 833
bone mineral density and, 709–710
metabolic aspects of, 710
Glucocorticoids, adrenal production of, 700–701
Glucose level, in diabetic ketoacidosis, 812, 814
in Type 1 diabetes, 777–778
secondary prevention and, 782
tertiary prevention and, 783
Glutamic acid decarboxylase (GAD), recombinant human, in Type 1 diabetes prevention, 777, 784, 786
Gluten, Type 1 diabetes prevention and, 781
Glycemic control, in diabetes. See also *Glucose level.*
complementary and alternative therapies for, **791–810**. See also *Complementary and alternative medicine (CAM).*
Gonadal damage, fertility preservation with, 763–764, 767–768
Gonadal dysfunction, fertility preservation with, 763, 765–767
Gonadal dysgenesis, testicular biopsy for, 823
testis-specific protein Y-encoded positive, 824
with primary amenorrhea, pelvic duplex/color Doppler sonography of, 748–749
XY pure, hypergonadotropic hypogonadism related to, 725, 727
primary amenorrhea related to, 749
Gonadal dysplasia, fertility preservation for, 765–767
Gonadal failure, autoimmune, fertility preservation with, 763–764
hypergonadotropic hypogonadism related to, 729
Gonadal hypoplasia, fertility preservation for, 765–767
Gonadal shielding, during radiation therapy, for fertility preservation, 771
Gonadarche, physiology of, 719
Gonadectomy, for intersex disorders, 823
Gonadotropin production/action, abnormalities of, hypergonadotropic hypogonadism related to, 725–726
Gonadotropin releasing hormone (GnRH), in gonadarche physiology, 719
in hypogonadotropic hypogonadism, 720, 722–724
pulsatile administration of, for fertility preservation, 763–764, 771
Gonadotropin stimulation, intermittent, for fertility preservation, 763–764
Gonadotropin-releasing hormone agonist analogs, for idiopathic short stature, 818
for small for gestational age, 819
prior to radiation therapy, for fertility preservation, 771
*GPR54* gene, hypogonadotropic hypogonadism related to, 721–722
Granulomas, epithelioid, pituitary involvement of, imaging of, 691–692
Growth and development, congenital adrenal hyperplasia effect on, 702, 833
congenital hypothyroidism effect on, 831
constitutional delay of, consensus statement on, 815–818
hypogonadotropic hypogonadism vs., 720
delayed sexual, with primary amenorrhea, pelvic duplex/color Doppler sonography of, 747
of small for gestational age patient, early, 818–819
management to adulthood, 819–820
Growth hormone (GH), for small for gestational age, 819–820

in idiopathic short stature, as treatment, 817–818
alternatives to, 818
dosing and duration of, 817
monitoring of, 817–818
response to, 817
diagnostic screening of, 816

**H**

Hamartomas, tuber cinereum, pituitary, imaging of, 691–692
Hematometrocolpos, primary amenorrhea related to, duplex/color Doppler sonography of, 755
Herbal products, for diabetic ketoacidosis, 805
*Hesx1* gene, hypogonadotropic hypogonadism related to, 721–722
Hindbrain malformations, Chiari, pituitary involvement of, imaging of, 694–695
History taking. See *Family history; Medical history.*
HLA genotypes, in Type 1 diabetes, 778–779
primary prevention and, 780
secondary prevention and, 782
zinc impact on, 805
Hormonal diagnosis, of congenital adrenal hyperplasia, 705–706
Hormonal suppression, prior to radiation therapy, for fertility preservation, 771
Hormone profiling, in congenital adrenal hyperplasia screening, 832–833
Hormone replacement therapy, for congenital adrenal hyperplasia, 706, 708, 833
bone mineral density and, 709–710
metabolic aspects of, 710
stress dosing of, 708
for hypogonadism, in adolescent boys, 731–732
in adolescent girls, 730–731
for idiopathic short stature, 818
for intersex disorders, 823
Hormones, adrenal production of, 700–701
steroidal. See *Steroids.*
Hydration status, in diabetic ketoacidosis, 813–814
Hydrocolpos, primary amenorrhea related to, duplex/color Doppler sonography of, 754–755
Hydrocortisone, for congenital adrenal hyperplasia, 706, 708
bone mineral density and, 709
stress dosing of, 708
Hydrometrocolpos, primary amenorrhea related to, duplex/color Doppler sonography of, 754–755
Hygiene hypothesis, of Type 1 diabetes, 779
Hypergonadotropic hypogonadism, in adolescents, 724–729
acquired origins of, 728–729
causes of, 724–725
clinical manifestations of, 724–725
congenital origins of, 724–728
evaluation of, 729
summary overview of, 719, 732
treatment of, 730–732
with primary amenorrhea, pelvic duplex/color Doppler sonography of, 748–749

Hyperplasia, adrenal, steroid 21 hydroxylase deficiency in, **699–718**. See also *Congenital adrenal hyperplasia (CAH).*
Hypogenesis, callosal, of pituitary, imaging of, 694
Hypogonadism, in adolescents, **719–738**
evaluation of, 729
hypergonadotropic, 724–729
acquired origins of, 728–729
causes of, 724–725
clinical manifestations of, 724–725
congenital origins of, 724–728
with primary amenorrhea, pelvic duplex/color Doppler sonography of, 748–749
hypogonadotropic, 719–724
acquired origins of, 723–724
causes of, 719–721
clinical manifestations of, 719–721
congenital origins of, 720, 722–723
constitutional delay of growth and puberty in, 720
with primary amenorrhea, pelvic duplex/color Doppler sonography of, 747
intersex disorders and, 823
summary overview of, 719, 732
treatment of, 730–732
estrogen replacement for, 730–731
testosterone replacement for, 731–732
Hypogonadotropic hypogonadism, in adolescents, 719–724
acquired origins of, 723–724
causes of, 719–721
clinical manifestations of, 719–721
congenital origins of, 720, 722–723
gene defects in, 720–723
syndromes in, 723
constitutional delay of growth and puberty in, 720
evaluation of, 729
summary overview of, 719, 732
treatment of, 730–732
with primary amenorrhea, pelvic duplex/color Doppler sonography of, 747
Hypophyseal portal system, pituitary, imaging of, 674
Hypoplasia, adrenal, steroid 17 hydroxylase deficiency in, 833
callosal, of pituitary, imaging of, 694–695
gonadal, fertility preservation for, 765–767
uterine and ovarian, primary amenorrhea related to, 747
Hypospadias, with intersex disorders, 823–824
Hypothalamic amenorrhea, hypogonadotropic hypogonadism related to, 724
Hypothalamic disorders, fertility preservation with, 765, 771
hypogonadotropic hypogonadism as, 719. See also *Hypogonadotropic hypogonadism.*
Hypothalamic-pituitary dysfunction, fertility preservation with, 765, 771
Hypothalamic-pituitary region, imaging of, for pediatric disorders, 673–675. See also *Pituitary disorders.*
embryology in, 675–676
gadolinium enhancement of, 676–677, 681, 687
of water balance, 667

## I

Idiopathic short stature (ISS), 815–818
  assessment of, 816
  consensus statement on, 815
  definition of, 815–816
  diagnostic studies for, 816
  treatment of, 817–818
    growth hormone in, 817–818
      alternatives to, 818
    primary goal of, 817
Immunoassays, for congenital adrenal hyperplasia screening, 832
  for congenital hypothyroidism screening, 827–828
In vitro fertilization (IVF), for fertility preservation, 768
In vitro follicular maturation, for fertility preservation, 763, 767–768
Induction, of ovulation, in fertility preservation, 768
Inhibin B, as prepubertal fertility marker, 764–765
Insulin resistance, chromium lowering of, 804
Insulin secretion, in Type 1 diabetes, 778
    tertiary prevention and, 783
Insulin sensitivity, in Type 1 diabetes, 783
Insulin therapy, for diabetic ketoacidosis, 814–815
  in Type 1 diabetes prevention, 782–785
    complementary and alternative therapies vs., 805–806
Insulin-like growth factor (IGF)-1, in idiopathic short stature, as treatment, 817–818
    diagnostic screening of, 816
  small for gestational age and, 819–820
Intensive care unit (ICU), diabetic ketoacidosis management in, 813
Internal genitalia, congenital adrenal hyperplasia features of, 701–702
Intersex disorders, 820–824. See also *Disorders of sex development (DSDs).*
  assigning gender in newborns, 821–822
  consensus statement on, 820, 824
  criteria suggestive of, 821
  definitions for, 820–821
  diagnosis of, 821–822
  introduction to, 820
  long-term outcomes of, 823–824
  pseudointersex with primary amenorrhea vs., 749
  psychosocial management of, 821, 823–824
  sex steroid replacement for, 823
  surgical management of, 822–823
Intracytoplasmic sperm injection (ICSI), for fertility preservation, 770
Intravenous fluids, for diabetic ketoacidosis, 813–815
Isolated hypogonadotropic hypogonadism (IHH), in adolescents, 719–724

## K

*KAL-1* gene, hypogonadotropic hypogonadism related to, 720–722
Kallman syndrome, hypogonadotropic hypogonadism related to, 720–722
Kieler Model, of transitioning pediatric patient to adulthood, with congenital adrenal hyperplasia, 712

Klinefelter syndrome, fertility preservation with, 767
hypergonadotropic hypogonadism related to, 725

L

Laboratory evaluation, of congenital adrenal hyperplasia, 705–706
of hypogonadism, 729
of idiopathic short stature, 816
of intersex disorders, 821–822
of primary amenorrhea, 739–740
Langerhans cell histiocytosis (LCH), pituitary involvement of, imaging of, 692–693
Legal issues, of fertility preservation, 762
*LEP* gene, hypogonadotropic hypogonadism related to, 721–723
*LEPR* gene, hypogonadotropic hypogonadism related to, 721–723
Leptin defects, hypogonadotropic hypogonadism related to, 721–723
Leptin receptor defects, hypogonadotropic hypogonadism related to, 721–723
Levothyroxine, for congenital hypothyroidism, in newborns vs. young adults, 830
Libido, intersex disorders and, 823
Liquid chromatography-tandem mass spectrometry, in congenital adrenal hyperplasia screening, 832–833
Luteinizing hormone (LH), as prepubertal fertility marker, 764–765
in gonadarche physiology, 719
in hypergonadotropic hypogonadism, 725–726

M

Magnetic resonance imaging (MRI), of brain, for pediatric water balance disorders, 667
of hypothalamic-pituitary region, for pediatric disorders, 673–675
of water balance, 667
technique for, 676
ovarian, in fertility preservation, 765
pelvic, for primary amenorrhea, 742, 746
Magnocellular pathway, of pituitary, imaging of, 673
Malignancy(ies), pediatric, fertility preservation with, gonadal shielding during at-risk therapy, 771
outcome studies of, 764–765
trends of, 761–764
intersex disorders and, 823–824
Mayer-Rokitansky-Küster-Hauser syndrome, primary amenorrhea related to, duplex/color Doppler sonography of, 756–757
McCune-Albright syndrome, pituitary involvement of, imaging of, 693–694
Medical history, in diabetic ketoacidosis, 813
in hypogonadism, 729
in idiopathic short stature, 817–818
in intersex disorders, 821
in primary amenorrhea, 739–740
Menarche, in Turner syndrome, fertility preservation and, 766–767
Mental retardation, congenital hypothyroidism and, 831
Metabolic disorders, congenital adrenal hyperplasia treatment and, 710
small for gestational age and, 819
Type 1 diabetes and, 777–778

Microadenomas, pituitary, imaging of, 685–687
Midline lesions, associated pituitary, imaging of, 693–695
Mineralocorticoid replacement therapy, for congenital adrenal hyperplasia, 708, 833
stress dosing of, 708
Mineralocorticoids, adrenal production of, 700–701
Molecular genetics, of congenital adrenal hyperplasia, 705, 707, 831–833
of hypergonadotropic hypogonadism, 724–728
of hypogonadotropic hypogonadism, 720–723
Monoclonal antibodies, in Type 1 diabetes prevention, 783, 786
Müllerian ducts, primary amenorrhea and, duplex/color Doppler sonography of, 752–754
Multiplex systems, for congenital hypothyroidism screening, 827–828
Mycophenolate mofetil (MMF), in Type 1 diabetes prevention, 786

## N

Nephrogenic diabetes insipidus (NDI), as pediatric disorder, 664
X-linked as, 664–666
Nephrogenic systemic fibrosis (NSF), imaging of, 677
Neurohypophyseal bright spot, of pituitary, imaging of, 683–684
Neurohypophysis, of pituitary, imaging of, 673
Neurophysin-vasopressin (NP-VP) complex, imaging of, 683
Newborn screening, for endocrinopathies, **827–837**
congenital adrenal hyperplasia, 831–834
false-positive results of, 832
improvement strategies for, 832–833
protocols for, 832
treatment of, 833–834
trends in, 831–832
congenital hypothyroidism, 827–831
false-positive results of, 828
genetics of, 830
incidence of, 829–830
protocols for, 828–829
technology for, 828
treatment and outcomes of, 830–831
trends in, 827–828
summary overview of, 827
Nicotinamide, for diabetes mellitus, 793–795
clinical trials of, 796
Nicotinamide plus vitamin D, for diabetes mellitus, 795, 797
Nicotinamide plus vitamin E, for diabetes mellitus, 794, 797–798
Noonan's syndrome, primary amenorrhea related to, 749
Nuclear receptor mutations, hypogonadotropic hypogonadism related to, 720–721

## O

Obstruction, uterine/vaginal, with primary amenorrhea, pelvic duplex/color Doppler sonography of, 752–757
Omega-3 fatty acids, for diabetes mellitus, 801
clinical trials of, 798
Type 1 diabetes prevention and, 781

Oocyte banking, for fertility preservation, in pediatrics, 762–763
Oocyte production, in fertility preservation, attainment of potential, 762
Oophoropexy, prior to radiation therapy, for fertility preservation, 771
Optic chiasm, in pituitary imaging, 679
Oral contraceptives, for congenital adrenal hyperplasia, 708
Osteopenia, congenital adrenal hyperplasia treatment effect on, 709–710
Osteoporosis, congenital adrenal hyperplasia treatment effect on, 709–710
Otelixizumab, in Type 1 diabetes prevention, 784
Ovarian failure, autoimmune, fertility preservation with, 763–764
    hypergonadotropic hypogonadism related to, 729
Ovarian hypoplasia, primary amenorrhea related to, 747
Ovarian tissue cryopreservation, for fertility preservation, 763, 768–770
Ovarian tissue transplantation, for fertility preservation, 767–768
Ovary(ies), duplex/color Doppler sonography of, normal anatomy in, 743–746
  volume of, premenarchal vs. menstrual, 744–746
Ovulation induction, in fertility preservation, 768
Oxandrolone, for idiopathic short stature, 818

**P**

Pancreatic transplantation, for Type 1 diabetes, 786–787
Pars intermedia cysts, imaging of, 689
Parvocellular pathway, of pituitary, imaging of, 673–674
Pediatric disorders. See also *Adolescent disorders.*
  adrenal hyperplasia as, **699–718**
    clinical presentations of, 701–705
      classical vs. nonclassical, 699–700
      external genitalia and, 701
      fertility and, 703
      gender role behavior and, 702–703
      internal genitalia and, 701–702
      nonclassical symptoms in, 704–705
      postnatal effects and growth in, 702
      puberty and, 702
      salt wasting and, 703–704
      secondary sexual characteristics in, 702
    diagnosis of, 705–707
      hormonal, 705–706
      molecular genetics in, 705, 707, 833
    late-onset, 704–705
    newborn screening for, 831–834
    pathophysiology of, 700–701
    steroid 21 hydroxylase deficiency in, 699–700
    summary overview of, 699, 712
    treatment of, 706, 708–712
      bone mineral density in, 709–710
      during pregnancy, 710–711
      fertility and, 710–712
      gene therapy in, 834
      goal of, 706
      hormone replacement for, 706, 708, 833

metabolic aspects of, 710
prenatal, 711
stress dosing for, 708
surgery for, 708–709
transitioning to adulthood, 711–712
endocrinopathy screening for, **827–837**
congenital adrenal hyperplasia, 831–834
congenital hypothyroidism, 827–831
summary overview of, 827
hypogonadism as, **719–738**. See also *Hypogonadism.*
in Type 1 diabetes, secondary prevention and, 781–782
of water balance, **663–672**
diabetes insipidus as, 664–667, 669
acquired forms of, 667
diagnosis of, 667
genetics of, 664–666
management of, 665, 667, 669
presenting signs of, 665, 667
normal plasma osmolality regulation vs., 663–664
syndrome of inappropriate antidiuretic hormone secretion as, 668–670
acute vs. chronic, 669–670
causes of, 668–669
diagnosis of, 669
differential diagnosis of, 669
euvolemia in, 669
therapy for, 669–670
pituitary, imaging of, **673–698**
adenomas in, 685–687
associated midline lesions in, 693–695
cystic lesions in, 687–691
embryology in, 675–676
for water imbalance, 667
gland size and signal in, 679–685
normal findings vs., 673–675
sella appearance, 677–679
summary overview of, 695–696
suprasellar tumors in, 691
systemic conditions in, 691–693
technique for, 676–677
Pediatric endocrinology. See also *Endocrinopathies.*
consensus statements in, **811–825**
on diabetic ketoacidosis management, 812–815
on idiopathic short stature, 815–818
on intersex disorders management, 820–824
on small for gestational age management to adulthood, 818–820
summary overview of, 811–812
evidence-based medicine in, 811
fertility preservation considerations for, **761–775**. See also *Fertility preservation.*
Pelvis, duplex/color Doppler sonography of, for primary amenorrhea, abnormal findings with, 746–757
advantages of, 739, 741–742, 746–747, 757

Pelvis (*continued*)
normal anatomy findings vs., 742–746
technique for, 741–742
normal anatomy review for, of ovary, 743–746
of uterus, 742–743
of vagina, 743–744
Physical examination, for diabetic ketoacidosis, 813
for hypogonadism, 729
for idiopathic short stature, 817–818
for intersex disorders, 821
for primary amenorrhea, 740–741
Pituitary adenomas, imaging of, 685–687
Pituitary disorders, pediatric, fertility preservation with, 765, 771
hypogonadotropic hypogonadism as, 719. See also *Hypogonadotropic hypogonadism.*
imaging of, **673–698**
adenomas in, 685–687
associated midline lesions in, 693–695
cystic lesions in, 687–691
embryology in, 675–676
for water imbalance, 667
gland size and signal in, 679–685
normal findings vs., 673–675
sella appearance, 677–679
summary overview of, 695–696
suprasellar tumors in, 691
systemic conditions in, 691–693
technique for, 676–677
Pituitary gland, pediatric, imaging of, abnormal findings with, 685–695
neurohypophyseal bright spot in, 683–684
normal findings with, 673–675, 677–679
postnatal progression in, 680
relative size in first 16 years, 681–682
size and signal in, 679–685
Plasma osmolality, in pediatric disorders, diabetes insipidus and, 665–667
normal regulation vs., 663–664
syndrome of inappropriate antidiuretic hormone secretion and, 668–670
Plasma renin activity (PRA), congenital adrenal hyperplasia treatment and, 708
Polycystic ovarian syndrome (PCOS), congenital adrenal hyperplasia associated with, 702–704
treatment of, 708, 833
with primary amenorrhea, pelvic duplex/color Doppler sonography of, 752
Posterior lobe, of pituitary, imaging of, 674
Posterior pituitary arterial supply, imaging of, 674
Postnatal growth, congenital adrenal hyperplasia effect on, 702
Prader-Willi syndrome (PWS), hypogonadotropic hypogonadism related to, 723
Prednisone, for congenital adrenal hyperplasia, 706
Pregnancy, congenital adrenal hyperplasia during, management of, 710–711
vitamin D supplements during, for Type 1 diabetes prevention, 801–802
vitamin E supplements during, for Type 1 diabetes prevention, 803
Prenatal period, congenital adrenal hyperplasia during, management of, 711

intersex disorders and, 821
Primary amenorrhea, **739–760**
definitions for, 739
duplex/color Doppler sonography for, abnormal findings with, 746–757
advantages of, 739, 746–747, 757
normal anatomy findings vs., 742–746
technique for, 741–742
with delayed sexual development, 747
with gonadal dysgenesis, 748–749
with hypergonadotropic hypogonadism, 748–749
with hypogonadotropic hypogonadism, 747
with pseudointersex, 749–752
with uterine/vaginal obstruction, 752–757
etiologies of, 740
medical evaluation of, 739–740
normal anatomy review for, 742–746
of ovary, 743–746
of uterus, 742–743
of vagina, 743–744
physical examination for, 740–741
puberty and, 740
summary overview of, 739, 757
Primary prevention, of Type 1 diabetes, 778–781
*Prop-1* gene, hypogonadotropic hypogonadism related to, 721–722
Protein exposures, cow's milk, Type 1 diabetes prevention and, 779–780
Pseudohermaphrodite, with primary amenorrhea, pelvic duplex/color Doppler sonography of, 749–752
Pseudohypoparathyroidism, hypergonadotropic hypogonadism related to, 726
Pseudointersex, with primary amenorrhea, pelvic duplex/color Doppler sonography of, 749–752
Psychosocial development, components of, 820–821
Psychosocial management, of intersex disorders, 821, 823–824
Puberty, congenital adrenal hyperplasia effect on, 702
constitutional delay of, hypogonadotropic hypogonadism vs., 720
disorders of, hypogonadism as, **719–738**. See also *Hypogonadism.*
primary amenorrhea as, **739–760**. See also *Primary amenorrhea.*
fertility preservation and, 761–772. See also *Fertility preservation.*
in small for gestational age patient, management of, 819–820
Pyridoxamine, for diabetes mellitus, 795, 800
Pyridoxamine plus folate, for diabetes mellitus, 797

## R

Radiation therapy, gonadal protection during, for fertility preservation, 771
hypergonadotropic hypogonadism related to, 728
Rathke cleft cysts (RCCs), imaging of, 687–688
Recombinant human glutamic acid decarboxylase, in Type 1 diabetes prevention, 777, 784, 786
Renin activity, plasma, congenital adrenal hyperplasia treatment and, 708
Rituximab, in Type 1 diabetes prevention, 786

## S


Salt wasting, steroid 21 hydroxylase deficiency and, 703–704
    treatment of, 708, 711, 833
Sarcoidosis, pituitary involvement of, imaging of, 691–692
Screening, for idiopathic short stature, 816
  for intersex disorders, 821–822
  newborn, for endocrinopathies, **827–837**. See also *Newborn screening.*
Secondary prevention, of Type 1 diabetes, 778–779, 781–782
Secondary sexual characteristics, congenital adrenal hyperplasia effect on, 701–702
Sella, pituitary, pediatric, coronal section, 677
      "empty," 690
      imaging of, 674, 677–679
Septo-optic dysplasia (SOD), pituitary involvement of, imaging of, 695
Sertoli/Leydig-cells, in Klinefelter syndrome, fertility preservation and, 767
17 hydroxylase deficiency, steroid, in adrenal hypoplasia, 833
Sex steroids, adrenal production of, 700–701
  replacement of, for intersex disorders, 823
Sexual characteristics, congenital adrenal hyperplasia effect on, secondary, 702
    virilization as, 701
Sexual development, delayed, with primary amenorrhea, pelvic duplex/color Doppler sonography of, 747
  disorders of. See *Disorders of sex development (DSDs); Intersex disorders.*
Sexual function/dysfunction, with intersex disorders, 823–824
Sexual orientation, psychosocial development and, 821
*SF-1* gene, hypogonadotropic hypogonadism related to, 720–721
Signaling system, in pituitary gland, embryology of, 675–676
    imaging of, 679–685
Small for gestational age (SGA), management to adulthood, 818–820
    consensus statement on, 818
    consequences of, 820
    definition of, 818
    early growth and development, 818–819
    endocrinopathies with, 819
    metabolic disorders with, 819
    of growth, 819–820
    of puberty, 819–820
Sodium level, in diabetic ketoacidosis, 813–814
Sonography, duplex/color Doppler, for primary amenorrhea, 741–757. See also *Duplex/color Doppler sonography.*
  ovarian, in fertility preservation, 765
Sperm banking, for fertility preservation, 764, 770
Sperm count, in fertility preservation, attainment of potential, 762
Sperm density, as prepubertal fertility marker, 764–765
Sperm injection, intracytoplasmic, for fertility preservation, 770
Spermatogenesis, in fertility preservation, attainment of potential, 762
Spermatogonial stem cell transplantation, for fertility preservation, 763, 770
Stalk, pituitary, imaging of, 674, 677–679
Stem cell transplantation, for Type 1 diabetes, 787
  spermatogonial, for fertility preservation, 763, 770
Steroid 17 hydroxylase deficiency, in adrenal hypoplasia, 833

Steroid 21 hydroxylase deficiency, in congenital adrenal hyperplasia, **699–718**
clinical presentations of, 701–705
classical vs. nonclassical, 699–700
external genitalia and, 701
fertility and, 703
gender role behavior and, 702–703
internal genitalia and, 701–702
nonclassical symptoms in, 704–705
postnatal effects and growth in, 702
puberty and, 702
salt wasting and, 703–704
secondary sexual characteristics in, 702
diagnosis of, 705–707
hormonal, 705–706
molecular genetics in, 705, 707, 833
late-onset, 704–705
newborn screening for, 831–834
pathophysiology of, 700–701
steroid 21 hydroxylase deficiency in, 699–700
summary overview of, 699, 712
treatment of, 706, 708–712
bone mineral density in, 709–710
during pregnancy, 710–711
fertility and, 710–712
gene therapy in, 834
goal of, 706
hormone replacement for, 706, 708, 833
metabolic aspects of, 710
prenatal, 711
stress dosing for, 708
surgery for, 708–709
transitioning to adulthood, 711–712
Steroid profiling, in congenital adrenal hyperplasia screening, 832–833
Steroids, adrenal production pathways of, 700–701
anabolic, for idiopathic short stature, 818
sex, adrenal production of, 700–701
replacement of, for intersex disorders, 823
Stress dosing, of corticosteroids, for congenital adrenal hyperplasia, 708
Suprasellar tumors, pituitary, imaging of, 691
Surgical management, of congenital adrenal hyperplasia, 708–709
of newborns, with intersex disorders, 822–823
Swyer syndrome, hypergonadotropic hypogonadism related to, 725, 727
primary amenorrhea related to, 749
Syndrome of inappropriate antidiuretic hormone secretion (SIADH), as pediatric disorder, 668–670
acute vs. chronic, 669–670
causes of, 668–669
diagnosis of, 669
differential diagnosis of, 669
euvolemia in, 669

Syndrome (*continued*)
therapy for, 669–670
Systemic conditions, pediatric, with pituitary disorders, imaging of, 691–693
Systemic fibrosis, nephrogenic, imaging of, 677

**T**

T4/TSH protocol, for congenital hypothyroidism screening, 827–829
Teplizumab, in Type 1 diabetes prevention, 784
Tertiary prevention, of Type 1 diabetes, 778–779, 783–786
Testes, removal of, with intersex disorders, 823
volume of, as prepubertal fertility marker, 764–765
Testicular adrenal rest tumor (TART), congenital adrenal hyperplasia associated with, 703–704, 708
Testicular biopsy, for intersex disorders, 823
Testicular damage, fertility preservation with, 763–764, 767–768
Testicular failure, autoimmune, fertility preservation with, 763–764
hypergonadotropic hypogonadism related to, 729
Testicular feminization, pelvic duplex/color Doppler sonography of, 749–751
Testicular regression sequence (TRS), hypergonadotropic hypogonadism related to, 725, 728
Testicular sperm extraction (TESE), for fertility preservation, 770
Testicular tissue cryopreservation, for fertility preservation, 763, 768, 770
Testicular tissue transplantation, for fertility preservation, 767–768
Testis-specific protein Y-encoded (TSPY) positive gonadal dysgenesis, 824
Testosterone, as prepubertal fertility marker, 764–765
Testosterone replacement, for hypogonadism, in adolescent boys, 731–732
for idiopathic short stature, 818
for intersex disorders, 823
Thiazide diuretics, for nephrogenic diabetes insipidus, 665
Thymoglobulin, in Type 1 diabetes prevention, 784
Thyroid dysgenesis, genetics of, 830
Transcription factor mutations, hypogonadotropic hypogonadism related to, 721–722
Transplantation, for fertility preservation, of ovarian or testicular tissue, 767–768
of spermatogonial stem cell, 763, 770
pancreatic, for Type 1 diabetes, 786–787
stem cell, for Type 1 diabetes, 787
Traumatic brain injury (TBI), hypogonadotropic hypogonadism related to, 723
Trial to Reduce IDDM in the Genetically at Risk (TRIGR), 780–781
TrialNet Study, on Type 1 diabetes prevention, 782, 785–786
TSH only protocol, for congenital hypothyroidism screening, 827–829
Tuber cinereum hamartomas, of pituitary, imaging of, 691–692
Tumors, central nervous system, hypogonadotropic hypogonadism related to, 723–724
intersex disorders and, 824
pituitary, imaging of, adenomas, 685–687
suprasellar, 691
Turner syndrome (TS), fertility preservation and, 763, 765–767
hypergonadotropic hypogonadism related to, 724–725
primary amenorrhea with, 748–749
21 hydroxylase deficiency. See *Steroid 21 hydroxylase deficiency.*
Type 1 diabetes (T1D), diabetic ketoacidosis with, 812–813

prevention of, **777–790**
"curing" established vs., 786–787
genetics and, 778–779
pathogenesis framework for, 777–778
primary strategies, 778–781
secondary strategies, 778–779, 781–782
targets for, 778–779
tertiary strategies, 778–779, 783–786
vitamin D for, 800–802
vitamin E for, 803
Type 2 diabetes (T2D), chromium for, 804
cinnamon for, 803–804
small for gestational age and, 819

## U

Ultrasound (US). See *Sonography.*
Unicornuate uterus, primary amenorrhea related to, duplex/color Doppler sonography of, 752–754
Urine osmolality, in pediatric disorders, diabetes insipidus and, 665, 667
normal regulation vs., 663–664
Uterine hypoplasia, primary amenorrhea related to, 747
Uterine obstruction, with primary amenorrhea, pelvic duplex/color Doppler sonography of, 752–757
Uterus, congenital anomalies of, primary amenorrhea related to, 752–757
duplex/color Doppler sonography of, normal anatomy in, 742–743

## V

Vagina, congenital anomalies of, primary amenorrhea related to, 752–757
duplex/color Doppler sonography of, normal anatomy in, 743–744
Vaginal atresia, primary amenorrhea related to, duplex/color Doppler sonography of, 753, 755
Vaginal dilatation, for intersex disorders, 822
Vaginal obstruction, with primary amenorrhea, pelvic duplex/color Doppler sonography of, 752–757
Vaginoplasty, for intersex disorders, 823
Venous drainage, of pituitary, imaging of, 674
Virilization, congenital adrenal hyperplasia features of, 701, 833
intersex disorders and, 822, 824
with primary amenorrhea, pelvic duplex/color Doppler sonography of, 751
Vitamin B, for diabetes mellitus, 795, 797, 800
Vitamin D, for diabetes mellitus, 800–802
clinical trials of, 797
Type 1 diabetes prevention and, 779, 781
Vitamin D plus nicotinamide, for diabetes mellitus, 795, 797
Vitamin E, for diabetes mellitus, 802–803
clinical trials of, 798
Vitamin E plus nicotinamide, for diabetes mellitus, 794, 797–798

W

Water balance, as pediatric disorder, **663–672**
diabetes insipidus in, 664–667, 669
acquired forms of, 667
diagnosis of, 667
genetics of, 664–666
management of, 665, 667, 669
presenting signs of, 665, 667
normal plasma osmolality regulation vs., 663–664
syndrome of inappropriate antidiuretic hormone secretion in, 668–670
acute vs. chronic, 669–670
causes of, 668–669
diagnosis of, 669
differential diagnosis of, 669
euvolemia in, 669
therapy for, 669–670

X

X chromosome abnormalities, hypergonadotropic hypogonadism related to, 725–726
X-linked nephrogenic diabetes insipidus (XNDI), as pediatric disorder, 664–666
XY pure gonadal dysgenesis, hypergonadotropic hypogonadism related to, 725, 727
primary amenorrhea related to, 749

Z

Zinc, for diabetes mellitus, 804–805

**United States Postal Service**

## Statement of Ownership, Management, and Circulation
## (All Periodicals Publications Except Requestor Publications)

1. Publication Title: Endocrinology and Metabolism Clinics of North America
2. Publication Number: 0 0 0 - 2 7 5
3. Filing Date: 9/15/09
4. Issue Frequency: Mar, Jun, Sep, Dec
5. Number of Issues Published Annually: 4
6. Annual Subscription Price: $242.00
7. Complete Mailing Address of Known Office of Publication (*Not printer*) (*Street, city, county, state, and ZIP+4®*)
   Elsevier Inc.
   360 Park Avenue South
   New York, NY 10010-1710
   Contact Person: Stephen Bushing
   Telephone (Include area code): 215-239-3688
8. Complete Mailing Address of Headquarters or General Business Office of Publisher (*Not printer*)
   Elsevier Inc., 360 Park Avenue South, New York, NY 10010-1710
9. Full Names and Complete Mailing Addresses of Publisher, Editor, and Managing Editor (*Do not leave blank*)
   Publisher (*Name and complete mailing address*)
   John Schrefer , Elsevier, Inc., 1600 John F. Kennedy Blvd. Suite 1800, Philadelphia, PA 19103-2899
   Editor (*Name and complete mailing address*)
   Rachel Glover, Elsevier, Inc., 1600 John F. Kennedy Blvd. Suite 1800, Philadelphia, PA 19103-2899
   Managing Editor (*Name and complete mailing address*)
   Catherine Bewick, Elsevier, Inc., 1600 John F. Kennedy Blvd. Suite 1800, Philadelphia, PA 19103-2899
10. Owner (*Do not leave blank. If the publication is owned by a corporation, give the name and address of the corporation immediately followed by the names and addresses of all stockholders owning or holding 1 percent or more of the total amount of stock. If not owned by a corporation, give the names and addresses of the individual owners. If owned by a partnership or other unincorporated firm, give its name and address as well as those of each individual owner. If the publication is published by a nonprofit organization, give its name and address.*)

| Full Name | Complete Mailing Address |
|---|---|
| Wholly owned subsidiary of | 4520 East-West Highway |
| Reed/Elsevier, US holdings | Bethesda, MD 20814 |

11. Known Bondholders, Mortgagees, and Other Security Holders Owning or Holding 1 Percent or More of Total Amount of Bonds, Mortgages, or Other Securities. If none, check box → ☐ None

| Full Name | Complete Mailing Address |
|---|---|
| N/A | |

12. Tax Status (*For completion by nonprofit organizations authorized to mail at nonprofit rates*) (*Check one*)
   The purpose, function, and nonprofit status of this organization and the exempt status for federal income tax purposes:
   ☐ Has Not Changed During Preceding 12 Months
   ☐ Has Changed During Preceding 12 Months (*Publisher must submit explanation of change with this statement*)

PS Form **3526**, September 2007 (Page 1 of 3 (Instructions Page 3)) PSN 7530-01-000-9931 **PRIVACY NOTICE**: See our Privacy policy in www.usps.com

13. Publication Title: Endocrinology and Metabolism Clinics of North America
14. Issue Date for Circulation Data Below: September 2009

| 15. Extent and Nature of Circulation | | | Average No. Copies Each Issue During Preceding 12 Months | No. Copies of Single Issue Published Nearest to Filing Date |
|---|---|---|---|---|
| a. Total Number of Copies (*Net press run*) | | | 2532 | 2226 |
| b. Paid Circulation (By Mail and Outside the Mail) | (1) | Mailed Outside-County Paid Subscriptions Stated on PS Form 3541. (*Include paid distribution above nominal rate, advertiser's proof copies, and exchange copies*) | 932 | 872 |
| | (2) | Mailed In-County Paid Subscriptions Stated on PS Form 3541 (*Include paid distribution above nominal rate, advertiser's proof copies, and exchange copies*) | | |
| | (3) | Paid Distribution Outside the Mails Including Sales Through Dealers and Carriers, Street Vendors, Counter Sales, and Other Paid Distribution Outside USPS® | 809 | 769 |
| | (4) | Paid Distribution by Other Classes Mailed Through the USPS (e.g. First-Class Mail®) | | |
| c. Total Paid Distribution (*Sum of 15b (1), (2), (3), and (4)*) → | | | 1741 | 1641 |
| d. Free or Nominal Rate Distribution (By Mail and Outside the Mail) | (1) | Free or Nominal Rate Outside-County Copies Included on PS Form 3541 | 87 | 68 |
| | (2) | Free or Nominal Rate In-County Copies Included on PS Form 3541 | | |
| | (3) | Free or Nominal Rate Copies Mailed at Other Classes Through the USPS (e.g. First-Class Mail) | | |
| | (4) | Free or Nominal Rate Distribution Outside the Mail (Carriers or other means) | | |
| e. Total Free or Nominal Rate Distribution (Sum of 15d (1), (2), (3) and (4) | | | 87 | 68 |
| f. Total Distribution (Sum of 15c and 15e) → | | | 1828 | 1709 |
| g. Copies not Distributed (See instructions to publishers #4 (page #3)) → | | | 704 | 517 |
| h. Total (Sum of 15f and g) | | | 2532 | 2226 |
| i. Percent Paid (15c divided by 15f times 100) → | | | 95.24% | 96.02% |

16. Publication of Statement of Ownership
   ☐ If the publication is a general publication, publication of this statement is required. Will be printed in the **December 2009** issue of this publication.  ☐ Publication not required

17. Signature and Title of Editor, Publisher, Business Manager, or Owner
   Stephen R. Bushing - Subscription Services Coordinator
   Date: September 15, 2009

I certify that all information furnished on this form is true and complete. I understand that anyone who furnishes false or misleading information on this form or who omits material or information requested on the form may be subject to criminal sanctions (including fines and imprisonment) and/or civil sanctions (including civil penalties).

PS Form **3526**, September 2007 (Page 2 of 3)